T0155909

Lecture Notes in Computer Science 13705

More information about this series at https://link.springer.com/bookseries/558

Agma Traina · Hua Wang · Yong Zhang ·
Siuly Siuly · Rui Zhou · Lu Chen (Eds.)

Health Information Science

11th International Conference, HIS 2022 Virtual Event, October 28–30, 2022 Proceedings

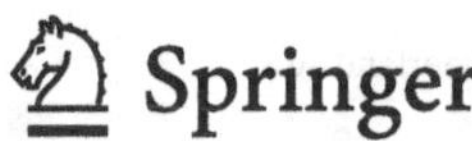

Editors
Agma Traina
University of São Paulo
São Carlos, Brazil

Hua Wang
Victoria University
Melbourne, VIC, Australia

Yong Zhang
Tsinghua University
Beijing, China

Siuly Siuly
Victoria University
Footscray, VIC, Australia

Rui Zhou
Swinburne University of Technology
Hawthorn, VIC, Australia

Lu Chen
Swinburne University of Technology
Hawthorn, VIC, Australia

ISSN 0302-9743 ISSN 1611-3349 (electronic)
Lecture Notes in Computer Science
ISBN 978-3-031-20626-9 ISBN 978-3-031-20627-6 (eBook)
https://doi.org/10.1007/978-3-031-20627-6

This Springer imprint is published by the registered company Springer Nature Switzerland AG
The registered company address is: Gewerbestrasse 11, 6330 Cham, Switzerland

Preface

The International Conference Series on Health Information Science (HIS) provides a forum for disseminating and exchanging multidisciplinary research results in computer science/information technology and health science and services. It covers all aspects of health information sciences and systems that support health information management and health service delivery.

The 11th International Conference on Health Information Science (HIS 2022) was held in Biarritz, France, during October 28–30, 2022. Founded in April 2012 as the International Conference on Health Information Science and Their Applications, the conference continues to grow to include an ever broader scope of activities. The main goal of these events is to provide international scientific forums for researchers to exchange new ideas in a number of fields that interact in-depth through discussions with their peers from around the world. The scope of the conference includes (1) medical/health/biomedicine information resources, such as patient medical records, devices and equipment, software, and tools to capture, store, retrieve, process, analyze, and optimize the use of information in the health domain;(2) data management, data mining, and knowledge discovery, all of which play a crucial role in decision-making, management of public health, examination of standards, privacy and security issues; (3) computer visualization and artificial intelligence for computer-aided diagnosis; and (4) development of new architectures and applications for health information systems.

The conference solicited and gathered technical research submissions related to all aspects of the conference scope. All the submitted papers were peer-reviewed in a single-blind manner by at least three international experts drawn from the Program Committee. After the rigorous peer-review process, a total of 29 papers among the 54 submissions were selected on the basis of originality, significance, and clarity and were accepted for publication in the proceedings. The authors were from Australia, Bangladesh, Brazil, China, Iran, Iraq, Italy, the Netherlands, Switzerland, the UK, the USA, and Vietnam. The high quality of the program – guaranteed by the presence of an unparalleled number of internationally recognized top experts – is reflected in the content of the proceedings. The conference was therefore a unique event where attendees were able to appreciate the latest results in their field of expertise and to acquire additional knowledge in other fields. The program was structured to favor interactions among attendees coming from many different areas, scientifically and geographically, from academia and from industry.

Finally, we acknowledge all those who contributed to the success of HIS 2022 but whose names are not listed here.

October 2022

Agma Traina
Hua Wang
Yong Zhang
Siuly Siuly
Rui Zhou
Lu Chen

Organization

General Co-chairs

Yannis Manolopoulos	Open University of Cyprus, Cyprus
Yanchun Zhang	Victoria University, Australia

Program Co-chairs

Agma Traina	University of Sao Paulo, Brazil
Hua Wang	Victoria University, Australia
Yong Zhang	Tsinghua University, China

Coordination Chair

Siuly Siuly	Victoria University, Australia

Publicity Co-chairs

Enamul Kabir	University of Southern Queensland, Australia
Mirela Cazzolato	University of Sao Paulo, Brazil
Varun Bajaj	Indian Institute of Information Technology, India

Publication Co-chairs

Rui Zhou	Swinburne University of Technology, Australia
Lu Chen	Swinburne University of Technology, Australia

Website Co-chairs

Yong-Feng Ge	La Trobe University, Australia
Mingshan You	Victoria University, Australia

HIS Steering Committee Representative

Fernando Martin-Sanchez	Institute of Health Carlos III, Spain

Program Committee

Venkat Achalam	CHRIST (Deemed to be University), India
Ashik Mostafa Alvi	Victoria University, Australia
Ömer Faruk Alçin	Bingol Üniversitesi, Turkey
Mirela Teixeira Cazzolato	University of São Paulo, Brazil
Lu Chen	Swinburne University of Technology, Australia
Soon Chun	City University of New York, USA
Thomas M. Deserno	TU Braunschweig, Germany
Mohammed Diykh	University of southern Queensland, Australia
Yong-Feng Ge	La Trobe University, Australia
Zhisheng Huang	Vrije Universiteit Amsterdam, The Netherlands
Md Rafiqul Islam	University of Technology Sydney, Australia
Enamul Kabir	University of Southern Queensland, Australia
Smith Khare	Shri Ramdeobaba College of Emgineering and Management, India
Fátima L. S. Nunes	University of São Paulo, Brazil
Shaofu Lin	Beijing University of Technology, China
Gang Luo	University of Washington, USA
Jiangang Ma	Federation University Australia, Australia
Muhammad Tariq Sadiq	University of Lahore, Pakistan
Siuly Siuly	Victoria University, Australia
Paolo Soda	Università Campus Bio-Medico di Roma, Italy
Le Sun	Nanjing University of Information Science and Technology, China
Lili Sun	University of Southern Queensland, Australia
Weiqing Sun	University of Toledo, USA
Supriya Supriya	Victoria University, Australia
Md. Nurul Ahad Tawhid	Victoria University, Australia
Agma Traina	University of Sao Paulo, Brazil
Hua Wang	Victoria University, Australia
Kate Wang	RMIT University, Australia
Jiao Yin	Victoria University, Australia
Mingshan You	Victoria University, Australia
Guoqiang Zhang	UTHealth, USA
Rui Zhou	Swinburne University of Technology, Australia

Additional Reviewer

Deserno Thomas

Contents

Applications of Health and Medical Data

Applications of Health and Medical Data

Evidence Extraction to Validate Medical Claims in Fake News Detection

Pritam Deka(✉), Anna Jurek-Loughrey, and Deepak P

Queen's University, Belfast, UK
{pdeka01,a.jurek}@qub.ac.uk, deepaksp@acm.org

Abstract. Fact-checking of online health information has become necessary due to the increasing usage of internet by people searching for medical advice. There is a plethora of false information available to the public, which can put people in harm's way. In order to aid the fact-checking process, recent research has leveraged the advancements made in NLP and deep learning techniques. Majority of the existing technology relies on the existence of labelled data, which is very limited. In this work we explored an unsupervised approach to identifying evidence sentences, which is the key task in claims verification process. We show by performing experiments on a publicly available dataset that our method achieves performance comparable to that of state-of-the-art supervised techniques. We also show how our proposed method can be adapted in cases where labelled data is available.

Keywords: Health misinformation · Fact-checking · Unsupervised learning · Evidence retrieval

1 Introduction

Fake news prevailing online is not a new phenomenon and has been around for quite sometime. However, with the increasing usage of internet, the rise of fake news has been more apparent since recent times. It particularly gained popularity during the 2016 US presidential election, which saw a huge trend in online fake news circulation [1]. It has become a serious problem in the world which is capable of jeopardising democracy, snatching freedom of expression of journalism and toppling market economy [43]. In order to tackle the problem of fake news, recent advancements in the field of machine learning and NLP have been used. However, the primary focus of most studies has been political news. There are different sub tasks within the broader aspect of fake news detection using AI. One of these is fact-checking of information. There has been a surge in research related to fact-checking with the public release of datasets such as Politifact [37], RumourEval [11,16], Claimbuster [18], FEVER [35], FEVEROUS [2]. However, these datasets mostly cater to general fact-checking that also includes political news fact-checking. This is markedly different from the fact-checking of

A. Traina et al. (Eds.): HIS 2022, LNCS 13705, pp. 3–15, 2022.
https://doi.org/10.1007/978-3-031-20627-6_1

health information which is garnering more attention since the Covid-19 pandemic [15,22]. Fact checking of online health information requires domain expertise, unlike general fact checking. It is also a time consuming process due to the fact that experts need to assess health related claims based on existing medical information available via medical databases such as PubMed. Recent advancements in NLP and machine learning has helped in boosting research related to this problem. However, the shortage of appropriate publicly available datasets limits the posibility of applying machine learning for the health related fact-checking task.

In order to address this challenge, we propose an unsupervised learning approach to retrieve evidence sentences for such claims from PubMed abstracts. This task is designed to be part of a pipeline for predicting veracity of medical claims which follows the retrieval of PubMed abstracts as evidence for such claims. We evaluate our method on a publicly available dataset and show that our method is comparable with the state-of-the-art supervised methods.

Task Definition
The task is defined as follows: For a list of claims and a set of relevant PubMed abstracts for each claim, the task is to identify the evidence sentences within those abstracts. Given a claim c and a set of relevant abstracts $A = [a_1, \ldots a_n]$, the goal is to find the evidence sentences from within those abstracts for the claim.

2 Related Work

In this section we will hereby discuss the recent research in the space of medical evidence retrieval, which is predominantly based on the application of transformer neural networks [36]. [38] released SCIFACT, a publicly available dataset for health/medical fact checking. They proposed a method that uses a RoBERTa-large [27] encoder for the task of evidence retrieval where abstracts for each claim are first extracted from a corpus using TF-IDF similarity. After that, for the sentence selection the RoBERTa-large encoder is used which is fine-tuned on SCIFACT.

VerT5erini [29] used a T5 (Text-To-Text Transfer Transformer) [30] model for the abstract retrieval and sentence selection. For identifying abstracts the authors proposed a one-stage as well as a two-stage model where the first stage in both the approaches used the BM25 algorithm to extract a list of k abstracts. For the two-stage method, they have used a T5 re-ranker to re-rank the list of k abstracts. For sentence selection, they again used the T5 model fine-tuned on SCIFACT. Their proposed method outperformed the approach of [38] in both abstract retrieval and sentence selection.

Another model named PARAGRAPH-JOINT [25] used BioSentVec [9] for retrieving the abstracts instead of using TF-IDF similarity. Sentence embedding is computed for each claim and each abstract using BioSentVec and cosine similarity is used to find out the top k most similar abstracts for each claim.

They used a RoBERTa-large encoder for the sentence selection task fine-tuned on SCIFACT.

ARSJOINT [42] also used BioSentVec [9] to first select the top k similar abstracts for further processing. This was done to minimize the total number of candidate abstracts and remove non-relevant abstracts. They experimented with RoBERTa-large and BioBERT-large [23] where both models were fine-tuned on the SCIFACT dataset. Their proposed method jointly learns all three tasks of abstract retrieval, sentence selection, and label prediction. They also proposed a regularization which is based on the divergence between the abstract retrieval sentence attention and the sentence selection outputs. They showed using experimental results that their proposed method performed better than the baseline models which were chosen.

The above works use a three step approach of abstract retrieval, evidence sentence selection and label prediction using the selected evidence sentences. However, the difference between them is the way the evidence sentences are selected. VerT5erini selects the evidence sentences by using each sentence independently whereas PARAGRAPH-JOINT and ARSJOINT uses the abstracts for evidence sentence selection using pooling and self-attention. Unlike previous approaches, MULTIVERS [39] uses a weakly-supervised approach where training is done using available scientific documents. Instead of encoding claims and abstracts separately, their method encodes both claims and abstracts using a Longformer [5] architecture which allows longer documents to be encoded without any information loss. For choosing candidate abstracts, they follow the two-stage methodology of VerT5erini. Once the candidate abstracts are selected, sentence selection is performed as a binary classification task and label prediction as a 3-way classification task. Their proposed method performed better than the baseline methods on both the abstract and sentence selection tasks evaluated on SCIFACT.

In our work, we have focused on the task of evidence sentence selection from candidate abstracts which are retrieved using a dense S-BERT [31] fine-tuned model. Our approach is different from these works, as we have explored an approach of selecting the evidence sentences from the candidate abstracts using evidence-based medicine (EBM) concepts combined with knowledge from BERT based models. The method can be used in an unsupervised way without the need for data labels relevant to the evidence sentence extraction task, however it can also be adapted in situations where labelled data is available.

3 Proposed Method

The proposed method is a two-stage approach with the assumption that evidence statements are usually sentences that reports the outcomes of a randomized controlled trial (RCT) including findings and results. RCTs belong to the highest level of EBM practice in terms of gathering evidence in a systematic manner [7]. The first stage of the method consists of selecting the sentences from the abstract, which are the most similar to the claim. The second stage uses a classifier to classify the sentences from the first stage as evidence or not evidence sentences. The proposed method is shown in Fig. 1.

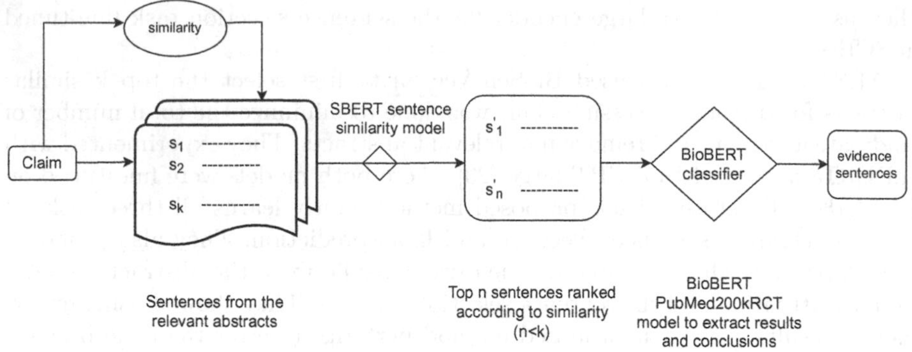

Fig. 1. Proposed method

3.1 Stage One (Selecting Similar Sentences)

The first stage of the method consists of using the S-BERT [31] framework to find sentences similar to the claims using cosine similarity between the embeddings of the claims and the sentences of the abstract. S-BERT uses siamese network architecture to fine tune BERT models in order to generate robust sentence embeddings which can be used with common similarity measures such as cosine similarity in a computationally efficient way. The idea behind using S-BERT is that claims will have reasonable level of similarity with the evidence sentences. By finding the most similar sentences first, we reduce the number of sentences that will then be used in the next stage of the method. Once we have the most similar sentences, these are then passed through the classifier to find only the relevant sentences. As the base model which is passed to the S-BERT framework, we have used SapBERT [26] which is a self aligning pretraining scheme using PubMedBERT [17] and UMLS data, a repository containing biomedical and health vocabulary. [31] have shown that using S-BERT to fine-tune BERT-based models over NLI (Natural Language Inference) and STS (Sentence Textual Similarity) data produces better sentence embeddings. Therefore, we have used the S-BERT[1] framework to fine-tune the SapBERT model using NLI and STS data. For NLI training, we have used the SNLI [6], MultiNLI [40], SCITAIL [21], SCINLI [33] and MedNLI [32] datasets where contradictions are taken as negatives and entailments as positives using a multiple negatives ranking loss function [19]. This loss function minimizes the negative log probability of the softmax-normalized scores for positives and negatives while training. For any batch k, if there are $x = \{x_1, x_2 \ldots x_k\}$ positives and $y = \{y_1, y_2 \ldots y_k\}$ negatives then the loss function [19] is represented by

$$\lambda = -\frac{1}{k}\sum_{n=1}^{k}\left[A(x_n, y_n) - log\sum_{m=1}^{k} e^{A(x_m, y_m)}\right] \tag{1}$$

[1] https://www.sbert.net/.

For the STS training, we have used the STS-B [8] dataset. We also experimented with different BERT-based models for comparison with SapBERT, including BioBERT [23], PubMedBERT [17], SciBERT [4], BERT [13], RoBERTa [27] and DistilBERT [34] using the same fine-tuning approach. These fine-tuned models were then used to find the semantic similarity between the claims and the extracted sentences and then sorted according to the descending order of cosine similarity.

3.2 Stage Two (Classifying Sentences)

The second stage involves using a classifier in order to classify the sentences from the first stage as in EBM, evidences are usually reported in the form of findings or results and also conclusions from RCTs [3]. In order to identify the results/findings/conclusions in an RCT, we have utilised a BERT-based architecture by approaching it as a classification task of the sentences in an RCT. For training such a classifier, we have leveraged a publicly available dataset, PubMed200kRCT [12] which consists of approximately 200,000 abstracts of structured randomized controlled trials, totalling 2.3 million sentences. Each sentence of each abstract is labelled with their role in the abstract using one of the following classes: BACKGROUND, OBJECTIVE, METHOD, RESULT, or CONCLUSION. The idea behind using this dataset is to train a transformer model so that it can identify the sentences in any RCT abstract according to the classes. Such a trained model is effective for any abstract without the need for any further training and hence any training data, which means that our model remains unsupervised for any future applications. We also share the model publicly in Huggingface[2] to aid further research work. The pseudo code for the whole approach is given in Algorithm 1.

Algorithm 1. Claim evidence retrieval

Input: List of p claims, $C = [c_1, c_2, c_3 \dots c_p]$ and a list of n sentences for each claim, $S = [s_1, s_2, s_3 \dots s_n]$

Output: A list of evidence sentences for each claim, $S' = [s'_1, \dots s'_m]$ where $m < n$

Load the S-BERT model
for all claims c in C **do**
  $c \leftarrow get\_S - BERT\_vector(c)$
  $D \leftarrow get\_S - BERT\_vector(S)$
  $similarities \leftarrow cosine(c, D)$
  Sort $s_i \in S$ in descending order of *similarities*
  Retrieve the k most similar sentences from s_i where $s_k \subseteq s_i, k < i$
  $S' \leftarrow BioBERT\_Classifier(s_k)$, the final evidence sentences list
end for

[2] https://huggingface.co/pritamdeka/BioBert-PubMed200kRCT.

4 Experiments Evaluation

In this section, we describe the dataset and the details of the experimental evaluation, which is followed by results and discussion.

4.1 Dataset Details

For general health related claims, SCIFACT [38] provides claims and PubMed abstracts as the evidences to those claims. The dataset contains 1.4K scientific claims that are matched with a labelled evidence-containing corpus of around 5K abstracts. Within such abstracts, certain sentences are labelled which either SUPPORTS or REFUTES the claims. Due to these unique properties, this dataset is the most suitable for our work, which is why we have focused on this particular dataset.

4.2 Experimental Settings

The classifier was built using the PubMed200kRCT [12] dataset by leveraging the publicly available Huggingface's [41] transformers training script[3]. We use the BioBERT [23] model as the 5-class classifier. The training parameters used for the classifier include:

- Learning rate = 5e−5
- Loss function = contrastive loss
- Batch size = 64
- Saving and evaluation steps = 5K
- Maximum sequence length = 130

The selection of these parameters follow the original BERT paper [13]. The sentences from the first stage are passed through the classifier where we have used the TextClassificationPipeline class of Huggingface Transformers. This class offers a simple API for Text Classification. For using this class we call the TextClassificationPipeline() object with the model and the model tokenizer. After that, each sentence is passed to the object and the API then identifies the sentence accordingly. For our case, we select only the RESULTS and the CONCLUSION sentences as these form the evidence sentences [3].

4.3 Results and Discussion

For evaluation purposes, we have used the SCIFACT dataset [38]. First, we compare the performance of various S-BERT models for the first stage of our model. For evaluating the performance we use the micro f-1 score [38]. Precision and recall were calculated based on the correctly retrieved sentences and the available gold standard sentences [28].

[3] https://github.com/huggingface/transformers/blob/master/examples/pytorch/text-classification/run_glue.py.

The f-1 score is calculated on the average precision and recall values, which is a micro f-1 score. We experiment in different settings, which include using the top 2 and top 3 retrieved abstracts and then the top 2 and top 3 retrieved sentences from these abstracts for the various models. From Table 1 we can see that the SapBERT model performs the best. This can be attributed to the fact that this model leverages the biomedical ontologies of UMLS, providing better scores for similarities between the sentences. We can also see that the domain specific models (BioBERT, PubMedBERT, SciBERT) performs better than the generic domain BERT models. We can also see that f-1 scores for the top 2 abstracts is greater than using the top 3 abstracts which is why in our future experiments we will use the top 2 retrieved abstracts.

Table 1. S-BERT model comparison for the first stage of the method

Models	Top 2 abstracts		Top 3 abstracts	
	Top 2 sentences	Top 3 sentences	Top 2 sentences	Top 3 sentences
	F-1 score	F-1 score	F-1 score	F-1 score
RoBERTa-base-fine-tuned	0.359	0.351	0.346	0.329
BERT-base-uncased-fine-tuned	0.324	0.339	0.305	0.312
DistilBERT-base-uncased-fine-tuned	0.361	0.356	0.337	0.335
BioBERT-fine-tuned	0.386	0.358	0.384	0.347
PubMedBERT-fine-tuned	0.410	0.401	0.391	0.375
SciBERT-fine-tuned	0.407	0.382	0.386	0.363
SapBERT-fine-tuned	0.418	0.416	0.409	0.406

The best performing S-BERT model is chosen for further experiments and comparison with baselines. The baselines used are supervised models as there has been no work that uses unsupervised approaches in selecting the evidence sentences from the SCIFACT dataset. We have used the zero-shot VERISCI baseline [38] and the zero-shot MULTIVERS [39] baseline since these are a better comparison against our approach as we do not use the provided SCIFACT training file. The zero-shot VERISCI results were taken directly from [38] for the dev(development) set. The MULTIVERS [39] paper reports their results on the SCIFACT test set whose gold standard values are not available publicly. We have therefore calculated the precision, recall and micro f-1 score for the dev (development) set. The results were calculated by using the provided model checkpoints and scripts by the MULTIVERS team from their github repository[4]. They have used a Longformer [5] model as their base model and the zero shot models are fine-tuned models over FEVER [35] and FEVER+Adapt where Adapt is composed of two datasets, PUBMEDQA [20] and EVIDENCEINFERENCE [14,24].

[4] https://github.com/dwadden/multivers.

It should be noted that these methods have a different trade-off point while calculating the precision and recall. The results are shown below in Table 2. We have used the open retrieval format wherein the gold standard abstracts are not provided and the abstracts are first extracted using an MS-MARCO fine-tuned PubMedBERT model[5] which is taken from [10]. We take the top 2 abstracts retrieved and then take the top 3 sentences from the first stage of the method which are then fed to the classifier which then finally gives the evidence sentences. We calculate the precision, recall and micro f-1 from the final list of evidence sentences. It can be seen from the table that our approach performs better than the MULTIVERS models in terms of recall and f-1 score. The high precision of those models can be attributed to the fact that most of the claims do not retrieve the relevant evidence sentences which is why the recall is low but precision is high. In case of the VERISCI model, there is a low precision and high recall which means most of the claims retrieve sentences, however, many of them are not the evidences. In our case, our method retrieves evidence sentences for all claims, which is the reason for balanced precision and recall values with the highest recall and f-1 score. The high recall value shows that for most of the claims the gold sentence is retrieved correctly. The low precision is due to the fact that for all claims 3 sentences are retrieved. This is important to note as our approach does not use the provided labelled data of SCIFACT whereas the rest of the approaches uses it.

Table 2. Comparison of our approach with zero-shot baselines

Model	Precision	Recall	F-1
Zero-shot FEVER MULTIVERS	0.7727	0.0464	0.0876
Zero-shot FEVER+Adapt MULTIVERS	**0.8600**	0.1174	0.2067
Zero-shot VERISCI	0.2860	0.3850	0.3280
Our approach	0.4370	**0.4726**	**0.4541**

We also experimented with a binary classifier wherein the number of classes were reduced from 5 to 2. This was achieved by grouping the classes METHOD, BACKGROUND, OBJECTIVE into one class named as IRRELEVANT and grouping CONCLUSION and RESULT into a class named as RELEVANT. The classifier was built in the same way as the 5 class classifier using BioBERT. After that, both the 5-class and the binary classifier were evaluated following our method where the fine-tuned SapBERT model is used in the first stage to retrieve the top k sentences which are then passed to the classifier for the final evaluation. The results are shown below in Table 3. It can be seen from the table that the binary classifier performs expectedly better than the 5-class classifier.

[5] https://huggingface.co/pritamdeka/S-PubMedBert-MS-MARCO-SCIFACT.

Table 3. Comparison of the 5-class and Binary classifier

Top n sentences	Binary classifier			5-class classifier		
	P	R	F1	P	R	F1
3	0.446	0.475	0.460	0.437	0.472	0.454
5	0.372	0.564	0.448	0.358	0.565	0.438
10	0.224	0.622	0.329	0.217	0.623	0.322

4.4 Supervised Case

In case of available labelled data, a supervised approach can be taken. For this, we have fine-tuned the model using two different strategies, both of which use a triplet training format consisting of positives and negatives in order to provide robust training for the model. Since there are fewer positive examples, adding negatives while training the model better trains the model. Both strategies use the claims and the corresponding gold standard evidence sentence/sentences for each claim as positives. For the first strategy, negatives are chosen from the gold standard abstracts excluding the gold standard evidence sentences. For the second strategy, we have used lexical similarity using Okapi BM25 to retrieve the top 20 lexically similar sentences for each claim from the whole corpus of 5k abstracts. We train the fine-tuned SapBERT model on both the strategies using a multiple negatives ranking loss using the S-BERT framework. After that we use this model to retrieve the top k sentences for each claim which are then passed to the binary classifier for the final retrieval of evidence sentences. Note that the labelled data are used only in the first stage of our approach. The comparison of these approaches with the previous approach where we do not use labelled data is shown in Table 4. It can be inferred from this that such training strategies improve the quality of sentence embedding which ultimately leads to higher similarity scores between sentences. We can also see that using the top 2 sentences gives better results when we use the fine-tuned strategies.

Table 4. Comparison of two strategies of fine-tuned S-BERT models

Top n sentences	Binary classifier (Not fine-tuned S-BERT)			Binary classifier (Fined-tuned S-BERT in-batch negatives)			Binary classifier (Fine-tuned S-BERT BM25 negatives)		
	P	R	F1	P	R	F1	P	R	F1
2	0.447	0.384	0.413	0.564	0.534	0.546	0.556	0.517	0.535
3	0.449	0.475	0.459	0.468	0.588	0.521	0.479	0.569	0.520
5	0.372	0.564	0.448	0.335	0.629	0.438	0.353	0.629	0.452
10	0.224	0.622	0.329	0.202	0.675	0.311	0.215	0.679	0.327

4.5 Ablation Study

We have performed an ablation study in which we drop the METHOD class since it is similar to the RESULT class from the dataset and trained the BioBERT classifier on 4 classes instead of 5. We then compared the precision, recall and micro f-1 score for the top k retrieved sentences where $k = 3, 5, 10$. The results of the comparison are shown in Table 5. Based on the results, it can be seen that by removing the class METHOD, more sentences are classified as RESULT or CONCLUSION leading to a higher recall, which shows that some relevant sentences were incorrectly classified as METHOD earlier. But as the sentences have increased, the precision value has also gone down.

Table 5. Comparison of classifiers for ablation study

Top n sentences	Binary classifier			5-class classifier			4-class classifier		
	P	R	F1	P	R	F1	P	R	F1
3	0.447	0.475	0.459	0.437	0.472	0.454	0.408	0.484	0.443
5	0.372	0.564	0.448	0.358	0.565	0.438	0.335	0.570	0.422
10	0.224	0.622	0.339	0.217	0.623	0.322	0.210	0.673	0.320

We also experimented using the 5-class classifier to check how many evidence sentences were classified as only CONCLUSION and only RESULT. We perform the experiment for the top 3, 5 and 10 sentences. The results of the experiment are shown in Table 6. It can be seen that for both RESULT and CONCLUSION, the precision value decreases with an increase in the number of sentences. However, the recall value in both cases increases. We can also see from the comparison that the precision, recall and f-1 scores for only RESULT are much higher than only CONCLUSION. However, both of these classes are needed while training the classifier in order to have higher accuracy.

Table 6. Precision, recall and F1 score for RESULTS and CONCLUSIONS

Top n sentences	Only RESULT			Only CONCLUSION		
	P	R	F1	P	R	F1
3	0.362	0.332	0.346	0.165	0.127	0.144
5	0.343	0.400	0.369	0.161	0.154	0.157
10	0.254	0.449	0.324	0.128	0.179	0.149

From our experiments we have seen that using RCT structure can help in extracting evidence sentences for health related claims. This is in line with our assumption of using evidence-based medicine concepts for this task.

5 Conclusion

From our experiments and result analysis, we can see how our proposed method can be helpful in providing a way to retrieve evidence sentences for health-related claims in an unsupervised setting. We have shown that utilising RCT elements along with BERT-based domain-specific models can help extract evidence sentences in a transfer-learned way. We have also shown how our proposed method achieved better results than the supervised zero-shot learning methods evaluated in the same dataset. We have also shown how we can fine-tune S-BERT models for generating sentence embeddings using the available data that can help achieve better results. We also compared two different strategies of fine-tuning and showed that using a lexical similarity based fine-tuning yields better results. As future work, we would like to see how using such an approach can also be applied to other medical-related datasets. We also plan to use these evidence sentences to check whether these support or refute a claim, thereby providing a pipeline of automated fact checking.

References

1. Allcott, H., Gentzkow, M.: Social media and fake news in the 2016 election. J. Econ. Perspect. **31**(2), 211–36 (2017)
2. Aly, R., et al.: FEVEROUS: fact extraction and verification over unstructured and structured information. arXiv preprint arXiv:2106.05707 (2021)
3. Bauchner, H., Golub, R.M., Fontanarosa, P.B.: Reporting and interpretation of randomized clinical trials. JAMA **322**(8), 732–735 (2019)
4. Beltagy, I., Lo, K., Cohan, A.: SciBERT: a pretrained language model for scientific text. arXiv preprint arXiv:1903.10676 (2019)
5. Beltagy, I., Peters, M.E., Cohan, A.: LongFormer: the long document transformer. arXiv preprint arXiv:2004.05150 (2020)
6. Bowman, S.R., Angeli, G., Potts, C., Manning, C.D.: A large annotated corpus for learning natural language inference. arXiv preprint arXiv:1508.05326 (2015)
7. Burns, P.B., Rohrich, R.J., Chung, K.C.: The levels of evidence and their role in evidence-based medicine. Plast. Reconstr. Surg. **128**(1), 305 (2011)
8. Cer, D., Diab, M., Agirre, E., Lopez-Gazpio, I., Specia, L.: SemEval-2017 task 1: semantic textual similarity-multilingual and cross-lingual focused evaluation. arXiv preprint arXiv:1708.00055 (2017)
9. Chen, Q., Peng, Y., Lu, Z.: BioSentVec: creating sentence embeddings for biomedical texts. In: 2019 IEEE International Conference on Healthcare Informatics (ICHI), pp. 1–5. IEEE (2019)
10. Deka, P., Jurek-Loughrey, A., Deepak, P.: Improved methods to aid unsupervised evidence-based fact checking for online health news. J. Data Intell. **3**(4), 474–504 (2022)
11. Derczynski, L., Bontcheva, K., Liakata, M., Procter, R., Hoi, G.W.S., Zubiaga, A.: SemEval-2017 task 8: RumourEval: determining rumour veracity and support for rumours. arXiv preprint arXiv:1704.05972 (2017)
12. Dernoncourt, F., Lee, J.Y.: PubMed 200k RCT: a dataset for sequential sentence classification in medical abstracts. arXiv preprint arXiv:1710.06071 (2017)

13. Devlin, J., Chang, M.W., Lee, K., Toutanova, K.: BERT: pre-training of deep bidirectional transformers for language understanding. arXiv preprint arXiv:1810.04805 (2018)
14. DeYoung, J., Lehman, E., Nye, B., Marshall, I.J., Wallace, B.C.: Evidence inference 2.0: more data, better models. arXiv preprint arXiv:2005.04177 (2020)
15. Evanega, S., Lynas, M., Adams, J., Smolenyak, K., Insights, C.G.: Coronavirus misinformation: quantifying sources and themes in the COVID-19 'infodemic'. JMIR Preprints **19**(10), 2020 (2020)
16. Gorrell, G., Bontcheva, K., Derczynski, L., Kochkina, E., Liakata, M., Zubiaga, A.: RumourEval 2019: determining rumour veracity and support for rumours. arXiv preprint arXiv:1809.06683 (2018)
17. Gu, Y., et al.: Domain-specific language model pretraining for biomedical natural language processing. ACM Trans. Comput. Healthc. (HEALTH) **3**(1), 1–23 (2021)
18. Hassan, N., et al.: ClaimBuster: the first-ever end-to-end fact-checking system. Proc. VLDB Endow. **10**(12), 1945–1948 (2017)
19. Henderson, M., et al.: Efficient natural language response suggestion for smart reply. arXiv preprint arXiv:1705.00652 (2017)
20. Jin, Q., Dhingra, B., Liu, Z., Cohen, W.W., Lu, X.: PubMedQA: a dataset for biomedical research question answering. arXiv preprint arXiv:1909.06146 (2019)
21. Khot, T., Sabharwal, A., Clark, P.: SciTaiL: a textual entailment dataset from science question answering. In: Thirty-Second AAAI Conference on Artificial Intelligence (2018)
22. Kouzy, R., et al.: Coronavirus goes viral: quantifying the COVID-19 misinformation epidemic on twitter. Cureus **12**(3) (2020)
23. Lee, J., et al.: BioBERT: a pre-trained biomedical language representation model for biomedical text mining. Bioinformatics **36**(4), 1234–1240 (2020)
24. Lehman, E., DeYoung, J., Barzilay, R., Wallace, B.C.: Inferring which medical treatments work from reports of clinical trials. arXiv preprint arXiv:1904.01606 (2019)
25. Li, X., Burns, G.A., Peng, N.: A paragraph-level multi-task learning model for scientific fact-verification. In: SDU@ AAAI (2021)
26. Liu, F., Shareghi, E., Meng, Z., Basaldella, M., Collier, N.: Self-alignment pretraining for biomedical entity representations. arXiv preprint arXiv:2010.11784 (2020)
27. Liu, Y., et al.: RoBERTa: a robustly optimized BERT pretraining approach. arXiv preprint arXiv:1907.11692 (2019)
28. Powers, D.M.: Evaluation: from precision, recall and f-measure to ROC, informedness, markedness and correlation. arXiv preprint arXiv:2010.16061 (2020)
29. Pradeep, R., Ma, X., Nogueira, R., Lin, J.: Scientific claim verification with VerT5erini. arXiv preprint arXiv:2010.11930 (2020)
30. Raffel, C., et al.: Exploring the limits of transfer learning with a unified text-to-text transformer. arXiv preprint arXiv:1910.10683 (2019)
31. Reimers, N., Gurevych, I.: Sentence-BERT: sentence embeddings using Siamese BERT-networks. arXiv preprint arXiv:1908.10084 (2019)
32. Romanov, A., Shivade, C.: Lessons from natural language inference in the clinical domain. arXiv preprint arXiv:1808.06752 (2018)
33. Sadat, M., Caragea, C.: SciNLI: a corpus for natural language inference on scientific text. arXiv preprint arXiv:2203.06728 (2022)
34. Sanh, V., Debut, L., Chaumond, J., Wolf, T.: DistilBERT, a distilled version of BERT: smaller, faster, cheaper and lighter. arXiv preprint arXiv:1910.01108 (2019)
35. Thorne, J., Vlachos, A., Christodoulopoulos, C., Mittal, A.: FEVER: a large-scale dataset for fact extraction and verification. arXiv preprint arXiv:1803.05355 (2018)

36. Vaswani, A., et al.: Attention is all you need. Adv. Neural Inf. Process. Syst. **30**, 5998–6008 (2017)
37. Vlachos, A., Riedel, S.: Fact checking: task definition and dataset construction. In: Proceedings of the ACL 2014 Workshop on Language Technologies and Computational Social Science, pp. 18–22 (2014)
38. Wadden, D., et al.: Fact or fiction: verifying scientific claims. arXiv preprint arXiv:2004.14974 (2020)
39. Wadden, D., Lo, K., Wang, L.L., Cohan, A., Beltagy, I., Hajishirzi, H.: LongChecker: improving scientific claim verification by modeling full-abstract context. arXiv preprint arXiv:2112.01640 (2021)
40. Williams, A., Nangia, N., Bowman, S.R.: A broad-coverage challenge corpus for sentence understanding through inference. arXiv preprint arXiv:1704.05426 (2017)
41. Wolf, T., et al.: HuggingFace's transformers: state-of-the-art natural language processing. arXiv preprint arXiv:1910.03771 (2019)
42. Zhang, Z., Li, J., Fukumoto, F., Ye, Y.: Abstract, rationale, stance: a joint model for scientific claim verification. arXiv preprint arXiv:2110.15116 (2021)
43. Zhou, X., Zafarani, R.: A survey of fake news: fundamental theories, detection methods, and opportunities. ACM Comput. Surv. (CSUR) **53**(5), 1–40 (2020)

Detection of Obsessive-Compulsive Disorder in Australian Children and Adolescents Using Machine Learning Methods

Umme Marzia Haque[1(✉)], Enamul Kabir[1], and Rasheda Khanam[2]

[1] School of Mathematics, Physics and Computing, University of Southern Queensland, Toowoomba, Australia
{UmmeMarzia.Haque,enamul.kabir}@usq.edu.au, marziahaque202@gmail.com

[2] School of Business, University of Southern Queensland, Toowoomba, Australia
rasheda.khanam@usq.edu.au

Abstract. Obsessive-compulsive disorder (OCD) is extremely common, but early detection is difficult because symptoms do not appear until puberty. Therefore, it is crucial to identify the causes of this mental illness. Making an early and accurate diagnosis of OCD in children and adolescents is essential to preventing the long-term problems. Several studies have looked at ways to recognise OCD in children, but their accuracy was not very high and they only included a few features and participants. Therefore, the purpose of this study was to examine the detection of OCD utilising machine learning algorithms and 667 features from Young Minds Matter (YMM), Australia's nationally representative mental health survey of children and adolescents aged 4 to 17 years. According to the internal CV score of the Tree-based Pipeline Optimization Tool (TPOTClassifier), the performance of the suggested technique has been evaluated on the YMM dataset using three of the most optimal algorithms, including Random Forest (RF), Decision Tree (DT), and Gaussian Naïve Bayes (GaussianNB). GaussianNB outperformed all other methods in classifying OCD with 91% accuracy, 76% precision, and 96% specificity, despite significant variation in model performance.

Keywords: OCD · YMM · RF · DT · GaussianNB · TPOTClassifier

1 Introduction

A common psychiatric disorder that affects children and adolescents is obsessive compulsive disorder (OCD). This disease is among the top 10 global causes of years spent handicapped, underscoring how serious it is and the pain it causes [1]. About 500,000 Australians, or between 2–3% of the population, have OCD [2]. Many of the affected kids went through their early years without even being aware of their OCD and they continue to be untreated as a result. Even in the ideal circumstances, this challenge may arise because childhood trauma has a major effect on OCD even in the earliest stages, at infancy [3]. Early-stage detection of OCD is difficult since the symptoms do not seem

A. Traina et al. (Eds.): HIS 2022, LNCS 13705, pp. 16–25, 2022.
https://doi.org/10.1007/978-3-031-20627-6_2

to fully manifest until adolescence, despite the fact that it frequently starts in childhood or adolescence [4]. Because the parents, relatives, caregivers, or teachers are unable to comprehend the symptoms, this disease is commonly left untreated. As a result, many children and adolescents who would benefit from early diagnosis are denied it. These severe problems emphasise the importance of figuring out the root causes of this mental illness in children and adolescents so that we can help their parents or other responsible people involved in their social and intellectual development who might not be aware that their kids or students are affected by this mental illness or whether they should seek medical advice to start treatment as soon as possible. Previously, machine learning (ML) techniques have been applied in OCD detection, with 61 adolescents with 46 demographic and clinical baseline variables by Child and Adolescent Psychiatry Research Center in Stockholm, Sweden [5]. In [6], OCD was identified with 72% accuracy calculated from 68 drug naïve OCD patients of Chinese Han nationality. Ensemble method has been used for OCD detection from 330 Iranian adult patients with 86% accuracy using 36 number of features [7]. In [8], ML has been used with Support Vector Machine (SVM) for OCD detection with 296 individuals with 75.4% accuracy using 24 baseline variables. OCD has been identified using SVM from 6 motion parameters with 54 drug naïve Chinese OCD patients [9]. These previous research results show a good value with accuracy, but they have considered a small number of participants with few collections of demographic data. As a result, the detection accuracy may not be representative. When compared to their counterparts in the community, children and adolescents with OCD appear to be at a greater risk of suffering higher levels of psychosocial stress and adversity [10]. To the best of our knowledge, no study on Australian children and adolescents has been undertaken to identify OCD using a precisely constructed dataset like Young Minds Matter (YMM) [11]. To overcome the methodological constraints of dataset imbalance of the previous research, this study will deal with 1011 cases of participants aged from 4 to 17 years using a large dimensional YMM dataset of 667 features. In this research, the performances of 32 machine learning algorithms have been evaluated to find out the most optimize result suited with the target dataset.

1.1 Contribution and Organization of the Paper

In this research, the YMM dataset, widely collected national representative Australian child and adolescents survey of mental health and wellbeing will be used to make the following indicators:

1. Identify the actual signs or symptoms of OCD that children and adolescents in Australia are encountering.
2. Evaluate the supervised models' performances in terms of measuring accuracy, sensitivity, specificity, precision, area under curve (AUC) and receiver operating characteristic curve (ROC) score and k-fold cross validation score.
3. Show the most significant features that contribute to OCD.

The remaining paper is presented as follows: Sect. 2 contains a detailed overview of the proposed methodology. Section 3 includes a full overview of the experimental method and results. Conclusions and future work are mentioned in Sect. 4.

2 Proposed Methodology

To investigate the performances of suggested ML algorithms in this research, data processing has been performed to set the target variable and feature selection from the source dataset (Fig. 1).

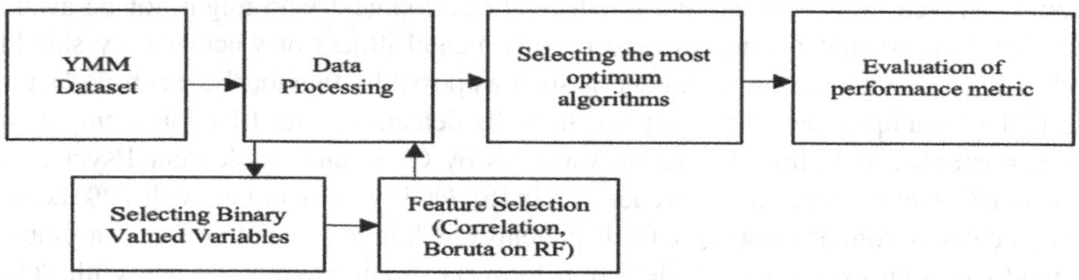

Fig. 1. The proposed approach for OCD detection

2.1 Dataset

Young Minds Matter (YMM), a nationally cross-sectional dataset is organised by the University of Western Australia (UWA) for the Telethon Kids Institute [12]. This survey has been conducted in collaboration with Roy Morgan Research. The YMM was the second Australian Child and Adolescent Survey of Mental Health and Wellbeing, conducted in 2013–14 that collected data from a diverse, nationally representative survey of 4–17 years children and adolescents and their parents or caregivers, including information about their mental disorders, child's learning, social conditioning, and healthy environment. This dataset can be accessed by contacting the Australian Data Archive (ADA) at the specified address (https://dataverse.ada.edu.au). In YMM, a multi-stage, area-based random sample procedure has been conducted. It has been developed to represent Australian families with children and teenagers. If a family had more than one eligible child, the survey has been performed to one of them at random. The survey included 6,310 parents/careers (55% of eligible households) of adolescents aged 4 to 17. The Diagnostic Interview Schedule for Children Version 4 (DISC-4) has been used in this dataset as a validated instrument for diagnosing mental health issues in children based on the Diagnostic and Statistical Manual of Mental Disorders Version 4 (DSM-4) criteria [12]. To overcome the methodological constraints of imbalance dataset from the previous research [13], this study will deal with 1011 cases of participants aged from 4 to 17 years using a large dimensional YMM dataset of 667 features. From the parent reported data, these 1011 individuals have been selected based on their mental health status that have been considered with these variables (child or adolescent went to doctor, mental health professional, psychiatrist, psychologist).

2.2 Data Processing

Target Variable
The factors informing the state of OCD confirmed by a doctor or mental health professional, as well as the continuation of OCD diagnosis, have been chosen for measuring the target variable. If any of these factors has a true value, the target feature is validated as OCD = 1, otherwise it is nonOCD = 0.

Feature Selection
Other than the target variable, all variables that inform the OCD confirmed by a doctor or professional mental health care professional have been excluded from the training set as they have been considered for measuring the target variable. After careful observation of data cleaning in order to accelerate data insights, 667 categorical variables with 'Yes' and 'No' values have been identified out of 2622 variables from the dataset. The response categories 'Do not know,' 'Refused,' and 'Missing' have been consciously eliminated from the analysis. The Pearson correlation of these 667 independent factors with the target outcome has been calculated. The Variables with a low correlation with the target variable have been eliminated. As correlated variables, might lead to misleading feature importance, a range was manually identified from the high correlated variables with the OCD target variable. A set of correlated values between the given variables and the target variable has been chosen. The best subset of 57 input features has been picked at a stage where the Root Mean Square Error and coefficient of determination are the lowest and highest (0.24, 0.27).

2.3 Methodology

The best algorithm for accurately identifying depression in Australian children and adolescents has been identified using The YMM dataset, which has been used to compare the performances of 32 ML algorithms [13]. The performance of 32 algorithms was evaluated, and the most accurate diagnosis for OCD, ADHD, and SAD with the best algorithm was determined using the same process. At first, using the Python 3.7.3 sci-kit-learn package, the Random Forest (RF) classifier has been implemented with the Boruta method for unbiased and stable selection by partitioning the entire dataset into training and test datasets with 57 high correlated features. The second step is to implement the Tree-based Pipeline Optimization Tool (TPOTClassifier) to examine 32 machine learning supervised algorithms to choose the most suitable supervised learning models with the dataset. After choosing the most significant features done by Boruta on RF, at the third step, the internal cv score of TPOTClassifier has been considered in order to pick appropriate supervised learning models and optimise their parameters [14]. Finally, according to the internal cv score of TPOTClassifier, the machine-learning algorithms such as RF, Decision Tree (DT), and Gaussian Naïve Bayes (GaussianNB) have been selected to find the most optimum result for this model.

ML Algorithms
Boruta Algorithm

Boruta is a wrapper method based on RF. It determines the relevance and importance of characteristics in respect to the target variable by deleting unsuitable features [15, 16].

Random Forest (RF)
The RF builds multiple decision trees and then combines them to produce a more accurate and dependable prediction. These number of trees and maximum tree depth in an RF algorithm are hyper-parameters that indicate how many interactions in the model are evaluated [17].

Tree-Based Pipeline Optimization Tool (TPOTClassifier)
The TPOTClassifier is a machine-learning algorithm which can determine the optimal parameters and model ensembles using genetic programming. It includes supervised classification models, preprocessors, selection techniques, and any other science-learn API-assessment estimators or transformers [18].

Decision Tree (DT)
The DT is divided into decision as class labels and leaf nodes as characteristics. The inside nodes of the tree represent the test data or input pattern. The internal nodes give mutually exclusive and exhaustive results for each test data based on the divide and conquer idea [19, 20].

Gaussian Naïve Bayes (GaussianNB)
The GaussainNB applies the Naive Bayes method with a Gaussian distribution with no co variances to determine the probability among the values of features. The input feature values are represented as vectors, and instances are assigned as class labels [21].

Performance Measure
The performance of the suggested machine learning methods has been measured by collecting True Positive (TP), True Negative (TN), False Positive (FP), and False Negative (FN) results by the confusion matrix. The accuracy, precision, sensitivity, specificity and F1 score in each ML model have been determined following the equations:

$$\text{Accuracy Rate} = \frac{TP + TN}{TP + FP + TN + FN} \tag{1}$$

$$\text{Precision} = \frac{TP}{TP + FP} \tag{2}$$

$$\text{Sensitivity} = \frac{TP}{TP + FN} \tag{3}$$

$$\text{Specificity} = \frac{TN}{TN + FP} \tag{4}$$

$$\text{F1score} = \frac{2 * Precision * Recall}{Precision + Recall} \tag{5}$$

3 Experimental Results and Discussion

In the YMM dataset, a minority class is observed to have 73 'OCD' class, however a majority class is regarded to have 938 'NonOCD,' resulting in an entirely imbalanced dataset encompasses 1011 cases [22]. The RF classifier has been applied with Boruta algorithm by partitioning dataset into training (70% observations) and test (30% observations) datasets, yielding 6 input features for OCD among top ranked 57 features shown in Table 1.

Table 1. Most significant 6 input features

#	OCD questionnaires Training set size: 707 Test set size: 304	Frequency Proportion	
		OCD	nonOCD
1	Not simply excessive worries about real-life problems	56.67%	43.33%
2	Attempts to ignore or suppress thoughts	37.84%	62.16%
3	Washing	100%	0%
4	Aimed at preventing or reducing stress	68.75%	31.25%
5	Checking: Distress, time-consuming, or interferes with functioning	71.79%	28.21%
6	Counting: Distress, time-consuming, or interferes with functioning	90%	10%

Using the sci-kit-learn module, the confusion matrices presented in Table 2 have been created by applying all three approaches such as RF, DT and GaussianNB to detect OCD.

Table 2. Accuracy, precision, specificity and sensitivity of RF, DT and GaussianNB

Disease	Models	Accuracy	Precision	Specificity	Sensitivity	F1 score
OCD	RF	0.92	0.57	0.97	0.36	0.44
	DT	0.92	0.54	0.97	0.32	0.40
	GaussianNB	0.91	0.76	0.96	0.50	0.60

Table 2 shows the accuracy, precision, specificity, sensitivity and F1 scores of different ML algorithms. The AUC and ROC scores of these 3 algorithms have been shown in Fig. 2.

All the ROC (AUC) values shown in Fig. 2 are within the acceptable range (>0.70, <0.80), and is slightly lower than the outstanding score of 0.80 [23]. From these performance metric, GaussianNB outperformed RF and DT in terms of detecting OCD, except the accuracy score. The K-Fold cross validation scores have been shown in Table 3.

Table 3 summarises the results of K-fold cross-validation for 3-fold, 5-fold, and 10-fold repetitions. Though RF scores the best in all terms of K-fold cross validation

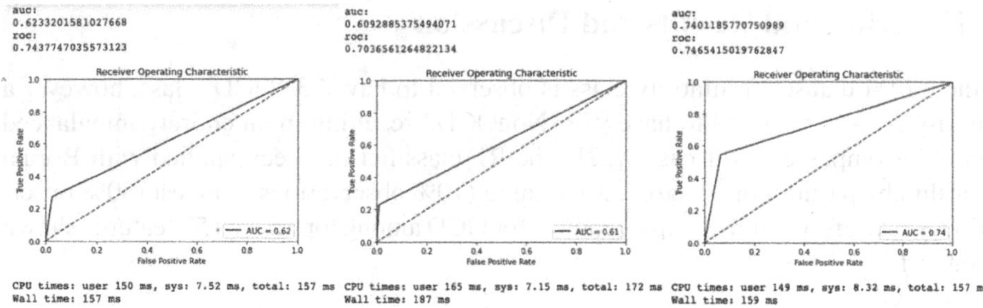

Fig. 2. AUC and ROC scores for a) RF, b) DT and c) GaussianNB

Table 3. Result of K-Fold cross validation of OCD detection

Disease	Models	3-fold	5-fold	10-fold
OCD	RF	0.9335	0.9330	0.9352
	DT	0.9317	0.9267	0.9146
	GaussianNB	0.8262	0.8315	0.8244

scores, the GaussianNB performs well in terms of precision (76%), sensitivity (50%), and F1 score (60%). GaussianNB has a specificity of 96%, which is somewhat lower than RF (97%). However, the sensitivity, which is a significant indication for reliably identifying positive cases, is much higher for GaussianNB (50%) than for RF (36%). In circumstances of classification imbalance of the sample dataset, the best model is the one with the highest F1 score to predict the actual positive cases, even if its accuracy is lower [24]. GaussianNB has the highest F1 score in OCD identification. Table 4 shows how the decision has been determined for 5 sample test cases with the fitted GaussianNB model in OCD prediction using the most significant input features.

It is critical to comprehend the causes of OCD in children and adolescents in order to effectively and quickly diagnose it for earlier detection and treatment. To identify significant patterns between input features with target domain in order to make adequate decisions, machine learning models need training data from a large dimensional dataset. In this study, YMM, Australia's most recent nationally representative mental health survey of children and adolescents has been used [11, 12]. The top 57 high correlated features from 667 binary valued variables have been identified form this large dimensional dataset. Moreover, this target variable in this dataset is also confirmed by a doctor, a mental health expert, and the status of OCD diagnosis. As a result, in the Australian context, this model can predict OCD in children and adolescents with 91% accuracy as well 96% specificity using the most significant 6 features. These 6 features have also been identified as important predictors of OCD symptoms in the previous research [25–27].

Table 4. Prediction of OCD in child and adolescence

Not simply excessive worries about real-life problems	Attempts to ignore or suppress thoughts	Washing	Aimed at preventing or reducing stress	Checking: Distress, time-consuming, or interferes with functioning	Counting: Distress, time-consuming, or interferes with functioning	Predicted OCD
1	0	1	0	0	0	1
1	1	0	0	0	1	1
1	0	0	1	0	0	0
1	0	1	1	1	1	1
1	0	1	0	1	0	1

* Note: 1 = yes, 0 = no.

4 Conclusion

The social and intellectual growth of children and adolescents, as well as their general wellbeing, depend on the early identification and treatment of OCD. GaussianNB has been discovered to be an effective and accurate classifier for diagnosing OCD using YMM, a large dimensional dataset on the mental health of children and adolescents in Australia. The performances of all three algorithms (RF, DT, and GaussianNB) in terms of confusion matrix parameters, K-fold cross validation results, scores of AUC, and ROC have shown the capabilities of TPOTClassifier in our model. The results of this model also show how the YMM dataset has a substantial predictive impact on OCD. There are several existing predictive models for OCD detection; however, this model is more accurate and instructive in predicting child and adolescent OCD in the Australian context due to its large dimensional dataset, optimal feature set, and most importantly, high precision, specificity, and F1 score in prediction. Therefore, this model can serve as the foundation for the identification of OCD in children and adolescents. In order to identify whether a child has OCD or not, the most prevalent six input features have been identified as questionnaire items for children, their parents, or carers. This approach can help them identify the condition early and start treatment as soon as feasible to prevent long-term obstacles.

Statements and Declarations. We confirm that all authors declare that they have no competing interests. The paper has been seen and approved by all authors and that they agree on the order of authorship. We ensure that this manuscript has not been published elsewhere and is not under consideration by another conference. All authors have read and approved the manuscript and agreed to be accountable for all aspects of the work.

References

1. Murray, C.J., Lopez, A.D., World Health Organization: The global burden of disease: a comprehensive assessment of mortality and disability from diseases, injuries, and risk factors in 1990 and projected to 2020: summary. World Health Organization (1996)
2. Burke, R.: The Lava Tube: A Christian's Personal Journey with Obsessive Compulsive Disorder. Wipf and Stock Publishers (2017)
3. Larson, S., et al.: Chronic childhood trauma, mental health, academic achievement, and school-based health center mental health services. J. Sch. Health **87**(9), 675–686 (2017)
4. Bloch, M.H., et al.: Adulthood outcome of tic and obsessive-compulsive symptom severity in children with Tourette syndrome. Arch. Pediatr. Adolesc. Med. **160**(1), 65–69 (2006)
5. Lenhard, F., et al.: Prediction of outcome in internet-delivered cognitive behaviour therapy for paediatric obsessive-compulsive disorder: a machine learning approach. Int. J. Methods Psychiatr. Res. **27**(1), e1576 (2018)
6. Yang, X., et al.: Multivariate classification of drug-naive obsessive-compulsive disorder patients and healthy controls by applying an SVM to resting-state functional MRI data. BMC Psychiatry **19**(1), 1–8 (2019)
7. Hasanpour, H., et al.: Novel ensemble method for the prediction of response to fluvoxamine treatment of obsessive–compulsive disorder. Neuropsychiatr. Dis. Treat. **14**, 2027 (2018)
8. Askland, K.D., et al.: Prediction of remission in obsessive compulsive disorder using a novel machine learning strategy. Int. J. Methods Psychiatr. Res. **24**(2), 156–169 (2015)
9. Bu, X., et al.: Investigating the predictive value of different resting-state functional MRI parameters in obsessive-compulsive disorder. Transl. Psychiatry **9**(1), 1–10 (2019)
10. Findley, D.B., et al.: Development of the Yale Children's Global Stress Index (YCGSI) and its application in children and adolescents with Tourette's syndrome and obsessive-compulsive disorder. J. Am. Acad. Child Adolesc. Psychiatry **42**(4), 450–457 (2003)
11. Hafekost, K., et al.: Validation of the adolescent self-esteem questionnaire: technical report. Telethon Kids Institute and the Graduate School of Education, The University of Western Australia, Perth, Australia, vol. 15, no. 10, p. 2018 (2017)
12. Hafekost, J., et al.: Methodology of young minds matter: the second Australian child and adolescent survey of mental health and wellbeing. Aust. N. Z. J. Psychiatry **50**(9), 866–875 (2016)
13. Haque, U.M., Kabir, E., Khanam, R.: Detection of child depression using machine learning methods. PLoS One **16**(12), e0261131 (2021)
14. Le, T.T., Fu, W., Moore, J.H.: Scaling tree-based automated machine learning to biomedical big data with a feature set selector. Bioinformatics **36**(1), 250–256 (2020)
15. Kursa, M.B., Rudnicki, W.R.: Feature selection with the Boruta package. J. Stat. Softw. **36**(11), 1–13 (2010)
16. Kursa, M.B.: Boruta for those in a hurry (2020)
17. Breiman, L.: Random forests. Mach. Learn. **45**(1), 5–32 (2001)
18. Olson, R.S., et al.: Evaluation of a tree-based pipeline optimization tool for automating data science. In: 2016 Proceedings of the Genetic and Evolutionary Computation Conference (2016)
19. Laura, I., Santi, S.: Introduction to data science. In: Laura, I., Santi, S. (eds.) Introduction to Data Science: A Python Approach to Concepts, Techniques and Applications, pp. 1–4. Springer, Cham (2017). https://doi.org/10.1007/978-3-319-50017-1_1
20. Nilsson, N.J.: Introduction to Machine Learning (1997)
21. Kharya, S., Soni, S.: Weighted naive bayes classifier: a predictive model for breast cancer detection. Int. J. Comput. Appl. **133**(9), 32–37 (2016)

22. Japkowicz, N.: Learning from imbalanced data sets: a comparison of various strategies. In: AAAI Workshop on Learning from Imbalanced Data Sets. AAAI Press, Menlo Park (2000)
23. Mandrekar, J.N.: Receiver operating characteristic curve in diagnostic test assessment. J. Thorac. Oncol. **5**(9), 1315–1316 (2010)
24. Japkowicz, N., Shah, M.: Evaluating Learning Algorithms: A Classification Perspective. Cambridge University Press, Cambridge (2011)
25. McKay, D., et al.: A critical evaluation of obsessive–compulsive disorder subtypes: symptoms versus mechanisms. Clin. Psychol. Rev. **24**(3), 283–313 (2004)
26. Foa, E.B., et al.: The obsessive-compulsive inventory: development and validation of a short version. Psychol. Assess. **14**(4), 485 (2002)
27. Abramowitz, J.S., et al.: Symptom presentation and outcome of cognitive-behavioral therapy for obsessive-compulsive disorder. J. Consult. Clin. Psychol. **71**(6), 1049 (2003)

An Anomaly Detection Framework Based on Data Lake for Medical Multivariate Time Series

Peng Ren[1], Zhiyuan Tian[2](✉), Zeyu Wang[2], Xin Li[3], Xia Wang[4], Tao Zhao[5], and Ming Sheng[1]

[1] BNRist, DCST, RIIT, Tsinghua University, Beijing 100084, China
{renpeng,shengming}@tsinghua.edu.cn
[2] Beijing Institute of Technology, Beijing 100081, China
tian107@foxmail.com, wangzeyu@bit.edu.cn
[3] Beijing Tsinghua Changgung Hospital, School of Clinical Medicine, Tsinghua University, Beijing 100084, China
Horsebackdancing@sina.com
[4] Institute for Intelligent Healthcare, Tsinghua University, Beijing 100084, China
wangxia_dt@tsinghua.edu.cn
[5] Shangqiu Institute of Technology, Shangqiu 476000, China

Abstract. Anomaly detection of multivariate time series has become a critical task in the medical domain. With the quick development of medical devices, a large amount of multi-source heterogeneous multivariate time series data is produced. Traditional data platforms have difficulties to organize and explore these data. In addition, the high dimensionality of multivariate time series also makes it difficult for the detection process to capture the correlation between different features. In this paper, we propose an anomaly detection framework based on data lake for medical multivariate time series. Firstly, heterogeneous data are fused to provide a big wide table. Then we help the doctors to explore data, filter out related features and get a filtered dataset. To reduce redundant or noisy data in the filtered dataset, we refine it with Relief algorithm. Finally, we identify anomalies through a multi-scale convolutional recurrent encoder-decoder. Experiments on a synthetic dataset and a use case of heart sound recordings confirm the validity of our framework.

Keywords: Data lake · Heterogeneous medical data · Multivariate time series · Anomaly detection · Auto-encoder

1 Introduction

Anomalies are the values in a dataset that differ significantly from correctly sensed values, and detecting these anomalies is critical because the operators can take further actions to resolve underlying issues [1]. By utilizing anomaly detection, doctors could improve medical efficiency and help their scientific research [2]. However, data storage becomes a problem because a large amount of multi-source heterogeneous multivariate time series

A. Traina et al. (Eds.): HIS 2022, LNCS 13705, pp. 26–33, 2022.
https://doi.org/10.1007/978-3-031-20627-6_3

data is produced. Traditional methods have two difficulties in the medical anomaly detection: identifying really related and useful features and the lack of a powerful data platform. To deal with data issues, Dixon [3] first proposes the concept of data lake, making the efficient data storage ability reality.

The doctors' knowledge can help more accurate feature extraction and selection in medical anomaly detection. Many works have confirmed the usefulness of empirical knowledge in feature selection [4, 5]. In medical domain, rich empirical knowledge from doctors could directly help select useful features, so we design an interface for doctors to contribute their prior knowledge, inspired by HKGB [6].

A lot of the anomaly detection researches focus on IoT data. He et al. [7] propose a framework for arrhythmia detection from IoT-based ECGs, which consists of a data cleaning module and a heartbeat classification module. Hill and Minsker [8] propose an approach for outlier detection in environmental sensor data. In the medical domain, Haque et al. [9] develop techniques to detect false alarms in medical sensor networks. However, most of these techniques cannot capture the sequential correlation in multivariate time series.

This paper proposes an anomaly detection framework for medical multivariate time series. By integrating the whole process based on the data lake platform [10], this framework could help medical workers detect anomalies of patients efficiently. We use data lake to store and integrate multi-source heterogeneous data. Different formats of structured and unstructured data are transformed into one unified format as a wide table. After that, doctors could use their empirical knowledge to select the useful features in the table. Finally, after further refining process, we utilize deep learning methods to conduct anomaly detection for multivariate time series data.

Our contributions are as follows:

1. We propose an anomaly detection framework based on data lake for medical multivariate time series. Unstructured data and structured data are merged into a wide table so that we could use them to explore essential features.
2. We develop a data exploration method and a data refining method to get proper features. With empirical knowledge of doctors, useful features and appropriate time length could be extracted.
3. We develop two medical anomaly detection methods. Both methods are based on encoder-decoder, which addresses the problem of sequential correlation by implementing system signature matrix.

In the rest of the paper, we will first discuss related work in Sect. 2. Then, we briefly introduce the workflow and architecture of our proposed framework in Sect. 3. The next three sections introduce details of the framework and Sect. 7 describes a case study. Finally, Sect. 8 concludes the paper.

2 Related Work

Literature related to anomaly detection frameworks include two aspects, which are anomaly detection frameworks and anomaly detection methods. Few researches focus on the medical domain and they often ignore the usage of empirical knowledge. Besides, they have relatively low accuracy on the multivariate time series data.

Anomaly detection frameworks in medical domain have not been fully explored in previous researches. Laptev et al. [11] propose a generic anomaly detection framework. However, they use traditional methods to detect anomalies and do not have the data exploration process. Venkataraman et al. [12] propose a black box anomaly detection framework that can be applied to a variety of data sources. This framework uses less efficient data storage tool and does not consider empirical knowledge in specific domains. Siuly et al. [13] develop a framework that can use EEG data to automatically distinguish mild cognitive impairment patients from healthy control subjects, but they ignore empirical knowledge, either. A summary of related work on anomaly detection frameworks is shown in Table 1.

Table 1. Summary of anomaly detection frameworks

Name	Heterogeneous data	Big data platform	Data exploration	Deep learning methods
EGADS [11]	×	√	×	×
TrafficComber [12]	√	×	×	×
Automatic framework [13]	×	×	√	√
Our work	√	√	√	√

As for the models, previous researches have tried to develop several methods to solve the problem of anomaly detection of time series data. We focus on the deep learning methods. Based on the multi-scale encoder-decoder model, Zhang et al. [14] introduce the concept of system signature matrix to capture the correlation between multivariable time series. Kieu et al. [15] use a sparse connected recurrent neural network to construct an auto-encoder. Adam et al. [16] propose an approximate projection automatic encoder (APAE) to obtain better reconstruction output. Most of the above researches are uninterpretable data-driven methods. On the contrary, knowledge-driven methods are highly interpretable and context-aware, which consist of two steps: knowledge acquisition and knowledge transformation [17, 18]. The combination of data-driven methods and knowledge-driven methods could develop a more efficient and interpretable technique.

Overall, previous methods have space for improvement due to the high-dimensional characteristics of multivariate time series data and the ignorance of empirical knowledge.

3 Proposed Framework

We propose an anomaly detection framework for medical multivariate time series based on data lake. This framework utilizes a data lake platform to realize data fusion and data exploration. In this section, we first introduce the workflow of the framework and then present key system design.

The workflow is depicted in Fig. 1. Multi-source heterogeneous data produced in various medical processes are merged by the data fusion module. Then, we invite doctors to conduct the data exploration process. After this process, we obtain a unified wide table consisting of different features in different periods. Then, in data refining, we conduct data preprocessing and obtain training and evaluation datasets. Finally, we use deep learning methods to detect anomalies. It is noteworthy that we conduct feature selection in data refining process, so the outcome of anomaly detection could reversely generate knowledge that is ignored by doctors.

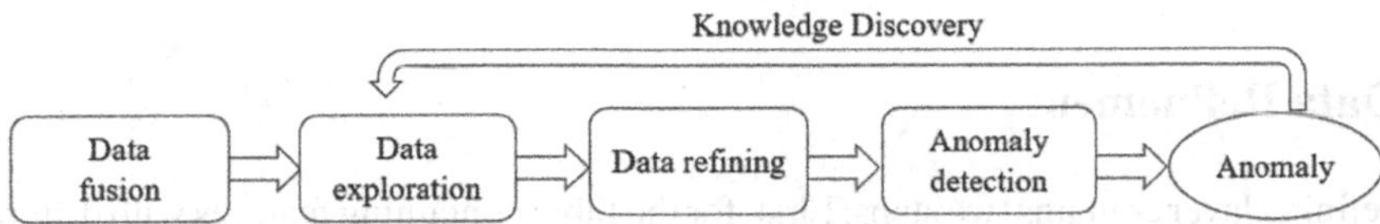

Fig. 1. Workflow of anomaly detection

The architecture of the proposed framework is presented in Fig. 2. There are four layers: data fusion layer, data exploration layer, refining layer and application layer, which correspond to the above work flow step. We will discuss details of these layers in the next following three sections.

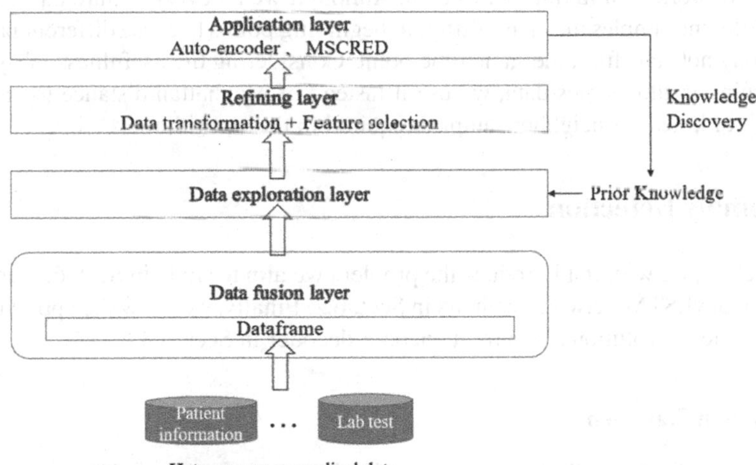

Fig. 2. Architecture of anomaly detection framework

4 Data Fusion and Exploration

We extend Delta Lake, a famous opensource data lake, to provides scalable and persistent storage capacity for medical multi-source heterogeneous data [10]. Through data fusion, more useful features and longer time periods can be merged. We use a unified concept for representation and adopt a new management mode for structured data and unstructured data.

After the fusion of multi-source data in data lake, we obtain a wide table. However, although this table has many features, some features are useless for further study, which increases workload and decreases efficiency. Moreover, some irrelevant features may reduce the significance of those vital features and cause misjudgments. Therefore, we need to conduct data exploration to reduce the dimensionality and simplify the table. Doctors can click any part of the table according to their need to merge, delete or interpolate any column or row in the table. Eventually, the simplified form serves in the platform as a new input for the subsequent refining layer.

5 Data Refinement

The refining layer contains two steps. First, for the table containing features with different time periods, we split individuals into different tables and transform them into training and evaluation datasets. Second, we use Relief algorithm to conduct further feature selection.

Relief algorithm is considered to be one of the most effective feature selection methods because of its simplicity and effectiveness. This paper uses this algorithm as the main method in the refining layer. However, it is worth noting that we have made some improvements. The distance in the original Relief algorithm uses the Manhattan distance that may not work well in time series data. Although we let every feature has the same length, different samples may have different beginning points because different patient's disease may not start from the same time point. Considering the usefulness of dynamic time warping in time series data, we use it instead of Manhattan distance to calculate the search of k-nearest neighbor samples required in the algorithm.

6 Anomaly Detection

In this section, we will first introduce the problem we aim to study in Sect. 6.1, and then show the ConvLSTM network methods in Sect. 6.2. Finally, we show the application of the multiscale convolutional recurrent encoder-decoder in Sect. 6.3.

6.1 Problem Statement

Definition 1: Given a collection of time series X_i = (x1, ..., xn) $\in R^{n*T}$, i = 1, ...m, where m is the number of samples, n is the number of features, T is the maximum of time steps, and X_i is the historical data of sample i, medical anomaly detection aims at finding anomaly events at certain time steps.

The method used in this paper is an unsupervised method, where the auto-encoder model lies in the core to model multivariate time series data and find abnormal patterns.

6.2 Convolutional LSTM Based Auto-encoder (CLBA)

Auto-encoder could be used to detect anomalies by comparing the reconstruction error. We use a CNN(Convolutional Neural Network) and a LSTM network as the encoder. CNN is mostly used for the recognition of two-dimensional data. Time series data contain sample information and characteristic information of each sample, which is similar to a two-dimensional picture. Therefore, we use a convolutional layer as the encoder. In this work, we use a Rectified Linear Unit (ReLU) as the activation function and 256 convolutional kernels with a size of 5 * 5. In addition, the same padding module is used.

CNN can capture the correlation between different time series, but the temporal dependency on the same time series has not been recognized. Temporal dependency is a major challenge for the anomaly detection of time series data. Considering the excellent performance of the LSTM model in pattern recognition of time series data, we add a LSTM network after the convolution layer to capture the temporal dependency of multivariate time series. In this work, we use an LSTM network with 256 hidden layers to receive input from the convolutional layer.

To decode the output from the previous LSTM layer and obtain the reconstructed error, we use a fully connected layer as the decoder layer. We maintain the output dimension exactly the same as the input of the whole network, so we could compare the output with the original data via the L-2 norm.

6.3 Multi-scale Convolutional Recurrent Encoder-Decoder (MSCRED)

We further extend CLBA to multi-scale convolutional recurrent encoder-decoder [14]. First, we introduce the concept of the system characteristic matrix. We can use the paired inner product of the subsequences of two time series to express the correlation between them. By selecting the length of different subsequences, we can not only use this signature matrix to model the correlation between two time series but also make the model more robust to the input noise.

After obtaining the system signature matrix, we can input the multi-scale system signature matrix into the convolutional encoder. Instead of using one layer, multi-layer convolution is conducted. The spatial feature maps generated by convolutional encoder is temporally dependent on previous time steps. We use an attention-based ConvLSTM to adaptively select relevant hidden states across different time steps. This improvement allows the model to capture the temporal information in the time series. The ConvLSTM layer is between the encoder and decoder. A specific explanation of this model can be found in previous research [14]. Correspondingly, we use the same size convolutional decoder to substitute the fully connected layer, as illustrated in the previous section. The final output of the decoder has the same size as the input matrices.

Finally, we design experiments to demonstrate that MSCRED's performance in anomaly detection and robustness to noise. A synthetic dataset that includes 30 time series is used, which is generated by trigonometric function and Gaussian noise. We compare MSCRED with five baseline methods of four categories, i.e., classification model, density estimation model and temporal prediction model. The result is shown in Table 2 and demonstrates the effectiveness of MSCRED.

Table 2. Anomaly detection results on synthetic data

Method	Synthetic data		
	Pre	Rec	F1
OC-SVM	0.14	0.44	0.22
DAGMM	0.33	0.20	0.25
HA	0.71	0.52	0.60
ARMA	0.91	0.52	0.66
LSTM-ED	1.00	0.56	0.72
MSCRED	**1.00**	**0.80**	**0.89**

7 Case Study

We use a heart sound recordings dataset from the PhysioNet/CinC Challenge 2016 [19]. The data are sourced from several contributors around the world, collected in either a clinical or nonclinical environment, from both healthy subjects and pathological patients.

After initial data fusion in the data lake, it is the doctors' work to conduct the data exploration process. Doctors use their empirical knowledge to determine which features are useful. In this case, to determine the most useful features to diagnose which patient has cardiac disease, doctors will select the typical four locations, which are the aortic area, pulmonic area, tricuspid area and mitral area. The sensors in these locations are chosen. After the data exploration process, we obtain a unified wide table consisting of features. Then, the data transformation module in the refining layer transforms the table into a training dataset and an evaluating dataset. By using Relief algorithm, we have access to refined features. Finally, by utilizing auto-encoder based methods in the application layer, we obtained the anomalies, i.e., in this case, the patients who had cardiac disease.

8 Conclusion

This paper proposes an anomaly detection framework for medical multivariate time series data based on data lake. Doctors and other related medical workers could use flexible query interface to explore useful features and obtain an efficient time series dataset. By using Relief as the refining algorithm, we can conduct a preprocessing task before anomaly detection to get proper features. Finally, we propose two auto-encoder based methods to complete anomaly detection. Several methods are combined to provide more accurate feature selection. Conversely, the results of anomaly detection can provide practical information about useful time length and features. Thus, this framework could help doctors both in clinical practice and scientific research. In the future, we will try to enhance the interpretability of the anomaly detection model.

Acknowledgement. This work was supported by National Key R&D Program of China (2020AAA0109603).

References

1. Chandola, V., Banerjee, A., Kumar, V.: Anomaly detection: a survey. ACM Comput. Surv. (CSUR) **41**(3), 1–58 (2009)
2. Qiao, Z., He, J., Cao, J., Huang, G., Zhang, P.: Multiple time series anomaly detection based on compression and correlation analysis: a medical surveillance case study. In: Sheng, Q.Z., Wang, G., Jensen, C.S., Xu, G. (eds.) APWeb 2012. LNCS, vol. 7235, pp. 294–305. Springer, Heidelberg (2012). https://doi.org/10.1007/978-3-642-29253-8_25
3. Dixon, J.: Pentaho, Hadoop, and Data Lakes, October 2010. https://jamesdixon.wordpress.com/2010/10/14/pentaho-hadoop-and-data-lakes/
4. Yamada, M., Kimura, A., Naya, F., et al.: Change-point detection with feature selection in high-dimensional time-series data. In: Twenty-Third International Joint Conference on Artificial Intelligence (2013)
5. He, W., Wang, Z., Jiang, H.: Model optimizing and feature selecting for support vector regression in time series forecasting. Neurocomputing **72**(1–3), 600–611 (2008)
6. Yong, Z., Ming, S., Rui, Z., et al.: HKGB: an inclusive, extensible, intelligent, semi-auto-constructed knowledge graph framework for healthcare with clinicians' expertise incorporated. Inf. Process. Manag. **57**(6), 102324 (2020)
7. He, J., Rong, J., Sun, L., Wang, H., Zhang, Y., Ma, J.: A framework for cardiac arrhythmia detection from IoT-based ECGs. World Wide Web **23**(5), 2835–2850 (2020). https://doi.org/10.1007/s11280-019-00776-9
8. Hill, D.J., Minsker, B.S.: Anomaly detection in streaming environmental sensor data: a data-driven modeling approach. Environ. Model. Softw. **25**(9), 1014–1022 (2010)
9. Haque, S.A., Rahman, M., Aziz, S.M.: Sensor anomaly detection in wireless sensor networks for healthcare. Sensors **15**(4), 8764–8786 (2015)
10. Ren, P., Lin, W., Liang, Y., Wang, R., Liu, X., Zuo, B., Chen, T., Li, X., Sheng, M., Zhang, Y.: HMDFF: a heterogeneous medical data fusion framework supporting multimodal query. In: Siuly, S., Wang, H., Chen, Lu., Guo, Y., Xing, C. (eds.) HIS 2021. LNCS, vol. 13079, pp. 254–266. Springer, Cham (2021). https://doi.org/10.1007/978-3-030-90885-0_23
11. Laptev, N., Amizadeh, S., Flint, I.: Generic and scalable framework for automated time-series anomaly detection. In: Proceedings of the 21th ACM SIGKDD International Conference on Knowledge Discovery and Data Mining (2015)
12. Venkataraman, S., Caballero, J., Song, D., et al.: Black box anomaly detection: is it utopian? Irvine Is Burning 127 (2006)
13. Siuly, S., Alçin, Ö.F., Kabir, E., et al.: A new framework for automatic detection of patients with mild cognitive impairment using resting-state EEG signals. IEEE Trans. Neural Syst. Rehabil. Eng. **28**(9), 1966–1976 (2020)
14. Zhang, C., Song, D., Chen, Y., et al.: A deep neural network for unsupervised anomaly detection and diagnosis in multivariate time series data. In: The Thirty-Third AAAI Conference on Artificial Intelligence (2019)
15. Kieu, T., Yang, B., Guo, C., et al.: Outlier detection for time series with recurrent autoencoder ensembles. In IJCAI (2019)
16. Goodge, A., Hooi, B., Ng, S.-K., et al.: Robustness of autoencoders for anomaly detection under adversarial impact. In: IJCAI (2020)
17. Lykourentzou, I., Papadaki, K., Kalliakmanis, A., et al.: Ontology-based operational risk management. In: IEEE 13th Conference on Commerce and Enterprise Computing. IEEE (2011)
18. Glimm, B., Horrocks, I., Motik, B., et al.: HermiT: an OWL 2 reasoner. J. Autom. Reason. **53**(3), 245–269 (2014). https://doi.org/10.1007/s10817-014-9305-1
19. Liu, C., Springer, D., Li, Q., et al.: An open access database for the evaluation of heart sound algorithms. Physiol. Meas. **37**(12), 2181 (2016)

Anomaly Detection on Health Data

Durgesh Samariya(✉) and Jiangang Ma

School of Engineering, Information Technology and Physical Sciences,
Federation University, Churchill, VIC, Australia
{d.samariya,j.ma}@federation.edu.au

Abstract. The identification of anomalous records in medical data is an important problem with numerous applications such as detecting anomalous reading, anomalous patient health condition, health insurance fraud detection and fault detection in mechanical components. This paper compares the performances of seven state-of-the-art anomaly detection algorithms to do detect anomalies in healthcare data. Our experimental results in six datasets show that the state-of-the-art method of isolation based method iForest has a better performance overall in terms of AUC and runtime.

Keywords: Anomaly · Anomaly detection · Healthcare · Machine learning

1 Introduction

Anomalies (a.k.a outliers) are the data points that are different and rare compared to the majority of data points. The following are some of the definitions found in literature:

- "An outlying observation, or 'outlier', is one that appears to deviate markedly from other members of the sample in which it occurs." [10]
- "An outlier is an observation which deviates so much from the other observations as to arouse suspicions that it was generated by a different mechanism." [12]
- "Anomalies are patterns in data that do not conform to a well-defined notion of normal behaviour." [7]

Anomaly detection have wide range of real-world application domains.

- **Intrusion detection.** In this domain, network or a computer system's malicious activities are referred as outliers. In this domain outlier detection monitor and analyse network from intrusion.
- **Fault detection/diagnosis.** In this domain, outlier detection process monitor faults occurring in mechanical machines such as motors, generators.
- **Healthcare.** In this domain, outliers are often considered as unusual health conditions of patients. In healthcare, it is essential to detect such outliers; detecting such outlier gives time to provide appropriate treatment to patients before any serious health condition.

A. Traina et al. (Eds.): HIS 2022, LNCS 13705, pp. 34–41, 2022.
https://doi.org/10.1007/978-3-031-20627-6_4

Apart from these applications, anomaly detection can be used in many other applications as well. We redirect our readers to these works [7,13,19] for extensive list of application domains for anomaly detection.

The reminder of this paper is organized as follows. Section 2 presents key state-of-the-art anomaly detection methods used; the details of experimental setup, datasets, methods to generate synthetic datasets and the implementation of anomaly detectors is provided in Sect. 3. Section 4 presents experimental results and discussion followed by conclusion in Sect. 5.

2 Key State-of-the-Art Methods

2.1 *k* Nearest Neighbors (*k*NN)

The *k*-NN global anomaly score is a widely used technique among other distance-based methods [1]. As name suggest, firstly, such technique find the *k*-Nearest Neighbors of each data points. Once neighbors are found, they are used to calculate anomaly score. Their are two different ways to compute the anomaly score of a data point – (i) distance to its kth-nearest neighbor as used in [17] (ii) the average or median distance to its all *k*-nearest neighbors as computed in [2]. In this paper, we will using 3 variant of *k*NN which are *k*NN, Avg. *k*NN and Median *k*NN.

2.2 Local Outlier Factor (LOF)

The core idea of density-based outlier detection is, the density of the anomaly object is significantly different from the normal instance. The first local density-based approach, called LOF which is stands for **L**ocal **O**utlier **F**actor introduced by Breunig et al. (2000) [6], which is the widely used local outlier detection approach. For any data object, the LOF score is the ratio of the average local density of its *k*-nearest neighbours to its local density [7]. The LOF score of data object q is defined as follows:

$$\text{LOF}(q) = \frac{\sum\limits_{x \in N^k(q)} lrd(x)}{|N^k(q)| \times lrd(q)}$$

where $lrd(q) = \frac{|N^k(q)|}{\sum\limits_{x \in N^k(q)} max(dist^k(x,D), dist(q,x))}$, $N^k(q)$ is a set of k-nearest neighbours of q, $dist(q,x)$ is a distance between q and x and $dist^k(q,D)$ is the distance between q and its k-NN in D. The LOF score represents the sparseness of data object. Data objects with higher LOF values are considered as outliers.

2.3 Isolation Forest

Liu et al. (2008, 2012) [15,16] presented a framework, called **I**solation **Forest** or iForest, which isolates each data point by axis-parallel partitioning of the attribute space. To the best of my knowledge, iForest is the first technique that uses isolation mechanism to detect anomaly.

iForest builds an ensemble of trees called isolation tree (iTree). Each iTree is built using randomly selected subsample without replacement from the data set. At each node, a random split is performed on a randomly selected point from attribute space. The partition will terminate once all the nodes have only one data object or nodes reach the tree's height limit for iTree. The anomaly score for $q \in \mathcal{R}^d$ based on iForest is defined as:

$$\text{iForest}(q) = \frac{1}{t} \sum_{i=1}^{t} l_i(q)$$

where $l_i(q)$ is the path length of q in tree T_i.

2.4 Histogram Based Outlier Score

In 2012, Goldstein and Dengel [9] proposed a **H**istogram-**B**ased **O**utlier **S**core (HBOS). HBOS is a simple yet more intuitive statistical based outlier detection technique. The idea of HBOS is similar to the popular classification Naive Bayes algorithm. HBOS is a two stage process; in first stage, HBOS first creates histogram in each dimensions and in subsequent stage, anomaly score for each data objects computed as multiplication of the inverse probability density (total data points fall in bin or height of bin) in which data resides in each dimension. The idea of using histogram is quite popular in intrusion detection [8,21].

2.5 Sp

Rather than searching for k-nearest neighbour in data set, Sugiyama and Borgwardt (2013) [20] employs scoring measure based on the nearest neighbour ($k=1$) in random subsamples ($\mathcal{S} \subset D$). The Sp score of data object q is defined as follows:

$$\text{Sp}(q) = \min_{x \in \mathcal{S}} dist(q, x)$$

where $dist(q, x)$ is a distance between q and x.

In [20], authors have shown that, Sp perform better than state-of-the-art anomaly detector LOF and runs faster than LOF.

2.6 iNNE

Tharindu et al. (2014, 2017) [4,5] proposed iNNE, which is stands for **i**solation using **N**earest **N**eighbor **E**nsemble. The core idea behind iNNE is an anomaly far away from its nearest neighbor, and the inverse is true for the regular object. iNNE implementation is influenced by iForest and LOF. The critical difference between iNNE and iForest, iForest build tree from subspaces while iNNE builds hyperspheres using all dimension. Isolation score of q is defined as follows:

$$I(q) = \begin{cases} 1 - \frac{\tau(\eta_{cnn(q)})}{\tau(cnn(q))}, & if q \in \bigcup_{c \in \mathcal{S}} \mathcal{B}(c), \\ 1, & otherwise \end{cases}$$

where $cnn(q) = \arg\min_{c \in S}\{\tau(c) : q \in \mathcal{B}(c)\}$, $\mathcal{S}$ is set of randomly selected subsamples, $|\mathcal{S}| = \psi$, $\mathcal{B}(c)$ is a hypersphere centered at c with radius $\tau(c) = ||c - \eta_c||$, where η_c is nearest neighbour of c. The anomaly score for data object q is defined as:

$$\text{iNNE}(q) = \frac{1}{t}\sum_{i=1}^{t} I_i(q)$$

where $I_i(q)$ is isolation score based on subsample in i^{th} set.

2.7 SPAD

In an independent study, [3] have introduced **S**imple **P**robabilistic **A**nomaly **D**etector (SPAD) which is based on the histogram. The intuition behind SPAD is an anomaly is dramatically different than in a few features where it has low probability. SPAD score of any data object q is computed as follows.

$$\text{SPAD}(q) = \sum_{i=1}^{d} \log \frac{|H_i(q)| + 1}{N + b}$$

where $H_i(q)$ is the bin in which q fall into in dimension i. $|\cdot|$ is a cardinality of the set.

3 Experimental Evaluation

3.1 Datasets

We evaluate each of measure described in Sect. 2 using 8 datasets ranging from 80 to 7129 data samples and containing 8 to 259 features. All datasets are publicly available on the ODDS library[1] [18]. The summary of datasets used in this study is presented in Table 1. Our study assess the effectiveness of each model based on unseen data, thus it is require for each algorithms to support unseen data. We split each data set in 70% of training data and 30% of testing data.

[1] http://odds.cs.stonybrook.edu.

Table 1. Summary of the datasets.

Data set	#instances (n)	#dimensions (D)	#anomalies (%)
Annthyroid	7129	21	534 (7.47%)
Arrhythmia	452	259	206 (45.78%)
Cardio	2114	21	466 (22.04%)
Heart	224	44	10 (4.4%)
Thyroid	3772	6	93 (2.5%)
WBC	278	30	21 (4.48%)

3.2 Algorithm Implementation and Parameters

We used Java implementation of SPAD implementation, which is provided by the authors [3]. We implemented all other algorithms using PyOD [22] python library. We used default parameters of each algorithms as suggested in respective papers unless specified otherwise.

- kNN: size of nearest neighbour (k) = 5, metric = euclidean;
- LOF: size of nearest neighbour (k) = 10, metric = euclidean;
- iForest: number of sets t = 100, and sub-sample size ψ = 256;
- HBOS: number of bins = 10; alpha (α) = 0.1; tolerance = 0.5;
- Sp: sub-sample size ψ = 20; and
- iNNE: number of sets t = 100, and sub-sample size ψ = 8.

3.3 Evaluation Measures

We evaluate the effectiveness (performance) of the anomaly detector methods by comparing the area under the ROC curve (AUC) [11] for anomaly ranking produced by an anomaly detector. Anomaly detector with high AUC indicates better detection accuracy, whereas low AUC indicates low detection accuracy.

We perform all experiments in an unsupervised setting. Specifically, we trained and tested anomaly detectors on the same datasets. However, we assumed that label information is unavailable. We only used class label information to calculate AUC in the evaluation stage.

All experiments were conducted in a MacOS machine with a 2.3 GHz 8-core Intel Core i9 processor and 16 GB memory running on MacOS Monterey 12.4.

4 Experimental Results and Discussion

Table 2 shows AUC obtained by seven anomaly detection algorithms. Overall there are no measure which perform best in all datasets. iForest and SPAD perform best in two datasets where as kNN, HBOS, and iNNE perform best in only one data set. LOF and Sp perform poorly on each data set. iForest is either top performing measure or second on each data set except on WBC.

Table 2. AUC score comparison of kNN, LOF, iForest, HBOS, Sp, iNNE and anomaly detection methods on 6 real-world healthcare datasets. Best performing measure is bold faced.

Data set	kNN	LOF	iForest	HBOS	Sp	iNNE	SPAD
Annthyroid	0.61	0.63	0.66	0.55	0.49	0.53	**0.77**
Arrhythmia	0.74	0.72	0.81	**0.85**	0.76	0.79	0.80
Cardio	0.51	0.62	**0.69**	0.63	0.64	0.31	0.49
Heart	0.69	0.45	0.69	0.65	0.45	**0.72**	0.65
Thyroid	0.93	0.88	**0.99**	0.97	0.93	0.95	**0.99**
WBC	**0.98**	0.96	0.91	0.93	0.91	0.93	0.67

Table 3. Runtime comparison of kNN, LOF, iForest, HBOS, Sp, iNNE and anomaly detection methods on 6 real-world healthcare datasets. Runtimes are in seconds, fastest measure is underlined.

Data set	kNN	LOF	iForest	HBOS	Sp	iNNE	SPAD
Annthyroid	0.48	0.11	0.38	0.71	0.01	0.44	0.23
Arrhythmia	0.03	0.01	0.23	0.05	0.01	0.21	0.20
Cardio	0.08	0.02	0.25	0.01	<0.01	0.22	0.11
Heart	0.01	0.01	0.19	<0.01	<0.01	0.14	0.02
Thyroid	0.09	0.08	0.28	<0.01	<0.01	0.25	0.07
WBC	0.01	0.01	0.19	0.01	<0.01	0.14	0.04

Table 3 shows runtime comparison of seven anomaly detection algorithms. Overall, Sp is the fastest measure. However, it is worst performing measure. HBOS as is second fastest measure and in term of performance it is second best performing measure.

Figure 1 shows the critical difference diagram [14] over seven anomaly detection algorithms. As previously mentioned, the state-of-the-art anomaly detector iForest is top performing measure.

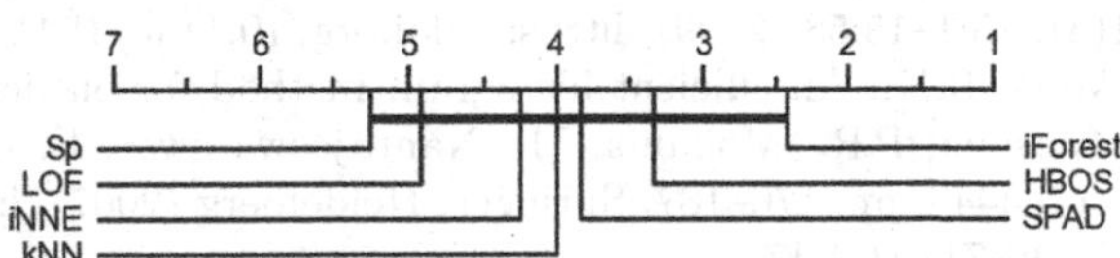

Fig. 1. Critical difference (CD) diagram of the post-hoc Nemenyi test ($\alpha = 0.05$).

5 Conclusion

This paper introduces seven state-of-the-art anomaly detection algorithms, which includes classic distance based kNN, density based LOF, SPAD, histogram based HBOS, sampling based Sp and isolation based iForest and iNNE. All measures have been evaluated on the seven real-world healthcare datasets obtained from the ODDS library. The area under curve (AUC) scores and runtime results shows that both iForest and HBOS have comparative performance than the other five anomaly measures.

Acknowledgments. This work is supported by Federation University Research Priority Area (RPA) scholarship, awarded to Durgesh Samariya.

References

1. Amer, M., Goldstein, M.: Nearest-neighbor and clustering based anomaly detection algorithms for rapidminer. In: Proceedings of the 3rd RapidMiner Community Meeting and Conference (RCOMM 2012), pp. 1–12 (2012)
2. Angiulli, F., Pizzuti, C.: Fast outlier detection in high dimensional spaces. In: Elomaa, T., Mannila, H., Toivonen, H. (eds.) PKDD 2002. LNCS, vol. 2431, pp. 15–27. Springer, Heidelberg (2002). https://doi.org/10.1007/3-540-45681-3_2
3. Aryal, S., Ting, K.M., Haffari, G.: Revisiting attribute independence assumption in probabilistic unsupervised anomaly detection. In: Chau, M., Wang, G.A., Chen, H. (eds.) PAISI 2016. LNCS, vol. 9650, pp. 73–86. Springer, Cham (2016). https://doi.org/10.1007/978-3-319-31863-9_6
4. Bandaragoda, T.R., Ting, K.M., Albrecht, D., Liu, F.T., Wells, J.R.: Efficient anomaly detection by isolation using nearest neighbour ensemble. In: 2014 IEEE International Conference on Data Mining Workshop, pp. 698–705 (2014). https://doi.org/10.1109/ICDMW.2014.70
5. Bandaragoda, T.R., Ting, K.M., Albrecht, D., Liu, F.T., Zhu, Y., Wells, J.R.: Isolation-based anomaly detection using nearest-neighbor ensembles. Comput. Intell. 1–31 (2017). https://doi.org/10.1111/coin.12156
6. Breunig, M.M., Kriegel, H.P., Ng, R.T., Sander, J.: LOF: identifying density-based local outliers. SIGMOD Rec. **29**(2), 93–104 (2000). https://doi.org/10.1145/335191.335388
7. Chandola, V., Banerjee, A., Kumar, V.: Anomaly detection: a survey. ACM Comput. Surv. **41**(3), 15:1–15:58 (2009). https://doi.org/10.1145/1541880.1541882
8. Gebski, M., Wong, R.K.: An efficient histogram method for outlier detection. In: Kotagiri, R., Krishna, P.R., Mohania, M., Nantajeewarawat, E. (eds.) DASFAA 2007. LNCS, vol. 4443, pp. 176–187. Springer, Heidelberg (2007). https://doi.org/10.1007/978-3-540-71703-4_17
9. Goldstein, M., Dengel, A.: Histogram-based outlier score (HBOS): a fast unsupervised anomaly detection algorithm. KI-2012: Poster and Demo Track, pp. 59–63 (2012)
10. Grubbs, F.E.: Procedures for detecting outlying observations in samples. Technometrics **11**(1), 1–21 (1969). https://doi.org/10.1080/00401706.1969.10490657
11. Hand, D.J., Till, R.J.: A simple generalisation of the area under the roc curve for multiple class classification problems. Mach. Learn. **45**(2), 171–186 (2001)

12. Hawkins, D.M.: Introduction. In: Hawkins, D.M. (ed.) Identification of Outliers, vol. 11, pp. 1–12. Springer, Dordrecht (1980). https://doi.org/10.1007/978-94-015-3994-4_1
13. Hodge, V., Austin, J.: A survey of outlier detection methodologies. Artif. Intell. Rev. **22**(2), 85–126 (2004). https://doi.org/10.1023/B:AIRE.0000045502.10941.a9
14. Ismail Fawaz, H., Forestier, G., Weber, J., Idoumghar, L., Muller, P.A.: Deep learning for time series classification: a review. Data Min. Knowl. Disc. **33**(4), 917–963 (2019)
15. Liu, F.T., Ting, K.M., Zhou, Z.H.: Isolation forest. In: 2008 Eighth IEEE International Conference on Data Mining, pp. 413–422 (2008). https://doi.org/10.1109/ICDM.2008.17
16. Liu, F.T., Ting, K.M., Zhou, Z.H.: Isolation-based anomaly detection. ACM Trans. Knowl. Discov. Data **6**(1), 3:1–3:39 (2012). https://doi.org/10.1145/2133360.2133363
17. Ramaswamy, S., Rastogi, R., Shim, K.: Efficient algorithms for mining outliers from large data sets. SIGMOD Rec. **29**(2), 427–438 (2000). https://doi.org/10.1145/335191.335437
18. Rayana, S.: ODDS library (2016). http://odds.cs.stonybrook.edu
19. Samariya, D., Thakkar, A.: A comprehensive survey of anomaly detection algorithms. Ann. Data Sci. (2021). https://doi.org/10.1007/s40745-021-00362-9
20. Sugiyama, M., Borgwardt, K.: Rapid distance-based outlier detection via sampling. In: Burges, C.J.C., Bottou, L., Welling, M., Ghahramani, Z., Weinberger, K.Q. (eds.) Advances in Neural Information Processing Systems, vol. 26, pp. 467–475. Curran Associates, Inc. (2013). https://proceedings.neurips.cc/paper/2013/file/d296c101daa88a51f6ca8cfc1ac79b50-Paper.pdf
21. Xie, M., Hu, J., Tian, B.: Histogram-based online anomaly detection in hierarchical wireless sensor networks. In: 2012 IEEE 11th International Conference on Trust, Security and Privacy in Computing and Communications, pp. 751–759. IEEE (2012)
22. Zhao, Y., Nasrullah, Z., Li, Z.: PyOD: a python toolbox for scalable outlier detection. J. Mach. Learn. Res. **20**(96), 1–7 (2019). http://jmlr.org/papers/v20/19-011.html

DRAM-Net: A Deep Residual Alzheimer's Diseases and Mild Cognitive Impairment Detection Network Using EEG Data

Ashik Mostafa Alvi[1(✉)], Siuly Siuly[1], Maria Cristina De Cola[2], and Hua Wang[1]

[1] Victoria University, Melbourne, VIC, Australia
ashik.alvi@live.vu.edu.au, {siuly.siuly,hua.wang}@vu.edu.au
[2] IRCCS Centro Neurolesi "Bonino-Pulejo", SS 113, Via Palermo C / da Casazza, 98123 Messina, Italy
mariacristina.decola@irccsme.it

Abstract. Mild Cognitive Impairment (MCI) and Alzheimer's diseases (AD) are two common neurodegenerative disorders which belong to the dementia family mostly found in elders. There is evidence that MCI may lead to Alzheimer's disease. Since there is no treatment for AD after it has been diagnosed, it is a significant public health problem in the twenty-first century. Existing classical machine learning methods fail to detect AD and MCI more efficiently and accurately because of their shallow and limited architecture. Electroencephalography (EEG) is emerging as a portable, non-invasive, and cheap diagnostic tool to analyze MCI and AD, whereas other diagnostic tools like computed tomography, positron emission tomography, mini-mental state examination, and magnetic resonance imaging are expensive and time-consuming. To address these obstacles, a deep residual Alzheimer's disease and MCI detection network (DRAM-Net) based framework has been introduced to detect MCI and AD using EEG data. This multi-class study contains EEG data collection, preprocessing (down-sampling, de-noising and temporal segmentation), DRAM-Net architecture to classify AD, MCI and normal subjects and experiment evaluation stages. Our proposed DRAM-Net framework has obtained 96.26% overall multiclass accuracy, outperforming existing multi-class studies, and also claimed accuracy of 96.66% for the normal class, 98.06% for the MCI class, and 97.79% for the AD class. This study will create a new pathway for future neuro-disease researchers and technology experts.

Keywords: Alzheimer's diseases · Mild cognitive impairment · EEG · Deep learning · Deep residual network

1 Introduction

Mild cognitive impairment (MCI) and Alzheimer's disease (AD) are linked to dementias induced by neurodegeneration. These neurological condition are mostly caused by the loss and dysfunction of neurons in the brain's cells. Symptoms of MCI and AD include

A. Traina et al. (Eds.): HIS 2022, LNCS 13705, pp. 42–53, 2022.
https://doi.org/10.1007/978-3-031-20627-6_5

memory loss, decreased vocabulary, and a decreased ability to perform accurate motor movements [1]. Approximately 50 million individuals worldwide are expected to suffer from dementia, and 60% of those instances are linked to Alzheimer's disease [3]. MCI is treated as the preliminary stage of AD [11]. People with AD or MCI have a wide variety of brain processes impaired, including memory and learning, as well as the ability to do complicated tasks like executive and motor skills and the ability to pay attention to others [2]. With age, the likelihood of experiencing it increases by a factor of 10 and often affects those over the age of 65 [4]. AD and MCI are currently untreatable and once diagnosed with AD, patients live 5–8 years [5, 19]. However, early detection may delay the progression of the disease and improve the quality of life for patients and their caregivers [24, 26].

Existing tools includes computed tomography, positron emission tomography, mini-mental state examination, and magnetic resonance imaging to detect MCI and AD are expensive, invasive and time consuming [12, 23]. Whereas, electroencephalography (EEG) is a newly emerged portable, low cost, easy to understand and access, and quick tool to identify neuro-disorders like AD and MCI [15]. EEG recordings retain the electrical movements in the cerebral cortex relative to time, which are the fundamental drivers for assessing neurological disorders. The procedure for capturing EEG data means placing electrodes on the scalp according to a specific design, with the international 10–20 system being the most popular set up [2]. In account of this, we have addressed the use of EEG as a useful approach for identifying MCI and AD at an earlier stage.

In order to identify MCI early and prevent it from progressing into AD or other cognitive diseases, several studies have been conducted in the last few decades. Morabito et al. [7] had performed a binary (AD vs MCI) epoch based classification using Convolutional Neural Network (CNN) with 11 MCI and 4 AD subjects. Recorded EEG data were preprocess by Power Spectral Density (PSD) and then a multi-dimensional CNN with *softmax* classifier model was employed to complete the binary classification. This effort gained accuracy rate up to 98.97% (95% confidence range: 98.68%–99.26%). A recent deep learning (DL) based approach [22] proposed two DL models: modified CNN and convolutional auto encoder (Conv-AE) neural network (NN) to differentiate 61 healthy volunteers (HVs), 56 MCI, and 63 AD participants. Time–frequency representation (TFR) with continuous wavelet transform (CWT) has been used for processing the EEG data prior to feed to the NNs. CNN and Conv-AE NN model achieved 92% and 89% average accuracy respectively. Ieracitano et al. [9] carried out an AD-MCI study with multiple machine learning (ML) methods [25, 27] with 63 AD, 63 MCI, and 63 HVs. CWT and higher order statistics (HOS) from the bispectrum (BiS) features were extracted and fed into Multi-Layer Perceptron (MLP), auto encoder (AE), Logistic Regression (LR), and Support Vector Machine (SVM). MLP outperformed rest of the ML [8, 20] classifiers used in this study with an accuracy of 89.22%. Another classical ML based effort [6, 10] with 109 participants (49 AD, 37 MCI, and 23 HVs) had been introduced where Fast Fourier Transform (FFT) and Discrete Wavelet Transform (DWT) were performed to obtain the spectrum features and denoising the signal. A Decision Tree (DT) with C4.5 algorithm was applied to perform the classification task and it received 83%, 92%, and 79% accuracy while differentiating HV vs AD, HV vs MCI, and MCI vs AD respectively. Pirrone et al. [2] proposed DT, SVM, and K-nearest neighbor (KNN) based AD-MCI study with 48 AD, 37 MCI, and 20 HVs and KNN remained at the top with 97%, 95%, 83%, and 75% accuracy (HV vs. AD, HV vs. MCI, MCI vs. AD, and HV vs. AD vs. MCI).

The studies we have reviewed have used the same multi-class EEG dataset that we have used. While analyzing these studies, we have concluded that most of the studies were conducted using classical ML algorithms [16, 18] and most importantly the multi-class performance is poor (below 90%). Classical ML algorithms have the tendency and limitation to overlook some important feature of the complex EEG data as their architecture do not allow them to capture those. To resolve these problems, we have come up with a DL based effort to not only enhance the performance but also extract those extra hidden complex features of EEG data which have significant involvement in classifier's learning rate. We have proposed a deep residual Alzheimer's disease and MCI detection network (DRAM-Net) framework consisting of four stages: EEG data collection, preprocessing, DRAM-Net architecture to identify MCI, AD, and Normal participants, and experiment evaluation. Below is the key contribution of this proposed DRAM-Net framework:

- For the first time, we have introduced a deep residual network, customly designed for AD-MCI detection
- Our experiment uses 5 s temporal segments and 5 s of EEG data is good enough to decide the patient's condition
- This proposed DRAM-Net framework has outperformed all the existing multi-class AD-MCI studies with this EEG dataset

The rest of the article has organized as following: Sect. 2 introduces the proposed DRAM-Net framework. Results and discussion are elaborated in Sect. 3. Finally, this study finishes with future study and conclusion in Sect. 4.

2 Proposed DRAM-Net Framework

This study represents a deep residual AD and MCI detection network (DRAM-Net) using EEG data. Figure 1 outlines the whole framework in a nutshell. This proposed DRAM-Net framework is made of four steps. In EEG data collection step, we gathered the raw EEG data of 109 subjects, Preprocessing: down-sampling, noise removing, and temporal segmentation are done to make sure the EEG data is clean and ready to feed to the network, DRAM-Net architecture where the preprocessed data are fed and the classifications are done, and finally the quality of the proposed model is checked in experiment evaluation step. A detailed talk about DRAM-Net is reported below.

2.1 EEG Data Collection

This multi-class study uses an EEG dataset containing 109 subjects enrolled in the IRCCS Centro Neurolesi "Bonino-Pulejo" [2, 10]. Among these 109 subjects, 49 AD, 39 MCI, and 23 HVs were present. The average age of patients with Alzheimer's disease and mild cognitive impairment is 78.4 6.4% and 74.1 9.4%, respectively, whereas the average age of healthy controls is 65.6 7.4%. The inclusion criteria were the diagnosis of AD or MCI, while the exclusion criteria were the existence of neurological or psychiatric illnesses that may cause cognitive imbalance, complicated systemic disorders, the presence of Epileptiform patterns in the EEGs, hydrocephalus, stroke, traumatic brain injuries, or other neurological abnormalities. The objective of this EEG recordings were explained to all the participants and everyone signed the consent form. Following the World Heath Organization's standard, the recording tool place and was approved by the local Ethics Committee of the RCCS Centro Neurolesi "Bonino-Pulejo". All the participants were in resting condition keeping their eyes closed. 19 electrodes (Fp1, Fp2, F3, F4, C3, C4, P3, P4, O1, O2, F7, F8, T3, T4, T5, T6, Fz, Cz and Pz) were placed across the scalp of each subject following the international 10–20 standard. The recording took place about 300 s for each subjects with a sampling frequency of 256 or 1024 Hz.

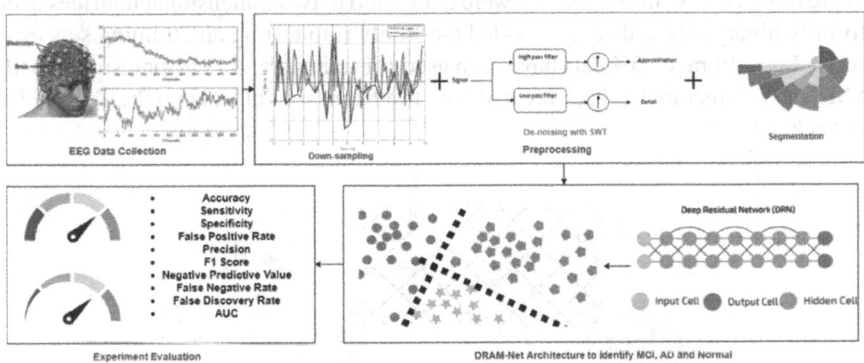

Fig. 1. DRAM-Net framework for AD, MCI, and normal subject's detection.

2.2 Preprocessing

Down-Sampling. Collected raw EEG data were not uniform in terms of sampling frequency. Therefore, we have made it uniform by down-sampling the sampling frequency to 256 Hz for all subjects using MATLAB.

Denoising with SWT. EEG recordings may be contaminated by a variety of factors, including electrode pops, eye blinks, outlier readings, power supply fluxes and interference (50 Hz), baseline drift, breathing patterns, and other electrical activities [13, 17, 21]. To remove these artifacts, Stationary Wavelet Transformation (SWT) has been applied to the down-sampled EEG recordings. A detailed description of this denosing process can be found in [1].

Temporal Segmentation. This study starts with an EEG dataset of 109 subject. However, just to increase the number of training and testing samples and also a quick efficient model, we have segmented the dataset. As mentioned in the EEG data collection step, each recording tool place for about 300 s. For this work, each subject's 300 s denoised recordings were segmented into 5 s chunks. After this segmentation process, 4525 AD, 3789 MCI, and 1663 HV temporal segments have been generated. All the newly created segments are stored as comma-separated values (CSV) files using MATLAB.

2.3 DRAM-Net Architecture to Identify AD, MCI, and HVs

This proposed DRAM-Net framework aims to discover AD, MCI, and HVs more accurately and efficiently. To ensure our objectives, the raw collected data have been properly preprocessed. We have introduced deep residual network for the first time with any EEG study and customly designed for AD, MCI, and HVs detection.

This classification process starts with importing all the temporal segments stored as CSV files. With the help of Python's Pandas library these CSV files and corresponding labels are inputted. All the dataframes were converted to two dimensional matrices using the NumPy library. Then, data are divided randomly into testing and training sets using the Scikit-Learn library. 85% data have been used for training and 15% for testing. Lastly, DRAM-Net architecture has been created with the Keras module having the TensorFlow as the backend.

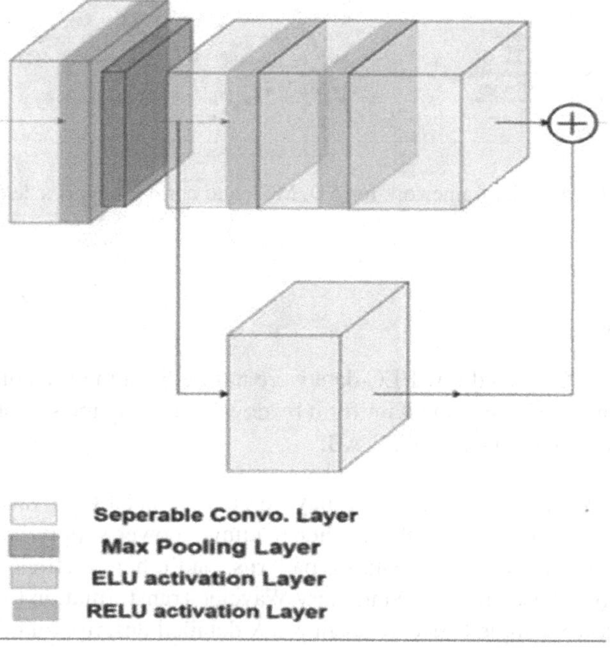

Fig. 2. Residual block of the proposed DRAM-Net.

DRAM-Net starts with a *SeparableConv2D* layer having 16 neurons. We have kept the kernel size and strides fixed for all the layers which are (4, 4) and (1, 1) respectively. A batch normalization has been performed using the *BatchNormalization()* function in the Keras library. A *ReLU* activation function has been added after that. There are four residual blocks present in our proposed DRAM-Net architecture. Figure 2 illustrates a single residual block. We have included a *MaxPooling2D* layer before and after each of those residual blocks. Each of these four residual block composed with 3 *SeparableConv2D* layers having 16, 32, 64, and 96 neurons respectively. Inside the residual block, *SeparableConv2D* layers are activated with *ELU* function. The final convolutional layer of each residual block is combined with the shortcut connection, and then a RELU activation layer is applied [14]. Lastly, a global average pooling function is carried out to create a 1D-vector, which is subsequently fed into a fully connected layer.

To stop over fitting, an early stopping set up has made by monitoring validation loss. *min_delta* and *patience* parameters havebeen holding 0.001 and 10 value respectively. The best model has been stored as hdf5 format. The batch size and number of epoch have been set to 32 and 150 respectively.

The training and testing process has been run on a Windows PC having 256 GB RAM, AMD Ryzen Threadripper PRO 3995WX 64-Cores 2.70 GHz processor, and NVIDIA RTX A6000 graphics card.

3 Results and Discussions

This study aims to establish a DL based method for efficient detection of AD, MCI, and HVs using EEG data. The preprocessing steps of this proposed study has produced 9977 temporal segments (4525 AD, 3789 MCI, and 1663 HVs). This has enabled us to have an accurate and efficient model as we have enough number of samples to extract the deep hidden features and use them while training the DRAM-Net.

Following (1), (2), (3), (4), (5), (6), (7), (8), (9), and (10) are the performance matrices used experiment evaluation where TP, TN, FP, and FN stands for true positive, true negative, false positive, and false negative respectively.

$$Accuracy = \frac{\mathrm{TP} + \mathrm{TN}}{TP + TN + FP + FN} \times 100 \tag{1}$$

$$Sensitivity = \frac{\mathrm{TP}}{TP + FN} \times 100 \tag{2}$$

$$Specificity = \frac{\mathrm{TN}}{TN + FP} \times 100 \tag{3}$$

$$False\ Positive\ Rate = \frac{\mathrm{FP}}{FP + TN} \times 100 \tag{4}$$

$$Precision = \frac{\mathrm{TP}}{TP + FP} \times 100 \tag{5}$$

$$F1\ Score = 2 \times \frac{Precision \times Sensitivity}{Precision + Sensitivity} \times 100 \tag{6}$$

$$Negative\ Predictive\ Value = \frac{\mathrm{TN}}{TN + FN} \times 100 \tag{7}$$

$$FalseNegativeRate = \frac{\text{FN}}{TP + FN} \times 100 \tag{8}$$

$$FalseDiscoveryRate = \frac{\text{FP}}{TP + FP} \times 100 \tag{9}$$

$$AUC = 1 - ROC \tag{10}$$

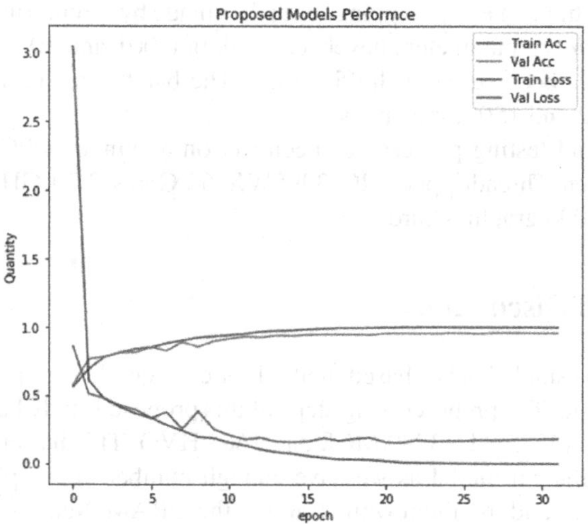

Fig. 3. Epoch vs overall accuracy of the proposed DRAM-Net.

Our proposed DRAM-Net framework took only 32 epochs to beat the existing efforts accuracy with the same EEG data set. Figure 3 shows the overall accuracy of DRAM-Net over 32 epochs. Initially, the accuracy was below 60%. As the learning rate increases, the accuracy grows. It is important to mention that the preprocessing steps have helped the DRAM-Net architecture to learn very quickly by removing the artifacts and extracting deep hidden important features.

After the splitting, there were 1497 samples in the testing set. Overall confusion matrix of the proposed DRAM-Net is portrayed in Fig. 4. 240, 537, and 664 samples have correctly identified as HVs, MCI, and AD respectively. And the misclassification rate is very low. Class wise performance report has been noted in Table 1, 2 and 3.

While classifying the normal subjects the accuracy has dropped a bit compared to the other two classes. Table 1 represents the performance report of normal class. DRAM-Net achieved 96.66% accuracy, 89.55% sensitivity, 98.21% specificity, 1.79% false positive rate (FPR), 91.60% precision, 90.57% F1 score, 97.73% negative predictive value (NPV), 10.45% false negative rate (FNR), 8.40% false discovery rate (FDR), and 93.88% area under the ROC (AUC) curve value.

DRAM-Net has performed so well while identifying MCI participants. Overall performance report of MCI class is reported in Table 2. DRAM-Net gained 98.06% accuracy,

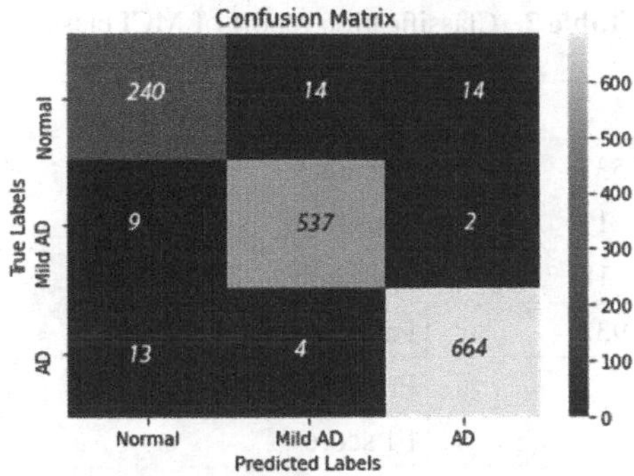

Fig. 4. Overall confusion matrix of the proposed DRAM-Net.

Table 1. Classification report of normal class.

Confusion matrix		Performance matrixes	
True positive	240	Accuracy	96.66%
True negative	1207	Sensitivity	89.55%
False positive	22	Specificity	98.21%
False negative	28	False positive rate	1.79%
		Precision	91.60%
		F1 score	90.57%
		Negative predictive value	97.73%
		False negative rate	10.45%
		False discovery rate	8.40%
		AUC	93.88%

97.99% sensitivity, 98.10% specificity, 1.90% FPR, 96.76% precision, 97.37% F1 score, 98.83% NPV, 2.01% FNR, 3.24% FDR, and 98.05% AUC.

Table 3 presents the overall classification report of AD class. While testing AD samples after model creation, DRAM-Net has received 97.80% accuracy, 97.50% sensitivity, 98.04% specificity, 1.96% FPR, 97.65% precision, 97.57% F1 score, 97.92% NPV, 2.50% FNR, 2.35% FDR, 97.77% AUC. Confusion matrix of AD class is also part of Table 3 where 664 samples were corrected identified as AD.

It is possible to visualize the effectiveness of a classification system by looking at the ROC curve. Figure 5 displays all the three ROC curves generated by each of the three classes. The green, blue, and yellow ROC curves are representing the normal class, MCI class, and AD class respectively.

This study has been conducted with 109 participants and our proposed DRAM-Net has achieved a satisfactory performance. From the literature, it can be found that most of the studies performed binary classification task using this multi-class dataset. When

Table 2. Classification report of MCI class.

Confusion matrix		Performance matrixes	
True positive	537	Accuracy	98.06%
True negative	11	Sensitivity	97.99%
False positive	18	Specificity	98.10%
False negative	931	False positive rate	1.90%
		Precision	96.76%
		F1 score	97.37%
		Negative predictive value	98.83%
		False negative rate	2.01%
		False discovery rate	3.24%
		AUC	98.05%

Table 3. Classification report of AD class.

Confusion matrix		Performance matrixes	
True positive	664	Accuracy	97.80%
True negative	17	Sensitivity	97.50%
False positive	16	Specificity	98.04%
False negative	800	False positive rate	1.96%
		Precision	97.65%
		F1 score	97.57%
		Negative predictive value	97.92%
		False negative rate	2.50%
		False discovery rate	2.35%
		AUC	97.77%

it comes to the multi-class classification, all the previous efforts failed to perform well. Moreover, the binary classification performances were not satisfactory. Previous efforts used classical ML methods like SVM, KNN, LR, and DT to perform this complex task. But the nature and pattern of EEG is too complex and it requires extra attention. In addition, classical ML efforts require extra steps to trim down the features for the classifier. And while doing this, important features got mixed and lost.

DL based methods are so advanced to take care of the feature extraction step by themselves. And connected hidden layers of DL methods allow to extract hidden complex feature from the EEG data. Our proposed DRAM-Net consisting of four hidden residual blocks which also have multiple *SeparableConv2D* layers are capable of trimming down important features from the non-stationary EEG data. A compassion of existing efforts

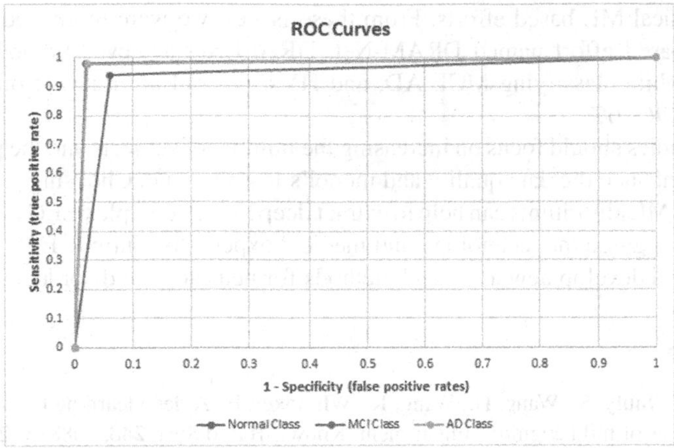

Fig. 5. ROC curves of normal, MCI, and AD classes. (Color figure online)

Table 4. Comparison with previous AD and MCI studies with same EEG dataset.

Efforts	Classes	Accuracy %
Morabito et al. [7]	AD vs MCI	98.97% (95% confidence range: 98.68%–99.26%)
Fouladi et al. [22]	HV vs MCI vs AD	92%
Ieracitano et al. [9]	HV vs MCI vs AD	89.22%
Fiscon et al. [10]	HV vs AD, HV vs MCI, and MCI vs AD	83%, 92%, and 79% respectively
Pirrone et al. [2]	HV vs AD, HV vs MCI, MCI vs AD, HV vs MCI vs AD	97%, 95%, 83%, and 75% respectively
Our proposed DRAM-net framework	**HV vs MCI vs AD**	**96.26%**

using the same EEG dataset with our proposed DRAM-Net has reported in Table 4. Morabito et al. [7] performed binary classification and it performed well, but did not solve the multi-class problem. Fouladi et al. [22], Ieracitano et al. [9], and Pirrone et al. [2] performed multi-classification and achieved 92%, 89.22%, and 75% respectively. On the other hand, our proposed DRAM-Net has outperformed achieved 96.66% for the normal class, 98.06% for the MCI class, 97.79% for the AD class, and 96.26% overall accuracy.

4 Future Study and Conclusion

Our proposed DRAM-Net framework focuses on efficient detection of MCI, AD, and HVs using EEG data. Previous efforts struggle to perform well while solving multi-class problem. And also, preprocessing steps are causing extra time and efforts for existing classical ML based efforts. From these issues, we were motivated and developed a DL based effort named DRAM-Net. DRAM-Net achieved 98.06%, 97.79%, and 96.66%while classifying MCI, AD, and HVs. Overall accuracy of our proposed framework is 96.26%.

Future studies should focus on increasing the number of subjects and the preprocessing steps to enhance the data quality and model's learning rate. Choosing a DL method over classical ML algorithms can help to extract deep hidden complex EEG data features. This effort will guide the technology and medical experts to continue EEG research to a new level and develop new ideas and methods for neurological disorders.

References

1. Alvi, A.M., Siuly, S., Wang, H., Wang, K., Whittaker, F.: A deep learning based framework for diagnosis of mild cognitive impairment. Knowl.-Based Syst. **248**, 108815 (2022)
2. Pirrone, D., Weitschek, E., Di Paolo, P., De Salvo, S., De Cola, M.C.: EEG signal processing and supervised machine learning to early diagnose Alzheimer's disease. Appl. Sci. **12**(11), 5413 (2022)
3. Patterson, C.: World Alzheimer report 2018. The state of the art of dementia research: new frontiers. Alzheimer's Disease International, London (2018)
4. Organization, W.H., et al.: Alzheimer's disease international. Dementia: a public health priority. World Health Org. **1**, 112 (2012)
5. Bracco, L., et al.: Factors affecting course and survival in Alzheimer's disease: a 9-year longitudinal study. Arch. Neurol. **51**(12), 1213–1219 (1994)
6. Alvi, A.M., Shaon, M.F.I., Das, P.R., Mustafa, M., Bari, M.R.: Automated course management system. In: 2017 12th International Conference for Internet Technology and Secured Transactions (ICITST), pp. 161–166. IEEE, December 2017
7. Morabito, F.C., Ieracitano, C., Mammone, N.: An explainable Artificial Intelligence approach to study MCI to AD conversion via HD-EEG processing. Clin. EEG Neurosci. (2021). https://doi.org/10.1177/15500594211063662
8. Alvi, A., Tasneem, N., Hasan, A., Akther, S.: Impacts of blockades and strikes in Dhaka: a survey. Int. J. Innov. Bus. Strat. **6**(1), 369–377 (2020)
9. Ieracitano, C., Mammone, N., Hussain, A., Morabito, F.C.: A novel multi-modal machine learning based approach for automatic classification of EEG recordings in dementia. Neural Netw. **123**, 176–190 (2020)
10. Fiscon, G., et al.: Combining EEG signal processing with supervised methods for Alzheimer's patients classification. BMC Med. Inform. Decis. Making **18**(1), 1–10 (2018)
11. Alvi, A.M., Siuly, S., Wang, H.: A long short-term memory based framework for early detection of mild cognitive impairment from EEG signals. IEEE Trans. Emerg. Top. Comput. Intell. (2022)
12. Alvi, A.M., Siuly, S., Wang, H.: Neurological abnormality detection from electroencephalography data: a review. Artif. Intell. Rev. **55**(3), 2275–2312 (2021). https://doi.org/10.1007/s10462-021-10062-8
13. Alvi, A.M., Siuly, S., Wang, H., Sun, L., Cao, J.: An adaptive image smoothing technique based on localization. In: Developments of Artificial Intelligence Technologies in Computation and Robotics: Proceedings of the 14th International FLINS Conference (FLINS 2020), pp. 866–873 (2020)
14. Chatterjee, C.C., Krishna, G.: A novel method for IDC prediction in breast cancer histopathology images using deep residual neural networks. In: 2019 2nd International Conference on Intelligent Communication and Computational Techniques (ICCT), pp. 95–100. IEEE, September 2019

15. Alvi, A.M., Siuly, S., Wang, H.: Developing a deep learning based approach for anomalies detection from EEG data. In: Zhang, W., Zou, L., Zakaria Maamar, Lu., Chen, (eds.) WISE 2021. LNCS, vol. 13080, pp. 591–602. Springer, Cham (2021). https://doi.org/10.1007/978-3-030-90888-1_45
16. Paul, S., Alvi, A.M., Nirjhor, M.A., Rahman, S., Orcho, A.K., Rahman, R.M.: Analyzing accident prone regions by clustering. In: Król, D., Nguyen, N.T., Shirai, K. (eds.) ACIIDS 2017. SCI, vol. 710, pp. 3–13. Springer, Cham (2017). https://doi.org/10.1007/978-3-319-56660-3_1
17. Alvi, A.M., Basher, S.F., Himel, A.H., Sikder, T., Islam, M., Rahman, R.M.: An adaptive grayscale image de-noising technique by fuzzy inference system. In: 2017 13th International Conference on Natural Computation, Fuzzy Systems and Knowledge Discovery (ICNC-FSKD), pp. 1301–1308. IEEE, July 2017
18. Paul, S., Alvi, A.M., Rahman, R.M.: An analysis of the most accident prone regions within the Dhaka Metropolitan Region using clustering. Int. J. Adv. Intell. Paradigms **18**(3), 294–315 (2021)
19. Helzner, E.P., Scarmeas, N., Cosentino, S., Tang, M., Schupf, N., Stern, Y.: Survival in Alzheimer disease: a multiethnic, population-based study of incident cases. Neurology **71**(19), 1489–1495 (2008)
20. Alvi, A.M., Tasneem, N., Hasan, M.A., Akther, S.B.: A study to find the impacts of strikes on students and local shopkeepers in Bangladesh. In: World Congress on Sustainable Technologies (WCST-2019) (2019)
21. Hasan, M.A., Tasneem, N., Akther, S.B., Das, K., Alvi, A.M.: An analysis on recent mobile application trend in Bangladesh. In: Barolli, L., Takizawa, M., Xhafa, F., Enokido, T. (eds.) WAINA 2019. AISC, vol. 927, pp. 195–204. Springer, Cham (2019). https://doi.org/10.1007/978-3-030-15035-8_18
22. Fouladi, S., Safaei, A.A., Mammone, N., Ghaderi, F., Ebadi, M.J.: Efficient deep neural networks for classification of Alzheimer's disease and mild cognitive impairment from scalp EEG recordings. Cogn. Comput. **14**, 1247–1268 (2022). https://doi.org/10.1007/s12559-022-10033-3
23. Alvi, A.M., Siuly, S., Wang, H.: Challenges in electroencephalography data processing using machine learning approaches. In: Hua, W., Wang, H., Li, L. (eds.) Databases Theory and Applications: 33rd Australasian Database Conference, ADC 2022, Sydney, NSW, Australia, September 2–4, 2022, Proceedings, pp. 177–184. Springer International Publishing, Cham (2022). https://doi.org/10.1007/978-3-031-15512-3_15
24. Vimalachandran, P., Liu, H., Lin, Y., Ji, K., Wang, H., Zhang, Y.: Improving accessibility of the Australian My Health Records while preserving privacy and security of the system. Health Inf. Sci. Syst. **8**(1), 1–9 (2020). https://doi.org/10.1007/s13755-020-00126-4
25. He, J., Rong, J., Sun, L., Wang, H., Zhang, Y., Ma, J.: A framework for cardiac arrhythmia detection from IoT-based ECGs. World Wide Web **23**(5), 2835–2850 (2020). https://doi.org/10.1007/s11280-019-00776-9
26. Lee, J., Park, J.S., Wang, K.N., Feng, B., Tennant, M., Kruger, E.: The use of telehealth during the coronavirus (COVID-19) pandemic in oral and maxillofacial surgery–a qualitative analysis. EAI Endorsed Trans. Scalable Inf. Syst. **9**(4), e10 (2022)
27. Pandey, D., Wang, H., Yin, X., Wang, K., Zhang, Y., Shen, J.: Automatic breast lesion segmentation in phase preserved DCE-MRIs. Health Inf. Sci. Syst. **10**(1), 1–19 (2022). https://doi.org/10.1007/s13755-022-00176-w

An Intelligence Approach for Blood Pressure Estimation from Photoplethysmography Signal

Shahab Abdulla[1], Mohammed Diykh[1,2,3](✉), Sarmad K. D. AlKhafaji[2], Atheer Y. Oudah[2,3], Haydar Abdulameer Marhoon[3,4], and Rand Ameen Azeez[5]

[1] UniSQ College, University of Southern Queensland, Toowoomba, Australia
{Shahab.Abdulla,Mohammed.Diykh}@usq.edu.au
[2] Department of Computer Sciences, College of Education for Pure Science, University of Thi-Qar, Nasiriyah, Iraq
Dr.sarmad@utq.edu.iq, Atheer@alayen.edu.iq
[3] Information and Communication Technology Research Group, Scientific Research Centre, Al-Ayen University, Nasiriyah, Iraq
Haydar@alayen.edu.iq
[4] Department of Information Technology, College of Computer Science and Information Technology, University of Karbala, Karbala, Iraq
[5] Directorate of Education, Iraqi Ministry of Education, Thi-Qar, Iraq

Abstract. Commercial cuff-based Blood pressure (BP) devices are mainly not suitable or portable. To ease the measurement of BP devices, we proposed a new model for BP estimation based on photoplethysmography (PPG) signal. PPG signals are segmented into cycles using an improved peak detection algorithm. Then, each segment is mapped into a graph. Graph wavelets transform (GWT) is applied to each segment. The spectral graph features are extracted and tested to assess the BP. A ridge regression is employed to evaluated the BP with the reference of PPG. A publica dataset is used to evaluate the proposed model. The proposed model achieved good results and the obtained results are promising in improving the accuracy of BP estimation.

Keywords: BP · GWT · Ridge regression · Segmentation · Peak detection algorithm

1 Introduction

According to the World Health Organization (WHO), cardiovascular disease is the leading factor of most death incidents in the world than other diseases [1]. Based on a report released by European Heart Journal an estimate of 4.1 million deaths annually due to cardiovascular that results from hypertension. Recent studies showed that the number of people who suffer from hypertension could be raised to 1.6 billion by 2030. Blood pressure (BP) is, one of hypertension's parameters, an important signal that provides significant information about human body for physicians and decision-makers [2–6]. Daily testing of BP can help early detection, control, and treatment of diseases related to

A. Traina et al. (Eds.): HIS 2022, LNCS 13705, pp. 54–63, 2022.
https://doi.org/10.1007/978-3-031-20627-6_6

BP such as hypotension [4]. BP level rises and drops according to human activities. Two factors are used to measure BP named a systolic blood pressure measures the pressure in vessels when a heart beats, and diastolic blood pressure measure the pressure when heart is rest.

Photoplethysmography (PPG) is a technique used to analyse pulse wave signals from blood volume changes of subcutaneous capillaries using a photoelectric sensor or even a consumer-level camera [3]. Recent years, many new methods of measuring BP using PPG technique without cuff have emerged. Among them, the method based on the pulse transit time (PTT) between PPG and ECG or between two PPG signals measured at different skin sites has been proved to be feasible [5–15].

In recent years, with the development of cuffless devices for the BP estimation and demands for more accurate BP devices, methods based on PPG signals have become a new research direction, and many works have been done to improve PB estimation performance. The earliest attempting work was proposed by Geddes et al. [15] explored the relation between PTT and BP. They found that there was a certain degree of linear correlation between PTT and BP. A combination of ECG and PPG signals has been adopted in more studies, for example Li et al. [3] took advantage of electrocardiogram (ECG) and PPG features to monitor systolic blood pressure and diastolic blood pressure levels. A bidirectional layer of long short-term memory was adopted as the first layer and a residual connection was added inside each of LSTM layers. They compared their results with several traditional machine learning methods. Alghamdi et al. [4] adopted oscillometric waveforms to predict BP. Oscillometric waveforms were partitioned into three periods from the starting of waveform to the systolic blood pressure, between systolic blood pressure and diastolic blood pressure, and diastolic blood pressure to the end of waveform. Senturk et al. [5] estimated BP using ECG and PPG signals. A 40 Hz low pass filter was applied to denoise ECG and PPG signals. In that study, Pan-Tomkins algorithm based on R-peak was utilised to segment ECG and PPG signals into intervals. Three types of features named chaotic, time domain, and frequency domain features were extracted and sent to a classifier to predict BP.

Linear or nonlinear regression-based approaches were other techniques used in BP estimation. In this way, several methods have been developed using different kinds of features extracted from ECG and PPG signals such as Pulse Transit Time (PTT), heart rate variability (HRV), etc. [6–10]. Wibmer et al. [8] examined the relation between PTT and BP. A linear and non-linear regression were employed to investigate the relation between the PTT and BP. They found that there were a significant, strong negative correlation between PTT and BP, and a weak relation between PTT and diastolic BP. Kachuee et al. [6] proposed a system based on regression technique for diastolic blood pressure (DBP), and mean arterial pressure (MAP), and BP estimation. Two different types of physiological features extracted from ECG and PPG were employed in that study. Sharifi et al. [1] utilised pulse transit time with photoplethysmogram (PPG) intensity ratio to estimate blood pressure (BP). They reported their results based on diastolic (Blood Pressure) BP, mean BP, and systolic BP. Mousavi et al. [2] proposed a model based on photoplethysmography (PPG) to predict mean arterial pressure, diastolic blood pressure and systolic blood pressure. Two algorithms named whole-based and parameter-based were suggested to extract features from PPG.

Recently, there is a trend of using deep learning models for BP estimation for example, Pan et al. [11] developed a deep learning-based technique for BP estimation. Frequency characteristics with temporal dependence of segmented Korotkoff sound (KorS) signals were adopted in that study. Miao et al. [12] designed a model based on fusion of a residual network and long short-term memory. Ghommem et al. [13] applied a deep learning model for temperature and pressure estimation using signal's characteristics. Su et al. [14] estimated BP using a deep recurrent neural network model consisting of multi-layered Long Short-Term Memory networks. Several features were extracted from PTT and PPG features, and they were fed to the recurrent neural network [6].

Based on the analysis above, the combination of handcrafted characteristics and machine learning approaches has become the focus of several research of BP estimation using single-channel PPG signal. However, the effectiveness of each feature and features combination needs in-depth research. The correlation among PPG features could have significant adverse effects on BP estimation. As a result, an intelligence system to remove redundant features, and extract the best combination of features from PPG to estimate BP could provide more accurate information on the level of BP than traditional approaches. In view of these limitations, we proposed a new model for BP estimation using single-channel PPG signal. First, PPG signals are pre-processed to remove noisy data, and segment PPG signals into intervals. Second, graph wavelet transform is applied to each interval to obtain the important features to estimate blood pressure. A regression technique is employed to compare the proposed model with the reference of PPG.

2 Methodology and Material

The overview of the framework of the proposed mode is shown in Fig. 2. The data pre-processing step is to guarantee that all the PPG signals used for BP estimation are in high quality. A public dataset is used to evaluate the proposed model.

2.1 Experimental Dataset

A publicly available dataset is used in this paper named UCI machine learning BP dataset (UCI-ML-BP). The dataset was collected from 12000 subjects. Each Sampled was composed of collected ECG, PPG and arterial blood pressure (ABP) signals. The data was sampled at a rate of 125 Hz with a temporal length 24 s. SBP and DBP values comprise of the labels of LASSO-LSTM model, which were obtained from the ABP signals. The approach used for extracting SBP and DBP named Locate peaks and troughs of each ABP signal. The average of peaks corresponds to SBP while that of troughs corresponds to DBP. The distribution of SBP and DBP values range from 73 mmHg to 199 mmHg and 50 mmHg to 148 mmHg respectively. Figure 1 shows the normal distribution of SBP, and DBP.

2.2 The Proposed Model

2.2.1 Pre-processing Phase

To build reliable BP estimation model, and improve the quality of PPG signals, a data pre-processing was applied to PPG signals. PPG signals contain irregular data that could

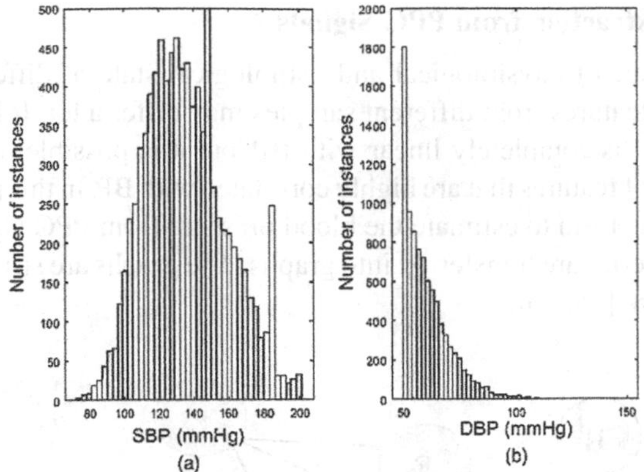

Fig. 1. Normal distribution of SBP and DBP

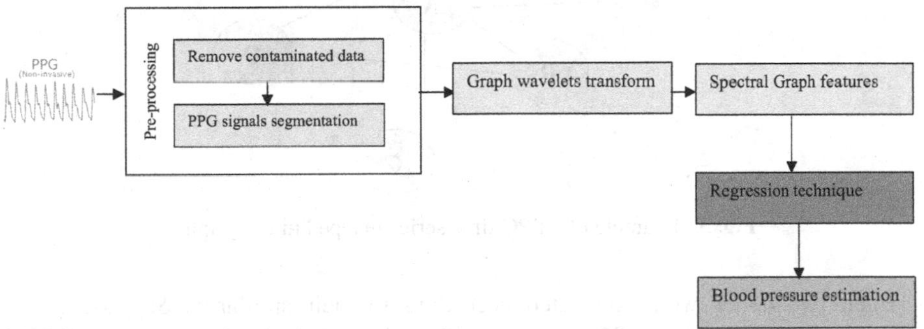

Fig. 2. Proposed model for blood pressure estimation

affect the performance of the proposed model. The following equation was applied to detect the contaminated PPG data.

$$SNR = \frac{\int_{p1}^{p2} d(f)df}{\int_{0}^{p1} d(f)df + \int_{p2}^{\infty} d(f)df} \tag{1}$$

where $d(f)$ denotes to the power spectrum density of a signal, $\int_{p1}^{p2} d(f)df$ is the signal energy. In this paper, we considered a threshold δ of 3.0, if the SNR of PPG signal is lower than δ, the signal is marked as noisy otherwise the signal is accepted and considered in the experiments. In addition to remove the baseline drift from PPG signals, smoothness priors' method is applied in this research.

To segment PPG signal into cycles, an improved peak detection algorithm was applied to PPG signals. In this paper, we considered that the value of main peak should not exceed 0.5 times of the maximum value of main peak of PPG signal.

2.2.2 Features Extraction from PPG Signals

Due to the difference of physiological and pathological state of different individuals, the extracted PPG features from different samples may differ a lot. It is difficult to find a single feature that is completely linear with BP, but it is possible to estimate BP by combining a series of features that are highly correlated with BP. In this paper, we applied a graph wavelet transform to estimate the blood pressure from PPG signals.

The PPG time series are transferred into graphs. The graphs are structured according to our previous work [15, 16].

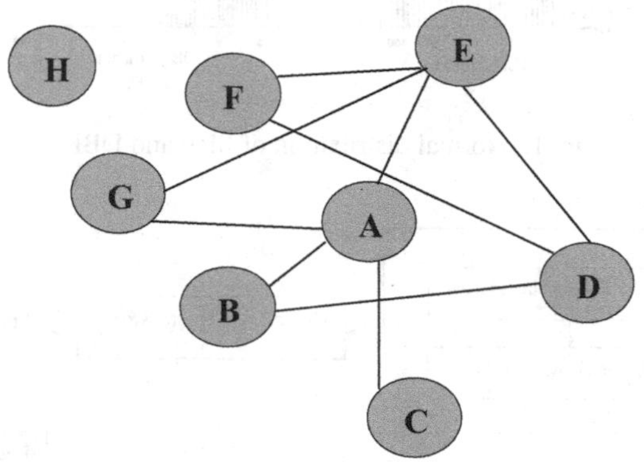

Fig. 3. Example of a PPG time series mapped into a graph

Each two nodes were connected according to their similarity. *Suppose* $X = \{x_1, x_2, x_3, \ldots\ldots, x_n\}$ is a PPG segment with n datapoints. Each data point of PPG segment was considered a node in a graph. For example, any pair of nodes (v_i, v_j) in a graph are connected based on the following equation

$$\left(v_i, v_j\right) \in E, ifd\left(v_i, v_j\right) \leq \delta \tag{2}$$

w here δ is threshold, Fig. 3 shows PPG segment being mapped as. The adjacency matrix and the Laplacian matrix are calculated for all nodes in graphs. The Laplacian matrix and adjacent matrix are symmetric. That means A $(v_i, v_j) =$ A (v_j, v_i).

In this paper, the low-pass and band-pass filters are applied to calculate eigenvector. The spectral graph coefficients and spectral graph wavelet coefficients are computed based on different scales. Then, they are used as the key features to estimate the PPG. We considered the Chebyshev polynomial approximation to avoid performing a full eigen-decomposition.

2.2.3 Spectral Graph Characteristics Analysis for Blood Pressure Estimation

The signal graph wavelet transform (GWT) was applied to PPG signals to obtain the desired information for blood estimation [16]. The PPG signal is decomposed into high-frequency components (wavelet coefficients), and low-frequency (scaling coefficients). The wavelet and scale function coefficients represented in Eqs. (11) and (12) are computed at scale t.

The spectral graph wavelet $\psi_{t,k}(m)$ at location k, scale t, $m \in$ V in the eigenspace of the graph Laplacian matrix is defined as.

$$\psi_{t,k}(m) = \sum_{n=1}^{N-1} g(t\lambda_n)x_n^*(k)x_n(m) \tag{3}$$

where g is a kernel function and behaves as a bandpass filter (0) $= 0$, $\lim x \to \infty g(o) = 0$, λ_k an eigenvector of a Laplacian matrix. The spectral graph wavelet coefficients of a signal $f \in \mathbb{R}^N$ represents as the projection of f onto the orthonormal Laplacian eigenvector space, and they are defined as:

$$W_f(t, k) =< \psi_{t,k}, f \geq \sum_{n=0}^{N-1} \psi_{t,k}^*(n)f(n) \tag{4}$$

As a result, the total energy of the wavelet and scaling function coefficients were considered as the essential characteristics to estimate blood pressure. Our results showed that the energy of the wavelet coefficients reflect the changes in PPG signals. We selected the total graph energy of the wavelet coefficients to estimate the blood pressure. The simulation results showed that the proposed model matched the PPG reference.

The number of the scale levels was investigated in this paper. We found that if the scale level was higher than 4 the wavelet coefficients did not reflect the significant information associated with blood pressure. As the result, we set the number of the scales $t = 3$.

At each step, the energy of the wavelet coefficients and scale coefficients for PPG segment were computed as follows:

- the energy of the wavelet coefficients and scale coefficients are calculated at each scale.

  Let $S_{it}$and W_{it} be the ith wavelet coefficients and scale coefficients at scale t, respectively. The total energy of the wavelet coefficients (EN_g) and the scale coefficients (EN_s) at scale t were calculated by the following equations.

$$EN_w = \sum_{i=1}^{n} (W_{it})^2 \tag{5}$$

$$EN_s = \sum_{i=1}^{n} (S_{it})^2 \tag{6}$$

- the average energy of the wavelet and scale coefficients are calculated by dividing EN_wandEN_s on the number of the wavelet and scale coefficients in the corresponding scale:

$$Av_{EN_W} = \frac{EN_w}{n} \tag{7}$$

$$Av_{EN_s} = \frac{EN_s}{n} \tag{8}$$

After the total energy of the wavelet and scaling coefficients are computed. Then, they were tested against the PPG reference. We noticed that the average energy of the wavelet coefficients (Av_{EN_W}) reflect a high matching with the reference values compared with the energy of the scaling coefficients (Av_{EN_s}).

2.3 Machine Learning Approach to Estimate Blood Pressure

Spectral graph characteristics were extracted from each PPG segments to estimate the blood pressure. The reference BP was compared with the proposed model to calculate the correlation degree. A multiple linear regression (MLR) was applied in this study to estimate the blood pressure [17–20]. It has been used to estimate cuffless BP, and depth of anaesthesia. The MLR started with selection random coefficients. Each predictor was linked with a coefficient. At each iteration, random error and the coefficients that refer to the difference between reference BP and the predicted were updated. The least square model was employed to minimize the squared error. The process of minimization of the squared error stayed until BP estimation was obtained.

3 Experimental Results

In this experiment the proposed model was compared with AAMI standard for blood pressure. Based on AAMI standard, the standard deviation of errors (SD) and ME for blood pressure should be lower than 8 mmHg, and 5 mmHg respectively. Table 1 shows the statistical comparison between the proposed model and the AAMI standard. It can be noticed that the proposed model complies with the standard of AAMI.

Table 1. Comparison between the proposed model with AAMI

		ME (mmHg)	SD (mmHg)	Subjects
The proposed mode	SBP	0.47	5.2	1800
	DBP	0.29	2.61	
AMMI	SBP AND DBP	<5	<8	>85

Another comparison was made with the Britain Hypertension Society (BHS). The results of comparisons were shown in Table 2. Based on the BHS, the proposed method achieved acceptable results for DBP and SBP based on the BHS standard.

The predicting DBP and SBP results of the proposed model were compared with four machine learning models, including SV, RF, and decision tree. Hold-out validation was considered to evaluate the proposed model by considering 70% of samples as the train set. The root mean square error and mean absolute error were calculated for each model by running each model seven times. The results of comparisons are shown in Table 3.

The performance of the proposed model was more significant than others. The RMSE and MAE of the proposed model the SBP estimation were 5.6 ± 3.4 and 3.8 ± 3.3

Table 2. Comparison between the proposed model with BHS

		≤5(*mmHg*)	≤10(*mmHg*)	≤15(*mmHg*)
Proposed model	SBP	72%	82%	96%
	DBP	76%	88%	97%
BHS	A	60%	85%	95%
	B	50%	75%	90%
	C	40%	65%	85%

Table 3. Performance evaluation comparison with different machine learning

		RF	SVM	Decision tree	The proposed model
SBP	MAE	4.3 ± 3.1	4.4 ± 2.6	5.2 ± 2.9	3.8 ± 3.3
	RMSE	6.7 ± 2.1	6.9 ± 3.4	7.1 ± 2.4	5.6 ± 3.4
DBP	MAE	5.4 ± 2.7	5.8 ± 2.4	6.8 ± 3.1	2.3 ± 2.2
	RMSE	7.8 ± 3.2	8.5 ± 3.0	7.8 ± 2.6	7.1 ± 3.0

Table 4. Performance comparison with previous studies for BP estimation

Authors	Dataset	Technique	Performance	
			SBP	DBP
El Hajj et al. [21]	MIMIC-II(UCI)	7 manual features based LSTM	SD = 4.73 Mean = 2.23	SD = 1.96 Mean = 1.59
Schlesinger et al. [22]	MIMIC-IIS	Spectrum bas CNN	SD = 8.65 Mean = 7.32	SD = 4.48 Mean = 3.91
Xing et al. [23]	Self-prepared	Manual features based random forest	0.45 ± 11.3	0.31 ± 8.55
The proposed model	UCI-ML-BP	Spectrum graph wavelet	SD = 5.2 Mean = 0.47	SD = 2.61 Mean = 0.29

respectively. While the RMSE and MAE of the proposed model for DBP estimation were 7.1 ± 3.0 and 2.3 ± 2.2 respectively.

3.1 Comparative Study with Different Feature Sets

Based on our knowledge, this is the first study that investigates spectral graph wavelet characteristics of PPG signals to estimate blood pressure. Table 4 reports the comparisons results among the proposed method with recent BP estimation studies. We found that there are many differences in dataset used, implementation and validation among the studies. It is hard to make a fair comparison. In addition, when making the comparison, trade-offs between performance, speed, and computational complexity measures should be taken into account. Our comparison focused on type of features, dataset, and BP estimation values. The proposed model was compared with studies in the Table 4. Most of the studies in literature used manual feature while the proposed model more effective features based approach compared to manual features based approach in which feature calculation, multiple peak detection, and validation algorithms were implemented. In addition, the proposed model achieved a good result compared with the previous studies.

4 Conclusions

In this study, we presented a new approach to estimate the blood pressure from PPG signals. The proposed method used graph wavelet transform technique to extract the desired features from PPG. The spectral graph characteristics were tested and evaluated based on a regression technique. Our work is a suitable tool to be used as an efficient cuff-less, and patient-friendly BP devices.

References

1. Sharifi, I., Goudarzi, S., Khodabakhshi, M.B.: A novel dynamical approach in continuous cuffless blood pressure estimation based on ECG and PPG signals. Artif. Intell. Med. **97**, 143–151 (2019)
2. Mousavi, S.S., Firouzmand, M., Charmi, M., Hemmati, M., Moghadam, M., Ghorbani, Y.: Blood pressure estimation from appropriate and inappropriate PPG signals using a whole-based method. Biomed. Signal Process. Control **47**, 196–206 (2019)
3. Li, Y.H., Harfiya, L.N., Purwandari, K., Lin, Y.D.: Real-time cuffless continuous blood pressure estimation using deep learning model. Sensors **20**(19), 5606 (2020)
4. Alghamdi, A.S., Polat, K., Alghoson, A., Alshdadi, A.A., Abd El-Latif, A.A.: A novel blood pressure estimation method based on the classification of oscillometric waveforms using machine-learning methods. Appl. Acoust. **164**, 107279 (2020)
5. Senturk, U., Polat, K., Yucedag, I.: A non-invasive continuous cuffless blood pressure estimation using dynamic recurrent neural networks. Appl. Acoust. **170**, 107534 (2020)
6. Kachuee, M., Kiani, M.M., Mohammadzade, H., Shabany, M.: Cuffless blood pressure estimation algorithms for continuous health-care monitoring. IEEE Trans. Biomed. Eng. **64**(4), 859–869 (2016)
7. Kim, J.S., Kim, K.K., Baek, H.J., Park, K.S.: Effect of confounding factors on blood pressure estimation using pulse arrival time. Physiol. Meas. **29**(5), 615 (2008)
8. Wibmer, T., et al.: Pulse transit time and blood pressure during cardiopulmonary exercise tests. Physiol. Res. **63**(3), 287–296 (2014)
9. Hennig, A., Patzak, A.: Continuous blood pressure measurement using pulse transit time. Somnologie - Schlafforschung Und Schlafmedizin **17**(2), 104–110 (2013)
10. Wong, M.Y.-M., Poon, C.C.-Y., Zhang, Y.-T.: An evaluation of the cuffless blood pressure estimation based on pulse transit time technique: a half year study on normotensive subjects. Cardiovasc. Eng. **9**(1), 32–38 (2009)
11. Pan, F., et al.: Development and validation of a deep learning-based automatic auscultatory blood pressure measurement method. Biomed. Signal Process. Control **68**, 102742 (2021)

12. Miao, F., et al.: Continuous blood pressure measurement from one-channel electrocardiogram signal using deep-learning techniques. Artif. Intell. Med. **108**, 101919 (2020)
13. Ghommem, M., Puzyrev, V., Najar, F.: Deep learning for simultaneous measurements of pressure and temperature using arch resonators. Appl. Math. Model. **93**, 728–744 (2021)
14. Su, P., Ding, X.R., Zhang, Y.T., Liu, J., Miao, F., Zhao, N.: Long-term blood pressure prediction with deep recurrent neural networks. In: 2018 IEEE EMBS International Conference on Biomedical & Health Informatics (BHI), pp. 323–328. IEEE, March 2018
15. Diykh, M., Li, Y., Wen, P.: EEG sleep stages classification based on time domain features and structural graph similarity. IEEE Trans. Neural Syst. Rehabil. Eng. **24**(11), 1159–1168 (2016)
16. Diykh, M., Li, Y., Wen, P., Li, T.: Complex networks approach for depth of anesthesia assessment. Measurement **119**, 178–189 (2018)
17. Diykh, M., et al.: Texture analysis based graph approach for automatic detection of neonatal seizure from multi-channel EEG signals. Measurement **190**, 110731 (2022)
18. Diykh, M., Miften, F.S., Abdulla, S., Saleh, K., Green, J.H.: Robust approach to depth of anaesthesia assessment based on hybrid transform and statistical features. IET Sci. Meas. Technol. **14**(1), 128–136 (2020)
19. Miften, F.S., Diykh, M., Abdulla, S., Siuly, S., Green, J.H., Deo, R.C.: A new framework for classification of multi-category hand grasps using EMG signals. Artif. Intell. Med. **112**, 102005 (2021)
20. Diykh, M., Abdulla, S., Saleh, K., Deo, R.C.: Fractal dimension undirected correlation graph-based support vector machine model for identification of focal and non-focal electroencephalography signals. Biomed. Signal Process. Control **54**, 101611 (2019)
21. El Hajj, C., Kyriacou, P.A.: Cuffless and continuous blood pressure estimation from PPG signals using recurrent neural networks. In: 2020 42nd Annual International Conference of the IEEE Engineering in Medicine & Biology Society (EMBC), pp. 4269–4272. IEEE, July 2020
22. Schlesinger, O., Vigderhouse, N., Eytan, D., Moshe, Y.: Blood pressure estimation from PPG signals using convolutional neural networks and Siamese network. In: ICASSP 2020–2020 IEEE International Conference on Acoustics, Speech and Signal Processing (ICASSP), pp. 1135–1139. IEEE, May 2020
23. Xing, X., Ma, Z., Zhang, M., Zhou, Y., Dong, W., Song, M.: An unobtrusive and calibration-free blood pressure estimation method using photoplethysmography and biometrics. Sci. Rep. **9**(1), 1–8 (2019)
24. Khare, S.K., Bajaj, V., Sengur, A., Sinha, G.R.: Classification of mental states from rational dilation wavelet transform and bagged tree classifier using EEG signals. In: Artificial Intelligence-Based Brain-Computer Interface, pp. 217–235. Academic Press (2022)
25. Khare, S.K., Bajaj, V.: A hybrid decision support system for automatic detection of Schizophrenia using EEG signals. Comput. Biol. Med. **141**, 105028 (2022)
26. Sharma, S., Khare, S.K., Bajaj, V., Ansari, I.A.: Improving the separability of drowsiness and alert EEG signals using analytic form of wavelet transform. Appl. Acoust. **181**, 108164 (2021)
27. Alsafy, I., Diykh, M.: Developing a robust model to predict depth of anesthesia from single channel EEG signal. Phys. Eng. Sci. Med. 1–16 (2022)
28. Majeed, R.R., Alkhafaji, S.K.: ECG classification system based on multi-domain features approach coupled with least square support vector machine (LS-SVM). Comput. Methods Biomech. Biomed. Eng. 1–8 (2022)

Tailored Nutrition Service to Reduce the Risk of Chronic Diseases

Jitao Yang(✉)

School of Information Science, Beijing Language and Culture University, Beijing 100083, China
yangjitao@blcu.edu.cn

Abstract. Chronic diseases such as cancer, stroke, hypertension, coronary heart disease, and diabetes seriously harm human health. According to the statistics of the World Health Organization (WHO), cancer is the leading cause of death in the world, and constitutes a great public health challenge for all the countries worldwide. To optimize the chronic prevention and control model, it is inevitable to strengthen the analysis of multi dimension data including multi omics' screening, physical examination, health condition and lifestyle data, to evaluate and identify high-risk groups effectively, and reduce the chronic disease risk through accurate, appropriate and effective intervention methods. In this paper, integrating genetic testing, physical examination, diet style, habits and customs, medical history, and exercise data together, we design and implement a personalized nutrition service that calculates the disease risk and nutrition requirement and then provides a tailored nutrition solution to reduce the risk of suffering from chronic diseases and the risk of death from chronic diseases.

Keywords: Chronic diseases · Genetic testing · Precision nutrition · Physical examination · Lifestyle

1 Introduction

Chronic diseases mainly include cancer, cardiovascular and cerebrovascular diseases, chronic respiratory diseases, diabetes, oral diseases, as well as endocrine, kidney, bone, and nerve diseases.

According to the statistics of the World Health Organization (WHO), in 2020, cancer caused the most death in the world [1], leading to nearly one-sixth deaths, the top 5 cancers causing of death in 2020 were: lung, colon and rectum, liver, stomach, and breast; in 2019, cancer was also the first or second leading cause of death in 112 countries and the third or fourth leading cause of death in 23 countries [2]. Cancer leads to a huge disease burden, which is not only one of the major causes of death in the world, but also an important factor hindering the extension of human life expectancy. The report "Global cancer statistics 2020: GLOBOCAN estimates of incidence and mortality worldwide for 36 cancers in 185 countries" [3,4] issued by the International Agency for Research on

A. Traina et al. (Eds.): HIS 2022, LNCS 13705, pp. 64–75, 2022.
https://doi.org/10.1007/978-3-031-20627-6_7

Cancer (IARC) pointed out that, the top ten cancers with the highest incidence rates in the global in 2020 are breast cancer, lung cancer, colorectal cancer, prostate cancer, gastric cancer, liver cancer, cervical cancer, esophageal cancer, thyroid cancer and bladder cancer; the top ten cancers with the highest mortality rates are lung cancer, colorectal cancer, liver cancer, gastric cancer, breast cancer, esophageal cancer, pancreatic cancer, prostate cancer, cervical cancer and leukemia. It is estimated that there will be 28.4 million new cancer cases in the world in 2040, an increase of 9.11 million cases compared with 2020, an increase of about 47%.

The Chinese cancer report "Cancer incidence and mortality in China, 2016" released by the National Cancer Center of China pointed out that [5], in 2016 there were about 4.064 million new cancer cases and 2.4135 million new cancer deaths in China. Lung cancer is a high-risk cancer with the highest incidence and mortality rates in China. The incidence rate of cancer in China continues to rise, higher in urban areas than in rural areas, and higher in men than in women. The cancer with the highest incidence rate in men is lung cancer (about 24.6% of the total number of male cancers), followed by liver cancer, gastric cancer, colorectal cancer and esophageal cancer. The cancer with the highest incidence rate in women is breast cancer (about 16.72% of the total number of female cancers), followed by lung cancer, colorectal cancer, thyroid cancer and gastric cancer. Affected by the population aging, the burden of colorectal cancer, prostate cancer and breast cancer will increase rapidly [6].

At present, the global cancer burden continues to grow, and the cancer mortality in many countries has surpassed the high mortality chronic diseases such as cardiovascular diseases (*e.g.*, stroke and coronary heart disease), which constitutes a great public health challenge.

The prevalence of cardiovascular diseases in China continues to rise, and the death of cardiovascular and cerebrovascular diseases accounts for the first place in the total death toll of urban and rural residents (46.66% in rural areas and 43.81% in urban areas) [7]. The annual incidence rate of stroke is 250/100000, the annual incidence rate of coronary heart disease is 50/100000, and the incidence rate of stroke is five times that of coronary heart disease. Stroke is the primary cause of death and disability for adults in China, and the number of stroke patients ranks first in the world.

Evidence based medicine research shows that hypertension is the most important risk factor for cardiovascular and cerebrovascular diseases in Chinese population. More than half of the occurrence and death of cardiovascular and cerebrovascular diseases are related to hypertension [8]. Control hypertension is the key to the prevention and treatment of cardiovascular and cerebrovascular diseases.

The risk factors of hypertension include genetic factors, age and a variety of unhealthy lifestyles. High sodium and low potassium diet is an important risk factor for hypertension in Chinese population. The risk of hypertension in overweight and obese people is 1.16–1.28 times that in normal weight people. Excessive drinking and long-term mental stress are risk factors for hypertension.

In addition, primary hypertension (H-type hypertension) with elevated blood homocysteine (Hcy) is an important factor leading to the high incidence and sustainable development of stroke in China. The proportion of H-type hypertension in Chinese patients with hypertension is about 80.3%. Folic acid supplementation to the person with the C677 T mutant of methylenetetrahydrofolate reductase (MTHFR)–a key enzyme in Hcy metabolism, can significantly reduce the risk of stroke (risk reduction of 21%, HR = 0.79, 95%CI: 0.69–0.93, P = 0.003) [9].

The death toll caused by chronic diseases accounts for 87% of the total death toll in China, and its disease burden accounts for 70% of the total disease burden in China, which has become a major public health problem affecting the national economic and social development.

To optimize the chronic disease prevention and control model, it is inevitable to strengthen the joint screening of multi omics, identify high-risk groups effectively, and reduce the chronic disease risk through accurate, appropriate and effective intervention methods. Therefore, in this paper, we proposed a personalized nutrition solution to reduce the incidence rate of chronic diseases based on the analysis of genetic data, physical examination data, and lifestyle data.

The paper is organized as follows, Sect. 2 introduces the relationship between chronic diseases and genes; Sect. 3 describes our tailored nutrition service for reducing chronic diseases that, Sect. 3.1 explains the genetic testing service, Sect. 3.2 explains how physical examination data were used in our model, Sect. 3.3 explains the implementation of lifestyle data in our model, Sect. 3.4 gives the tailored nutrition solution; Sect. 4 summarizes the paper and describes the future research directions.

2 Chronic Diseases and Genes

Genetic predisposition refers to the tendency that different populations or individuals are prone to certain polygenic diseases under the influence of external environment due to different genetic structures [10]. “Susceptibility” means that a certain group or individual is easy to develop into a certain disease, if an individual does not carry susceptibility locus, he/she has low disease risk, the more susceptibility loci an individual carries, the higher disease risk the individual has. The development of genome-wide association studies (GWAS) makes it possible to precisely prevent and control cancers. Recognize the genetic susceptibility of individuals or groups through extensive genetic testing, and to identify cancer risk factors, is a powerful means of primary cancer prevention.

For example, breast cancer, which has the highest female incidence rate in China, has been confirmed that about 10% of the patients are caused by pathogenic germline mutations of known breast cancer genes, which is called hereditary breast cancer. Up to now, it has been known that more than 10 genes’ pathogenic germline mutations are related to breast cancer [11]. Among them, BRCA1, BRCA2, TP53 and PALB2 are breast cancer genes with high penetrance, mutation carriers of the above genes increase the risk of breast cancer by at least five times [12]. In addition, many studies [13–15] show that, mutations at related loci of ZNF365, FGFR2, CASC16, ZC3H11A and other genes are obvious susceptibility factors for breast cancer in East Asian women; APOBEC3A, CCDC170, ESR1 and other genes are closely related to the occurrence, development and distal metastasis of breast cancer, and affect the treatment and prognosis of breast cancer patients.

With the acceleration of population aging and urbanization in China, the unhealthy lifestyle of residents has become increasingly prominent, and the incidence rate of cardiovascular disease has continued to increase. In 2020, there were about 330 million people suffering from cardiovascular diseases, including 13 million stroke, 11.39 million coronary heart disease, 8.9 million heart failure and 245 million hypertension. According to the prediction model of China's cardiovascular disease from 2015 to 2025, compared with maintaining the status quo, the treatment of patients with stage I and II hypertension can reduce 803000 cardiovascular events per year (i.e., reduce 690000 strokes and 113000 myocardial infarction) [16]. Individual's lifestyle and genetic background affect the incidence and progression of hypertension and cardiovascular diseases.

In recent years, genome-wide association studies (GWAS) of hypertension has reported more than 1000 blood pressure related genetic loci [17]. For example, the loci of rs17249754 (ATP2B1), rs880315 (CASZ1) and rs9910888 (CACNA1D) are closely related to systolic blood pressure [18], and the loci of rs7136259 (ATP2B1) and rs1378942 (CSK) are closely related to diastolic blood pressure [19].

Following a healthy lifestyle and reasonable nutrition supplementation can reduce the genetic risk of stroke, hypertension, coronary heart disease, Alzheimer's disease, diabetes, colorectal cancer, breast cancer and other diseases [20–23].

3 Tailored Nutrition Intervention

Through the genetic testing, we can screen the genetic susceptible population of the above diseases and the population carrying the nutrient metabolism disorder risk genes. By evaluating their susceptibility risk and nutrient deficiency level, we can determine the types and doses of nutritional supplements for personalized nutrition intervention, so that to realize the health management of high-risk groups, reduce the risk of diseases. For those who have suffered from diseases, our personalized solution can play the role of adjuvant therapy and improve prognosis.

For example, supplementing folic acid, vitamin C, selenium and other antioxidant nutrients can delay the progression of atrophic gastritis and reduce the risk of gastric cancer. Supplementing vitamin E can reduce the risk of gastric cancer. Vitamin B_2 supplementation can reduce the blood pressure of people with MTHFR 677TT genotype. Folic acid supplementation can reduce the risk of stroke. Zinc supplementation can improve dyslipidemia, reduce total cholesterol, low-density lipoprotein and triglyceride in blood lipids. Supplementing vitamin D and vitamin E can reduce the risk of colorectal cancer. Vitamin C supplementation can help improve vascular endothelial function. Vitamin E supplementation can reduce the risk of myocardial infarction. Selenium supplementation may reduce the risk of death from cardiovascular disease. Supplementing ganoderma lucidum triterpenoids and ganoderma lucidum polysaccharides can inhibit the proliferation of nasopharyngeal carcinoma, gastric cancer and colorectal cancer cells. Lycopene can induce apoptosis of gastric cancer cells, affect the production of reactive oxygen species by helicobacter pylori, and prevent oxidative damage.

3.1 Genetic Testing

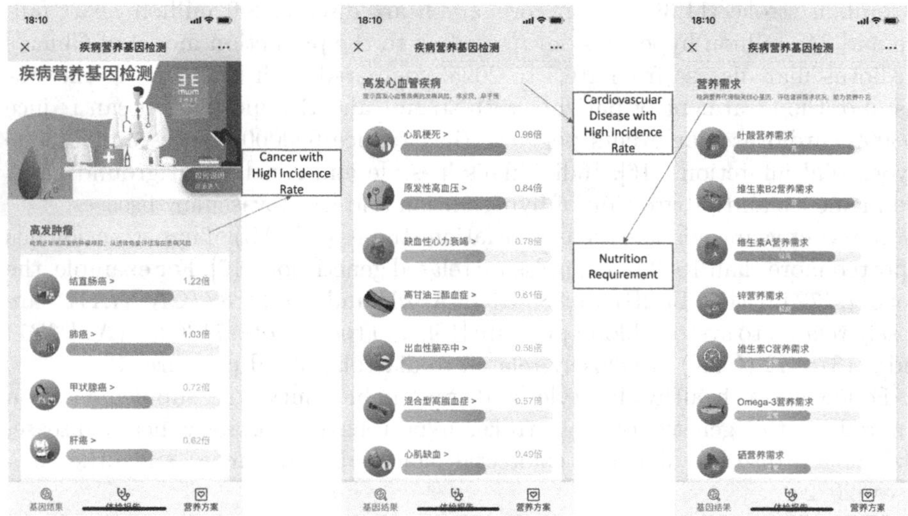

Fig. 1. The screen shots of the homepage of the disease and nutrition genetic testing report.

To evaluate individual's chronic disease risk and nutrition requirement, we developed a disease and nutrition genetic testing service, which includes three genetic testing item categories, *i.e.*, (1) Cancer with High Incidence Rate, (2) Cardiovascular Disease with High Incidence Rate, and (3) Nutrition Requirement. The disease and nutrition genetic testing report is demonstrated in Fig. 1:

- The "Cancer with High Incidence Rate" category tests the risk of cancers with high incidence rate in recent years, and assess the potential risk from a genetic perspective. As described in Fig. 1 left, it includes the genetic testing items of: colorectal cancer, lung cancer, carcinoma of thyroid, liver cancer, esophagus cancer, stomach cancer, and prostate cancer.
  For example, the colorectal cancer is one of the most common malignant tumors that seriously damage health and life span, its incidence rate and mortality rate are very high in the world. The incidence of colorectal cancer has certain genetic factors, about 1/3 of patients have genetic background,

and 5%–6% of patients can be diagnosed as hereditary colorectal cancer. The GREM1 gene encodes a member of the bone morphogenetic protein (BMP) antagonist family, which contains cystine junctions and usually forms homodimers and heterodimers. The antagonism of the secreted glycosylated protein encoded by this gene may be related to its direct binding with BMP protein. As an antagonist of BMP, the gene may play a role in regulating organogenesis, body formation and tissue differentiation. Genome wide association studies (GWAS) showed that the GREM1 gene's polymorphism is associated with the risk of colorectal cancer [24]. A large number of studies have shown the role of calcium in the prevention of colorectal cancer or its precursor adenoma.

Increased intake of calcium and vitamin D can reduce the risk of colorectal cancer [25], increased intake of dairy products and increased intake of vitamins B_2, B_6, B_{12} and folic acid can also reduce the risk of colorectal cancer.

- The "Cardiovascular Disease with High Incidence Rate" category tests the risk of cardiovascular disease with high incidence rate in recent years, so that to realize early detection and early intervention. As described in Fig. 1 middle, it includes the genetic testing items of: myocardial infarction, essential hypertension, ischemic heart failure, hypertriglyceridemia, hemorrhagic stroke, mixed hyperlipidemia, myocardial ischemia, and angina pectoris.

  For example, essential hypertension is a polygenic genetic disease caused by genetic and environmental factors, which can lead to changes in the function and structure of the heart and cardiovascular system.

  ATP2B1 [26] gene's encoding product is a plasma membrane calcium/calmodulin dependent ATPase expressed in vascular endothelial cells, which is mainly involved in the transfer of calcium ions from cytoplasm to extracellular. Animal experiments showed that compared with normotensive rats, the expression level of PMCA1 mRNA in aortic smooth muscle cells of spontaneously hypertensive rats increased, which was consistent with the regulatory role of ATP2B1 in blood pressure. The genetic variation of ATP2B1 gene can change the regulation of blood pressure by changing the structure of coding protein or the level of gene expression. ATP2B1 gene is considered to be related to systolic blood pressure, diastolic blood pressure and hypertension, and reaches the significant difference level of genome-wide association studies.

  DASH (Dietary Approaches to Stop Hypertension) diet [27] is an auxiliary diet for the treatment of hypertension introduced by the American Heart, Lung and Blood Institute in 1997, and has been adopted by major hospitals. This diet provides rich minerals such as potassium, calcium, magnesium and dietary fiber, increases the intake of high-quality protein and unsaturated fatty acids, reduces the intake of fat, especially saturated fatty acids and cholesterol, helps to expand blood vessels, reduces blood pressure, reduces the cholesterol level in the blood, and plays a role in preventing and treating atherosclerosis. In addition, patients with hypertension should have homocysteine (Hcy) test. If Hcy $\geq$ 15umol/L, they can be diagnosed as type H hypertension. Patients with H-type hypertension (especially MTHFR 677TT genotype carriers) can effectively reduce the level of homocysteine by properly supplementing folic acid and vitamin B_2, which can reduce blood pressure and prevent stroke to a certain extent.

– The "Nutrition Requirement" category tests the core genes related to nutrition metabolism, so that to evaluate nutrition requirement and support nutrition supplementation solutions. As described in Fig. 1 right, it includes the genetic testing items of: folic acid, vitamin B_2, vitamin A, zinc, vitamin C, omega-3, selenium, calcium, and vitamin D.

  For example, Zinc is one of the essential micronutrients for human body and the component of many important enzymes, it can not be synthesized in the body and can only be supplemented by external food. The effects of zinc on human body include: promoting growth, promoting sexual function development, promoting wound healing, improving immune ability, maintaining normal taste and appetite, maintaining normal dark vision ability, physiological regulation, etc.

  SLC30A8 [28] encodes zinc transporter 8, belonging to the zinc transport family ZnT family, which transfers zinc and other metal ions from the cytoplasm into the lumen or extracellular of intracellular organelles. The polymorphism of SLC30A8 gene will cause zinc deficiency and increase the risk of type II diabetes.

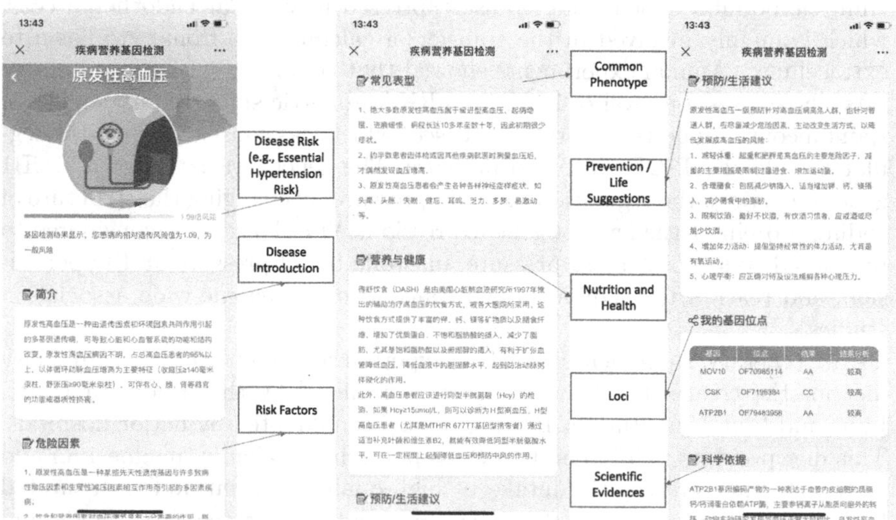

Fig. 2. The screen shots of the second level page of the disease and nutrition genetic testing report.

Click the genetic testing item name (*e.g.*, Essential Hypertension), a second level page will be opened as described in Fig. 2. The "Disease Risk" module gives the risk to have the disease; the "Disease Introduction" module introduces the disease; the "Risk Factors" module lists the factors that may cause the disease; the "Common Phenotype" module describes the symptoms of the disease; the "Nutrition and Health" module explains the relationship between nutrition and the disease; the "Prevention/Life Suggestion" module gives suggestions on how to prevent the happening of the disease; the "Loci" module lists the tested genes related to the disease; the "Scientific Evidences" module explains how the tested genes affect the disease.

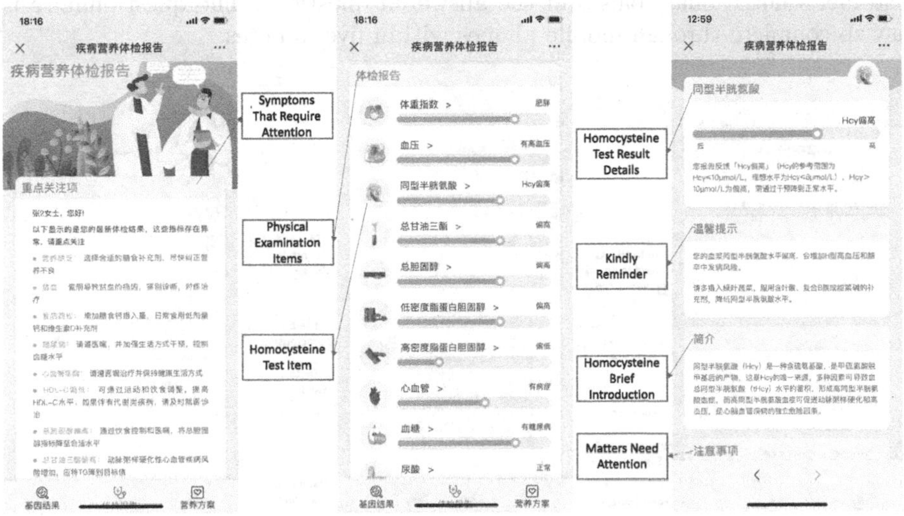

Fig. 3. The screen shots of the physical examination report

3.2 Physical Examination

To understand the current health status of customers, we suggest customers to provide physical examination data to our system. Figure 3 demonstrates the physical examination report.

Figure 3 left summarizes the symptoms that requires attention based on customer's physical examination data, and provides short advice for each symptom.

Figure 3 middle lists all the physical examination items that related to the diseases in the genetic testing report. Click the name of each physical examination item, more detail information will be displayed as described in Fig. 3 right.

In Fig. 3 right, using Homocysteine test item as an example, the first module gives the test result and relevant explanation, the second module is "kindly remainder" that gives some suggestions to decrease homocysteine level, the third module is "homocysteine brief introduction" that introduces homocysteine and its connections with disease, the fourth module is "matters need attention" that explains the factors (*e.g.*, polymorphism of genes) causing the increase of homocysteine level.

3.3 Health Condition and Lifestyle Evaluation

The physical condition, diet style, habits and customs, medical history, and nutritional goal are also important data to evaluate a person's nutrition requirement, therefore, we developed an online questionnaire (including food frequency questionnaire [29]). The questionnaire totally has more than one hundred questions, but will only pop out around 20 questions for each customer based on customer's nutritional goals and the answered questions. The questionnaire is easy to complete through mobile phones within five minutes.

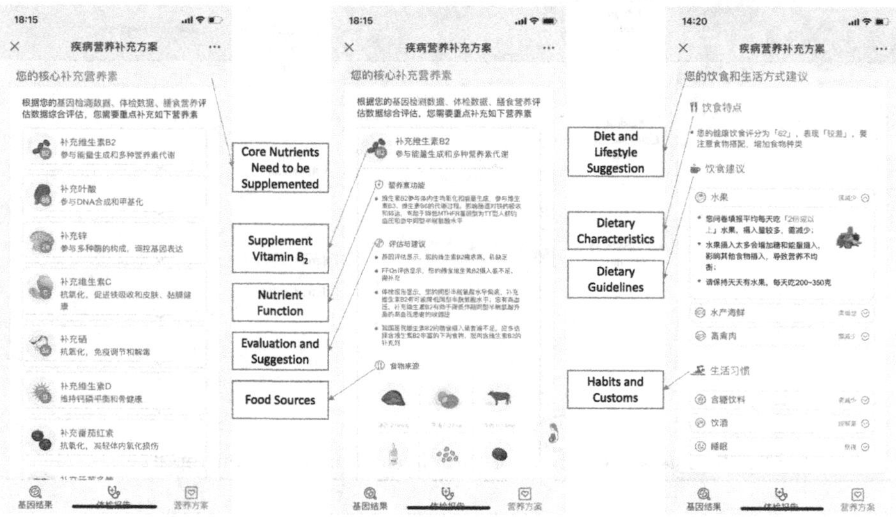

Fig. 4. The screen shots of the personalized nutrition report.

3.4 Tailored Nutrition

Combing genetic testing, physical examination, health condition and lifestyle data together, our personalized nutrition data model will compute a tailored nutrition solution for each customer, the report is described in Fig. 4.

Figure 4 left lists the core nutrients need to be supplemented, such as vitamin B_2, folic acid, zinc, vitamin C, selenium, vitamin D, lycopene, coriolus versicolor polysaccharide based on different customer's nutrition requirement.

Click the name of each nutrient, more information concerning why the nutrient should be supplemented will be displayed in a dropdown page as described in Fig. 4 middle, using vitamin B_2 as an example, the "nutrient function" module explains the function of vitamin B_2 and its relationship with diseases, the "evaluation and suggestion" module gives the evaluation basis (considering genetic, health condition and lifestyle, and physical examination data) and explains why vitamin B_2 should be supplemented, the "food sources" module suggests the foods rich in vitamin B_2 and lists the nutrients per 100g edible portion.

Figure 4 right provides diet and lifestyle suggestions. The "dietary characteristics" module summarizes the bad diet habits of the customer based on food frequency questionnaire's evaluation result. The "dietary guidelines" module gives detail suggestions on eating vegetables, fruits, livestock and poultry meat, aquatic products and seafood, and milk in daily life. The "habits and customs" module gives suggestions on control of sugary drinks, smoking and drinking and ensuring of adequate sleep and exercise.

4 Conclusions

Cancer, cardiovascular and cerebrovascular diseases, and other chronic diseases cause a great public health challenge in the world, therefore, it is necessary to carry out chronic disease screening, intervention and health management, so that to reduce the risk of suffering from chronic diseases, and reduce the risk of death from chronic diseases.

This paper implements a personalized nutrition intervention service, which integrates genetic testing data, individual physical examination results, and nutrition/metabolism status data, then evaluates an individual's chronic disease risk systematically, and further calculates a tailored nutrition intervention scheme for customer. The service will also regularly track and re-evaluate individual's risk status through regular physical examination, questionnaires, nutrition return visits and other means, and dynamically implement personalized health intervention closed-loop solutions.

In the coming years, with the development of large-scale clinical trials of precision nutrition, more and more data will be accumulated to build nutrition data analysis models and dynamic intervention suggestions. Precision nutrition interventions based on multi-omics will play a huge role in the primary prevention of cancer and other chronic diseases, and will explore new ways to reduce world's public health expenditure and improve people's life quality.

We are currently investigating to combine the data of wearable devices (especially sports watches) to our personalized nutrition model so that to provide more dynamic personalized nutrition solutions based individual's amount of exercise, intensity of exercise, sleep duration, deep sleep duration, apnea times, heart rate, heart rate variability, and etc.

Acknowledgment. This research project is supported by Science Foundation of Beijing Language and Culture University (supported by "the Fundamental Research Funds for the Central Universities") (Approval number: 22YJ080008).

References

1. World Health Organization (WHO): Cancer. https://www.who.int/news-room/fact-sheets/detail/cancer (2022). Accessed 4 Sept 2022
2. World Health Organization (WHO): Global health estimates: leading causes of death (2000–2019). https://www.who.int/data/gho/data/themes/mortality-and-global-health-estimates/ghe-leading-causes-of-death. Accessed 5 June 2022
3. Sung, H., Ferlay, J., Siegel, R.L., et al.: Global cancer statistics 2020: GLOBOCAN estimates of incidence and mortality worldwide for 36 cancers in 185 countries. CA Cancer J. Clin. **71**(3), 209–249 (2021)
4. International Agency for Research on Cancer: Global Cancer Observatory: Cancer Today (2020). https://gco.iarc.fr/today. Accessed 4 Sept 2022
5. Zheng, R., Zhang, S., Zeng, H., et al.: Cancer incidence and mortality in China, 2016. J. Natl. Cancer Center **2**(1), 1–9 (2022)
6. Feng, R.M., Zong, Y.N., Cao, S.M., Xu, R.H.: Current cancer situation in China: good or bad news from the 2018 Global Cancer Statistics? Cancer Commun. (Lond). **39**(1), 22 (2019)
7. Report on cardiovascular health and diseases in China 2020. Chin. J. Cardiovasc. Res. **19**(7), 582–590 (2021)
8. Chinese guidelines for the management of hypertension 2018. Chin. J. Cardiovasc. Med. **24**(01), 24–56 (2019)
9. Xu, X.: Interpretation of the "Expert consensus on diagnosis and treatment of H-type hypertension 2016". Chin. Circulation J. **31**(z2), 4 (2016)
10. Frank, S.A.: Genetic predisposition to cancer - insights from population genetics. Nat. Rev. Genet. **5**(10), 764–772 (2004)
11. Breast Cancer Association Consortium, Dorling, L., Carvalho, S., Allen, J., et al.: Breast cancer risk genes - association analysis in more than 113,000 women. N. Engl. J. Med. **384**(5), 428–439 (2021)
12. China Anti Cancer Association: Expert consensus on clinical diagnosis and treatment of familial hereditary tumors in China (2021 Edition) (1) - familial hereditary breast cancer. Chin. J. Clin. Oncol. **48**(23), 1189–1195 (2021)
13. Hsieh, Y.C., Tu, S.H., Su, C.T., et al.: A polygenic risk score for breast cancer risk in a Taiwanese population. Breast Cancer Res. Treat. **163**(1), 131–138 (2017)
14. Kim, Y.S., Sun, S., Yoon, J.S., et al.: Clinical implications of APOBEC3A and 3B expression in patients with breast cancer. PLoS ONE **15**(3), e0230261 (2020)
15. Wang, Q., Zhao, Y., Zheng, H., et al.: CCDC170 affects breast cancer apoptosis through IRE1 pathway. Aging (Albany NY) **13**(1), 1332–1356 (2020)
16. The Writing Committee of the Report on Cardiovascular Health and Diseases in China: Key points of report on cardiovascular health and disease report in China 2020. Chin. J. Cardiovasc. Med. **26**(03), 209–218 (2021)
17. Cabrera, C.P., Ng, F.L., Nicholls, H.L., et al.: Over 1000 genetic loci influencing blood pressure with multiple systems and tissues implicated. Hum. Mol. Genet. **28**(R2), R151–R161 (2019)
18. Hu, Z., Liu, F., Li, M., et al.: Associations of variants in the CACNA1A and CACNA1C genes with longitudinal blood pressure changes and hypertension incidence: the GenSalt study. Am. J. Hypertens. **29**(11), 1301–1306 (2016)
19. Cai, C., Liu, F.C., Li, J.X., et al.: Effects of the total physical activity and its changes on incidence, progression, and remission of hypertension. J. Geriatr. Cardiol. **18**(3), 175–184 (2021)

20. Whayne, T.F., Jr., Saha, S.P.: Genetic risk, adherence to a healthy lifestyle, and ischemic heart disease. Curr. Cardiol. Rep. **21**(1), 1 (2019)
21. Li, Y., Schoufour, J., Wang, D.D., et al.: Healthy lifestyle and life expectancy free of cancer, cardiovascular disease, and type 2 diabetes: prospective cohort study. BMJ **368**, l6669 (2020)
22. Lourida, I., Hannon, E., Littlejohns, T.J., et al.: Association of lifestyle and genetic risk with incidence of dementia. JAMA **322**(5), 430–437 (2019)
23. Pazoki, R., Dehghan, A., Evangelou, E., et al.: Genetic predisposition to high blood pressure and lifestyle factors: associations with midlife blood pressure levels and cardiovascular events. Circulation **137**(7), 653–661 (2018)
24. Whiffin, N., Hosking, F.J., Farrington, S.M., et al.: Identification of susceptibility loci for colorectal cancer in a genome-wide meta-analysis. Hum. Mol. Genet. **23**(17), 4729–4737 (2014)
25. Xu, Y., Qian, M., Hong, J., et al.: The effect of vitamin D on the occurrence and development of colorectal cancer: a systematic review and meta-analysis. Int. J. Colorectal Dis. **36**(7), 1329–1344 (2021)
26. Levy, D., Ehret, G.B., Rice, K., et al.: Genome-wide association study of blood pressure and hypertension. Nat. Genet. **41**(6), 677–687 (2009)
27. DASH Eating Plan. https://www.nhlbi.nih.gov/education/dash-eating-plan. Accessed 25 June 2022
28. Evans, D.M., Zhu, G., Dy, V., et al.: Genome-wide association study identifies loci affecting blood copper, selenium and zinc. Hum. Mol. Genet. **22**(19), 3998–4006 (2013)
29. Paillard, F., Flageul, O., Mahé, G., et al.: Validation and reproducibility of a short food frequency questionnaire for cardiovascular prevention. Arch. Cardiovasc. Dis. **114**(8–9), 570–576 (2021)

Combining Process Mining and Time Series Forecasting to Predict Hospital Bed Occupancy

Annelore Jellemijn Pieters and Stefan Schlobach(✉)

Vrije Universiteit Amsterdam, De Boelelaan 1105, 1081 HV Amsterdam, The Netherlands
k.s.schlobach@vu.nl

Abstract. This research investigates in how far AI methods can support the prediction of bed occupancy in hospital units based on individual patient data. We combine process mining and a Deep Spatial-Temporal Graph Modeling algorithm and show that this improves the performance of the prediction over existing approaches. To improve the model even more it is extended with knowledge available from patient records, like the day of the week, the time of the day, whether it is a vacation day or not and the amount of emergency cases per data point.

1 Introduction

Hospitals are more and more dealing with waits, delays and cancellations [8]. Sometimes hospitals can also get overflows of patients, which means that a hospital cannot handle the number of patients coming into that hospital anymore. Those problems used to be solved by adding more resources [10], such as beds, equipment or more staff. Nowadays those problems cannot be fixed that easily by adding resources for economic reasons. Moreover, research states that adding resources is not the best solution to the problem: instead literature shows that the focus should be on analysing how the patient moves through a hospital and optimising the capacity of bed occupancy.

When a patient goes to a hospital (s)he will follow a certain care pathway, e.g. starting the pathway with the emergency room for a broken leg. Hereafter the patient might need surgery, going to the operating rooms. After surgery (s)he will go to the post-anesthesia care unit to recover, and so the pathway grows, creating a so called *patient flow* through the hospital. According to research understanding this patient flow is crucial for reducing the overflows in a hospital [4,9,10,24].

Along with analysing the patient flows, the bed capacity management needs to be optimised as well. In a hospital there are a certain number of beds, though not always all the beds can be used. This can have several reasons, such as the absence of employees. For the hospital that we focused on, the beds are distributed over seventeen different departments, such as Day Care Unit for cancer, the General Care Unit hall B, the General Care Unit, the Post Anesthesia

A. Traina et al. (Eds.): HIS 2022, LNCS 13705, pp. 76–87, 2022.
https://doi.org/10.1007/978-3-031-20627-6_8

Care Unit level 3 or the Sleep Awake Unit, etc. The number of beds used on a day is determined by the number of employees working on that department that specific day. This means that each department has a number of beds available for patients, which varies per day.

To address this problem, this paper attempts to answer whether we can predict the bed occupancy of a hospital based on the previous and current occupancy? To answer this main research question, this study is divided into four sub-questions:

1. How to use Artificial Intelligence to find patient flows from patients in a hospital?
2. What methods perform best to predict bed occupancy of a hospital?
3. Can we improve existing bed occupancy perdition by combining process mining with a state-or-the-art forecasting algorithm?
4. Can we extend the forecasting model with domain knowledge in order to improve the performance of predicting bed occupancy?

Section 2 will present the relevant literature. Next, Sect. 3 describes the data that is used for this research, before the methodology of the different techniques is presented in Sect. 4. The experimental setup and the corresponding results are described in Sect. 5. The paper concludes in Sect. 6 with a discussion of the contributions and some recommendations, as well as the limitations of this research.

2 Theoretical Framework

Capacity Management. To get a grip on the occupation of the beds in a hospital, a hospital makes use of capacity management, which ensures that its capacity is used in an efficient and effective manner. There are three different kinds of capacity in a hospital; 1. Medical specialists, 2. Supporting personnel (e.g. nurses), 3. Resources (e.g. equipment or rooms). This paper focuses on resource capacity.

To use the capacity in a hospital efficiently, one needs to take into account the capacity management triangle. This triangle considers the variability, the capacity and the service times [13]. The variability includes fluctuations in the arrival times of a patient, the availability of the capacity and the duration of an appointment. The capacity means that there is a certain capacity level and utilization rate. The service times include waiting times, cancellations etc. Besides the triangle, there are four elements that put pressure on the capacity management; 1. Financial, 2. Institutional and social, 3. Clinical, 4. Professional [23]. By taking all of the mentioned above into account, the capacity management critically contributes to the effectiveness of a hospital.

Patient Flow. Investigating patient flows in hospitals is an important challenge for capacity management of hospitals. According to Walley and Steyn, around 60/70% of the patients in a hospital bed is getting active treatment and 40/30% of the patients in a hospital bed are waiting to see a doctor or they are waiting to get a sign that they are allowed to go home [26]. This poor patient flow is accompanied by eight problems according to Villa, Barbieri and Lega [23]: 1. There are not enough supplies, 2. Patients must wait for a long time, 3. Bottlenecks, 4. Resources that are not used in an efficient way, 5. Patients need to stay for a long time in hospitals, 6. Not a lot of productivity, 7. Clinical settings that are used inappropriate, 8. The variability of the workload.

A successful tool developed by Domova et al. visualises the patient flows in order to help the hospital improve and optimise the services that they offer [5]. Analysing patient flows is also successfully used for hospital planning [11] to improve the quality of the healthcare network. Another research that uses patient flows is a simulation model that is used to analyse the patient flows in a hospital in Hong Kong [20].

Forecasting Methods. Most current methods to predict the number of occupied beds in hospital use Support Vector Machines (SVM) [3,7], claiming that SVM are among the best algorithms for bed occupancy prediction in hospitals. More recently, neural networks are used for predictions [6,19,25], outperforming older algorithms they used. However, in those articles the research focuses on all departments as individuals, ignoring the relations and flows between the different departments. In this study, we considered a different prediction model, called Deep Spatial-Temporal Graph Modeling algorithm, which is currently used to predict traffic flows [28], and applied it to predict bed occupancy.

3 Data

For this study, data from a Dutch hospital was used. For every patient the actions or treatments that (s)he underwent is saved in an Electronic Health Record (EHR) The EHR software that is used by this hospital is HiX (Healthcare Information eXchange).

The dataset is retrieved from the EHR system with an SQL query that states: which bed is occupied at which moment for the last six years and by which patient. From this view an overview was created with two timestamps a day, 10:00 and 16:00. For every occupied bed there is more information about that patient collected, such as whether the patient was an emergency case, the intake type (for a day or longer) and the patient origin (from home, another hospital or somewhere else). First we performed data preprocessing and data cleaning based on an exploratory data analysis.

Exploratory Data Analysis. In the original dataset the first timestamp in the data is January, 1st 2016 and the last timestamp February, 11, 2022. On each day at 10:00 and at 16:00 an entry is created of which beds are occupied. This results in 857418 observations for 2.234 days. Because of relocation, with new departments being created, and missing values (patients being still in the hospital) the time range of the dataset is restricted to a range between 29-01-2017 and 01-01-2022.

We can see that there are 115971 different hospitalizations, for 61261 different patients. This means that some patients are hospitalized multiple times in this period. After removing departments that are not of interest for this research from the dataset, we obtain 110236 different hospitalizations for 60431 different patients. Hereafter, we are deleting missing values and convert NaN values to zero values if there are no patients in the hospital at that time.

The next step is to analyse the time series data. First we analysed trends, or pattern that can be found in the data. The second component is seasonality, which means that there are (predictable) changes which occur every year. Figures 1, 2 and 3 show original data, the trend and the seasonality. In Fig. 2 we can, first, see that in March 2020, the COVID-19 pandemic started, because at this point large fluctuations in the number of beds that are occupied starts.[1] Moreover, holidays in the Netherlands are visible in the Figure, leading to a decreased number of occupied beds.[2] Figure 3 shows seasonality in the data. The seasonality in this data is that during weekdays the number of beds that are occupied are higher than during the weekend. This is the case every week. This can be explained since there are no appointments or surgeries scheduled during the weekends.

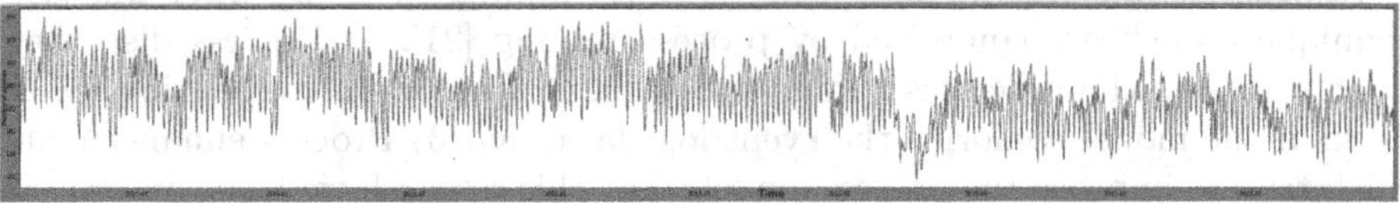

Fig. 1. Plot with the original data

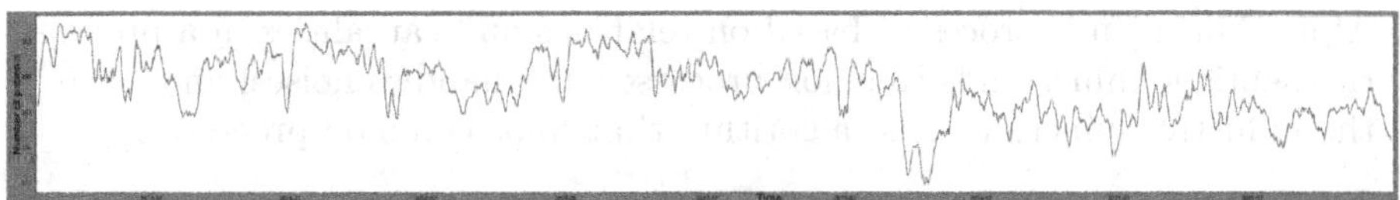

Fig. 2. Plot with the trend of the data

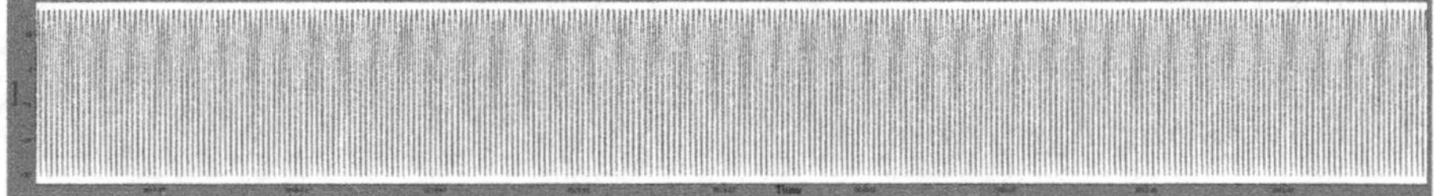

Fig. 3. Plot with the seasonality of the data

[1] Despite these fluctuations, we still chose to keep the data from when the pandemic started in the dataset, since COVID-19 is not completely gone yet, it is still possible that there are patients with COVID-19 in the hospital.

[2] We can see that during the Christmas holidays at the end of the year there is a decrease in occupied beds in the hospital. This is recurring every year.

4 Methods

The goal of this research is: Can we predict the bed occupancy of a hospital based on the currency occupancy? To do this, first the patient flow method is described, to solve the problem of finding the patient flows of the patients in a hospital. Then, we take a closer look at forecasting algorithms to find the bnest method to predict bed occupancy of a hospital.

4.1 Process Mining of Patient Flows

To determine the patient flow we apply process mining. Process mining is a method that is used to extract processes and insights from event logs [22]. Event logs are defined as: *"A set of process instances or traces, each of which contains a set of events. Events represent occurrences of process tasks or activities at a certain point in time"* [18]. The input for a process mining algorithm needs to have three different elements [17], a unique identifier, a timestamp and a name or description of the event.

In order to analyse the data using process mining, there are three different techniques which are comprised by process mining [21], 1) Process discovery, which discovers the processes behind the data, 2) Conformance checking which checks if the model conforms the event log data, and 3) Process enhancement, which tries to improve the process models. For this research we focus on process discovery, which takes event logs as input and creates a model without any a priori information. There are several different algorithms for process discovery [21].

1. Alpha Miner finds processes based on relations and causalities in a process,
2. the heuristic miner finds common processes and handles noises, and
3. the inductive miner, a sound algorithm that finds common processes.

The process models that are created using those algorithms from the event log data can be visualised in a directly follow graph (DFG) [14]. In the graph, each activity is visualised as a node and each relation is visualised as an edge between the nodes.

4.2 Forecasting Algorithm

Support Vector Machines. We use SVMs for regression in a variant called SVR, which is supervised machine learning algorithm based on finding optimal hyperplanes in a n-dimensional space, where n stands for the number of features or independent variables. By adapting the hyperplanes to a maximum margin, the error is reduced.

Deep Spatial-Temporal Graph Modeling. A forecasting method that takes into account the relations between the different hospital units is the Deep Spatial-Temporal Graph Modeling algorithm. Time series forecasting takes data of observations over time into account [2] and predicts values based on a series of historical observations. This algorithm takes a graph structure as input and takes spatial and temporal information into account [28]. The Deep Spatial-Temporal Graph Modeling model creates an adjacency matrix which will develop over time through training and node embedding. For an unweighted matrix the values are 1 or 0, where 1 means that the elements are connected and 0 means that the elements are not connected [27]. The weights in a matrix represent e.g. the strength of an edge (or 0 if there is no link).

A graph neural network architecture is used to model the different node-levels which are dynamic with the help of the relations between the different nodes. The model is heavily used in forecasting traffic speed flows [15]. To capture the relation between the spatial variables and the temporal variable they formally used graph convolution networks (GCN) and transformed it into recurrent neural networks (RNN).

For our research a different approach has been used, consisting of multiple spatial-temporal layers and one output layer [28]. Before the data is entering a spatial-temporal layer, the input data is transformed by a linear layer. After the linear layer the data goes on to the Spatial-Temporal layers, in which the first step is the Gated Temporal Convolution Module (Gated TCN), containing gating mechanisms where complex temporal dependencies in the data are learned. The Graph Convolution Layer (GCN) works together with the previous layer, the TCN layer, to keep the spatial-temporal dependencies of the data. Each of the Spatial-Temporal layers is connected with the output layer by skip connections [16].

Another component that is used is a stacked dilated 1D convolution component, this makes it possible to create a receptive field which can keep track of the amount of layers and increase exponentially with these number of layers. By using this algorithm the relation between the spatial and the temporal components can be observed.

As a baseline we use a majority baseline, which always predicts the most frequent class label in the dataset.

5 Experiments and Results

5.1 Modeling Hospital Patient Flows

In order to find the patient flows using process mining we used the Process Mining for Python (PM4Py) framework. The heuristic miner algorithm of this package is used acting on the Directly-Follows Graph and in this way the most common processes are found. For this part of the experimental setup the heuristic miner will be used to obtain the patient flows and visualise them. This algorithm is chosen since this algorithm has the goal to obtain the most common flows, which is what we want to obtain.

Results. Figure 4 shows the most common 0.0001% of the patient flows from the (whole) hospital. This 0.0001% is chosen as otherwise the graph would be too big to analyse, based on parameter tuning to keep overview small enough, while still providing an idea of how many different patient flows there are.

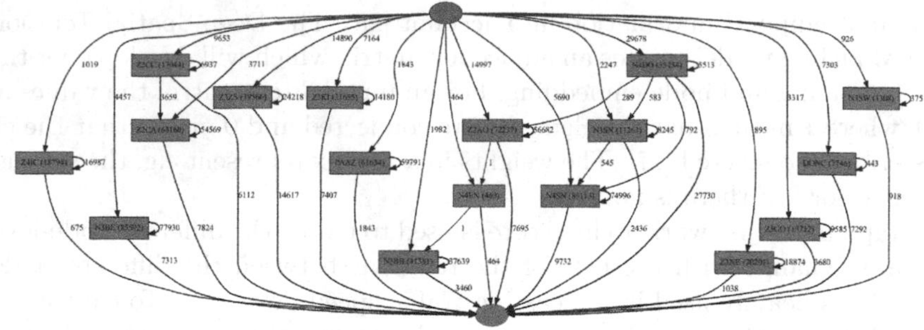

Fig. 4. 0.0001% most common patient flows in a hospital

The most common patient flows, are when patients are moving to another bed on the same department. A second movement that frequently occurs is the flow from the Cardiac Care Unit (Z3CC) to the Cardiology (Z2CA) unit. Another patient flow that occurs often is patients that move from the Day Care Unit (N4DO) to the Post Anesthesia Care Unit (N4SN).

Next to visualising the data we can also get a table with the most common patient flows in a hospital. An observation is that the most frequent flows in the department are from a department to itself, as visualised in Table 1. However also a movement from the Cardiac Care Unit to the Cardiology unit happens often in this timeframe.

Table 1. The 5 most common patient flows between two units

Number	Patient flows
1	Day Care Unit -> Day Care Unit
2	Care Suites Unit -> Care Suites Unit
3	Acute Medical Unit -> Acute Medical Unit
4	Children Ward -> Children Ward
5	Post Anesthesia Care Unit level 4 -> Post Anesthesia Care Unit level 4

Table 1 shows the place in the top 5 and the respective patient flow in the chosen time period. We can see that the patient flow is from Day Care Unit to Day Care Unit, which means that the patient is laying on the Day Care Unit and is moving to another bed in the time-frame. This happens 5062 times in almost five years, which is the highest number of all the patient flows.

5.2 Forecasting Bed Occupancy

In order to investigate which forecasting algorithm is performing best in predicting bed occupancy in a hospital compared Support Vector Regression (SVR) with the Deep Spatial-Temporal Graph Modeling algorithm and the baseline.

For the SVR algorithm we use default settings, including an rbf kernel, the gamma is scale and the probability is False. With the help of feature selection, we use features: the hour of the day, emergency or not, intake type (e.g. is it for a day or longer), and origin (e.g. from home or the emergency room) and the timestamp.

For the Deep Spatial-Temporal Graph Modeling algorithm we also used the default settings, i.e. only knowledge about the hour of the day. The sequence length is set to seven[3]. The algorithm is trained for 100 iterations.

The data is divided into a training set (70%) and a test set of 30% of the data. This experiment were evaluated by comparing Mean Absolute Error (MAE) [1] and and Root Mean Squared Error (RMSE) [12][4].

For all values that are predicted for each datapoint of the test set, the MAE and the RMSE are calculated. The mean of all those error scores is calculated in order to find the error rate for each different algorithm. Each experiment is repeated 20 times and the mean of the MAE and RMSE is calculated.

Results. In this subsection we show the results of the comparison between the SVR algorithm, the baseline and the Deep Spatial-Temporal Graph Modeling algorithms. In Table 2 the results of the forecasting with the different algorithms are shown. Table 2 shows that the baseline, non surprisingly, that always predicts random values has the highest MAE and RMSE scores. The second highest scores for the MAE and RMSE are obtained by the SVR algorithm. This means that the SVR algorithm is performing the second worst. Furthermore can we see that the values for the MAE and RMSE scores for the majority baseline are better than SVR, but worse than the mean Deep Spatial-Temporal Graph Modeling. This means that the Deep Spatial-Temporal Graph Modeling algorithm has the lowest error values for the MAE and RMSE and is performing the best.

Table 2. Different forecasting algorithms predicting the bed occupancy

	Mean MAE	Mean RMSE
SVR	2.7186	3.3218
Deep Spatial-Temporal Graph Modeling	**1.9189**	**2.5711**
Baseline majority	2.5133	2.9445

[3] A prediction looks at the number of patients of the last week (seven days).

[4]

$$MAE = (\frac{1}{n})\sum_{i=1}^{n}|F_t - A_i| \qquad RMSE = \sqrt{(\frac{1}{n})\sum_{i=1}^{n}(F_i - A_i)^2} \quad (1)$$

Where n is the number of observation, F_t is the predicted output value, A_t is the actual output value and t is the time point the value is predicted for.

5.3 Combining Patient Flows with A Forecasting Model

We now create a model that combines process mining and the Deep Spatial-Temporal Graph Modeling algorithm. To investigate this model different inputs for the Deep Spatial-Temporal Graph Modeling algorithm will be used, adjusting the adjacency matrix based on what was learned during process mining.

We compared four different inputs for the model, an empty adjacency matrix, where all values in the matrix are set to zero. The second input is an adjacency matrix with all values set to zero except for the diagonal row, those values are filled with ones. This diagonal input is chosen because of frequent flows within departments. The third input is an adjacency matrix filled with random values differing between zero and one. The fourth and last input is an adjacency matrix filled with the input retrieved from the process mining method. To find the correlations between the different departments, we divided the amount of occurrences of a flow by the total number of occurrences of all flows.

Results. Table 3 shows the comparison between the combination of process mining and Deep Spatial-Temporal Graph Modeling and models with other input.

Table 3. Comparison of various deep spatial-temporal graph modeling algorithm

	MAE	RMSE
Empty matrix	2.0121	2.6852
Diagonal matrix	1.9841	2.6548
Random matrix	1.9441	2.5967
Process mining matrix	**1.9189**	**2.5711**

Table 3 shows that when the process mining values are used as input for the model, the model has the lowest error values for the MAE and RMSE evaluation metrics and thus performs the best.

5.4 Model Extension with Knowledge

To extend the model created with the combination of process mining and Deep Spatial-Temporal Graph Modeling, we investigated if adding knowledge to the model improves the performance of the model. A set of interviews with hospital employees provided the following factors influencing the number of patients: 1. The time of the day, 2. The day in the week, 3. Vacation periods and 4. The amount of emergency cases on a day. Each of these statements was added to the model individually and in every possible combination.

Table 4 shows that the values are lower, when the knowledge about the time of day is added to the model. Besides this, we can see that the error is the lowest if the knowledge about the time in the day, the day in the week and vacation is added to the model.

Table 4. Model extension with knowledge

	MAE	RMSE
Time of the day	1.9189	2.5711
Day in the week	2.2165	2.8973
Vacation	2.3159	3.0507
Emergency	2.2215	2.9045
Time of the day - Day in the week - Vacation	**1.8564**	**2.4812**
Time of the day - Day in the week - Emergency	1.8928	2.5197
Day in the week - Vacation - Emergency cases	2.2342	2.8990
Time of the day - Day in the week - Vacation	1.9009	2.5282

6 Discussion

Conclusion. In this paper we have shown that Process Mining can be used in order to find the patient flows from the patients. By using a heuristic miner the patient flows can be analysed and visualised. We tested four different algorithms for predicting the bed occupancy of a hospital, showing that a Deep Spatial-Temporal Graph Modeling algorithm is performing best to predict the bed occupancy. Moreover, a model is made that combines process mining with Deep Spatial-Temporal Graph Modeling forecasting. Table 3 shows that this model has the lowest error values and thus is performing the best. Finally, we extended the model with domain knowledge and showed that adding time of the day always improves the model, and if this statement is missing, the results are getting worse. There is also found that overall the more statements added to the model, the better the model is performing. However, the combination of time of the day, day in the week and vacation day or not, is performing the best. We can conclude that the best way to predict hospital occupancy is by combining the patient flow algorithm with the Deep Spatial-Temporal Graph Modeling algorithm and extend this with knowledge about the time of the day, the day in the week and if it is a vacation day or not.

Limitations and Recommendations. While the literature suggests that SVR is the best performing method for bed prediction in hospitals, there has been no approach using Deep Spatial-Temporal Graph Modeling algorithm as of yet. However, there are limitations to this research, such as the time range of the data, which included the start of COVID-19. This results into big fluctuations the bed occupancy. However, we still chose to keep this data in the dataset, since COVID-19 is still in our lives and may still be there for a long period of time.

Another limitation is that this research is only performed on one dataset. For future research one can investigate this research on multiple datasets of different hospitals to see if the model created in this research, can also be utilized on different datasets.

Initially within this research we wanted to extend the model with knowledge about the diagnosis of each patient. However, access to more structured data (such as diagnostic knowledge using, e.g., ICD10 was not available at the time of this research). For future research this might be very interesting to focus on.

References

1. Akdemir, B., Çetinkaya, N.: Long-term load forecasting based on adaptive neural fuzzy inference system using real energy data. Energy Procedia **14**, 794–799 (2012)
2. Chatfield, C.: Time-Series Forecasting. Chapman and Hall/CRC (2000)
3. Daghistani, T.A., Elshawi, R., Sakr, S., Ahmed, A.M., Al-Thwayee, A., Al-Mallah, M.H.: Predictors of in-hospital length of stay among cardiac patients: a machine learning approach. Int. J. Cardiol. **288**, 140–147 (2019)
4. Dart, T., Cui, Y., Chatellier, G., Degoulet, P.: Analysis of hospitalised patient flows using data-mining. In: Studies in Health Technology and Informatics, pp. 263–268 (2003)
5. Domova, V., Sander-Tavallaey, S.: Visualization for quality healthcare: patient flow exploration. In: 2019 IEEE International Conference on Big Data (Big Data), pp. 1072–1079. IEEE (2019)
6. Gentimis, T., Ala'J, A., Durante, A., Cook, K., Steele, R.: Predicting hospital length of stay using neural networks on MIMIC III data. In: 2017 IEEE 15th International Conference on Dependable, Autonomic and Secure Computing, 15th International Conference on Pervasive Intelligence and Computing, 3rd International Conference on Big Data Intelligence and Computing and Cyber Science and Technology Congress (DASC/PiCom/DataCom/CyberSciTech), pp. 1194–1201. IEEE (2017)
7. Hachesu, P.R., Ahmadi, M., Alizadeh, S., Sadoughi, F.: Use of data mining techniques to determine and predict length of stay of cardiac patients. Healthc. Inform. Res. **19**(2), 121–129 (2013)
8. Hall, R.: Patient flow. AMC **10**, 12 (2013)
9. Hanne, T., Melo, T., Nickel, S.: Bringing robustness to patient flow management through optimized patient transports in hospitals. Interfaces **39**(3), 241–255 (2009)
10. Haraden, C., Resar, R.: Patient flow in hospitals: understanding and controlling it better. Front. Health Serv. Manag. **20**(4), 3 (2004)
11. Jay, N., Kohler, F., Napoli, A.: Using formal concept analysis for mining and interpreting patient flows within a healthcare network. In: Yahia, S.B., Nguifo, E.M., Belohlavek, R. (eds.) CLA 2006. LNCS (LNAI), vol. 4923, pp. 263–268. Springer, Heidelberg (2008). https://doi.org/10.1007/978-3-540-78921-5_19
12. Kalogirou, S.A.: Solar thermal systems: components and applications-introduction. Elsevier Ltd. (2012)
13. Klassen, R.D., Menor, L.J.: The process management triangle: an empirical investigation of process trade-offs. J. Oper. Manag. **25**(5), 1015–1034 (2007)
14. Leemans, S.J., Poppe, E., Wynn, M.T.: Directly follows-based process mining: exploration and a case study. In: 2019 International Conference on Process Mining (ICPM), pp. 25–32. IEEE (2019)
15. Li, Y., Yu, R., Shahabi, C., Liu, Y.: Diffusion convolutional recurrent neural network: data-driven traffic forecasting. arXiv preprint arXiv:1707.01926 (2017)
16. Liu, F., Ren, X., Zhang, Z., Sun, X., Zou, Y.: Rethinking skip connection with layer normalization. In: Proceedings of the 28th International Conference on Computational Linguistics, pp. 3586–3598 (2020)

17. Moeke, D.: De meerwaarde van process mining bij het optimaliseren van de patient flow (2021)
18. de Murillas, E., Reijers, H.A., van der Aalst, W.M.: Case notion discovery and recommendation: automated event log building on databases. Knowl. Inf. Syst. **62**(7), 2539–2575 (2020). https://doi.org/10.1007/s10115-019-01430-6
19. Pofahl, W.E., Walczak, S.M., Rhone, E., Izenberg, S.D.: Use of an artificial neural network to predict length of stay in acute pancreatitis. Am. Surg. **64**(9), 868 (1998)
20. Rado, O., Lupia, B., Leung, J.M.Y., Kuo, Y.-H., Graham, C.A.: Using simulation to analyze patient flows in a hospital emergency department in Hong Kong. In: Matta, A., Li, J., Sahin, E., Lanzarone, E., Fowler, J. (eds.) Proceedings of the International Conference on Health Care Systems Engineering. SPMS, vol. 61, pp. 289–301. Springer, Cham (2014). https://doi.org/10.1007/978-3-319-01848-5_23
21. Rojas, E., Munoz-Gama, J., Sepúlveda, M., Capurro, D.: Process mining in healthcare: a literature review. J. Biomed. Inform. **61**, 224–236 (2016)
22. Van Der Aalst, W.: Process mining. Commun. ACM **55**(8), 76–83 (2012)
23. Villa, S., Barbieri, M., Lega, F.: Restructuring patient flow logistics around patient care needs: implications and practicalities from three critical cases. Health Care Manag. Sci. **12**(2), 155–165 (2009). https://doi.org/10.1007/s10729-008-9091-6
24. Villa, S., Prenestini, A., Giusepi, I.: A framework to analyze hospital-wide patient flow logistics: evidence from an Italian comparative study. Health Policy **115**(2–3), 196–205 (2014)
25. Walczak, S., et al.: Predicting hospital length of stay with neural networks. In: FLAIRS Conference, pp. 333–337 (1998)
26. Walley, P., Silvester, K., Steyn, R., Conway, J.B.: Managing variation in demand: lessons from the UK national health service/practitioner application. J. Healthc. Manag. **51**(5), 309 (2006)
27. Weisstein, E.W.: Adjacency matrix (2007). https://mathworld.wolfram.com/
28. Wu, Z., Pan, S., Long, G., Jiang, J., Zhang, C.: Graph WaveNet for deep spatial-temporal graph modeling. arXiv preprint arXiv:1906.00121 (2019)

HGCL: Heterogeneous Graph Contrastive Learning for Traditional Chinese Medicine Prescription Generation

Zecheng Yin[1(✉)], Yingpei Wu[2], and Yanchun Zhang[1,3]

[1] Guangzhou University, Guangzhou, China
yinzecheng@e.gzhu.edu.cn
[2] Fudan University, Shanghai, China
ypwu16@fdu.edu.cn
[3] Pengcheng Lab, Shenzhen, China

Abstract. Traditional Chinese Medicine (TCM) is a highly empirical, subjective and practical discipline. Generating an appropriate prescription has been one of the most crucial components in building intelligent diagnosis systems that provide clinical decision support to physicians. While various machine learning models for prescription generation have been created, they suffer from specific limitations (e.g., data complexity and semantic ambiguity, lack of syndrome differentiation thinking, etc.). For handling these limitations, we propose a novel Heterogeneous Graph Contrastive Learning (HGCL) based model to conduct prescription generation with the idea of syndrome differentiation and treatment. Specifically, we first model the TCM clinical prescriptions as a Heterogeneous Information Network (THIN), and then explore node- and semantic-level contrastive learning on THIN, so as to enhance the quality of node representations for several downstream tasks such as node classification, prescription generation, etc. We conduct extensive experiments on three real TCM clinical datasets, demonstrating significant improvement over state-of-the-art methods, even though some of which are fully unsupervised.

Keywords: Heterogeneous graph · Data mining · Contrasitve learning · Representation learning

1 Introduction

Syndrome differentiation and treatment (Bian Zheng Lun Zhi) is one of the most important principles in the clinical practice of TCM. In TCM treatment, physicians first obtain the symptoms through the four diagnoses (i.e., observation, listening, questioning, and pulse analyses). By carefully analyzing these symptoms, physicians deduce the syndromes of the patient and then choose a set of suitable herbs as a formula to cure the syndromes [7].

The syndrome differentiation process, however, is particularly sophisticated. A symptom can show in a variety of syndromes, while a syndrome contains

A. Traina et al. (Eds.): HIS 2022, LNCS 13705, pp. 88–99, 2022.
https://doi.org/10.1007/978-3-031-20627-6_9

multiple symptoms [3,24]. Even for the same specific set of symptoms, different physicians may reach different syndromes, rendering it difficult to find criteria for syndrome differentiation [8]. These make the clinical diagnosis and treatment of TCM very difficult for physicians. Consequently, a study of the prescription generation with syndrome reasoning is needed to help TCM physicians prepare prescriptions and provide clinical decision support.

Several recent studies on TCM prescription generation have achieved encouraging results [10]. Topic-model based methods consider each prescription as a document with several latent topics where symptoms and herbs are viewed as a group of words respectively [26,27]. Unfortunately, the performance of these methods is limited by the sparsity of prescriptions [14]. Graph representation learning-based methods focus on learning low-dimensional embeddings of TCM entities, and then generating prescription based on these embeddings [8,14,15]. Because of being based on random walk-based skip-gram model or graph convolution network (GCN) [9], most of these methods fail to capture the global information of a graph and thus overlook much of high-order properties [13]. In summary, current TCM prescription generation models suffer from following limitations:

(1) Data complexity and semantic ambiguity. A TCM clinical prescription consists of three parts (i.e., a set of symptoms, herbs, and syndromes), implying the syndrome differentiation and treatment procedure. There are rich semantic relations among TCM entities, such as the herb compatibility, the generalization relation between symptoms and syndromes, and the evolutionary relation between symptoms. Considering entities of prescriptions in weak order, modeling the prescription text and extracting the semantic relation information between entities is a critical issue. **(2) Lack of syndrome differentiation thinking.** Most of the above-mentioned methods simply deliver a combination of herbs for the symptoms. The generation process is a black box lacking an explicit syndrome induction and not following the philosophy of syndrome differentiation and treatment.

To address these limitations, we propose a novel Heterogeneous Graph Contrastive Learning (HGCL) based model to conduct prescription generation with the philosophy of syndrome differentiation and treatment. Based on the constructed THIN, our HGCL framework is designed to optimize two objectives, namely node-level and semantic-level contrastiveness. Firstly, considering the skewed data distribution in THIN, we perform topology and feature augmentations on THIN and generate two correlated graph views. Then, a novel node-level contrastive loss tailored for THIN is proposed to maximize the agreement of node embeddings of these two views. The intuition behind is that modifying the graph structure and reducing the influence of high-degree nodes can help alleviate the degree biases, which guide the model to capture the structure information of THIN without the influence of skewed data distribution. Secondly, to capture high-order semantic information in heterogeneous graph, the semantic-level contrastive learning is conducted on THIN. We first generate meta-path instances including the positive and negative samples which contain rich and subtle semantic information in THIN, and then distinguish these samples with a innovative semantic-level contrastive learning. Our main contributions are summarized as follows:

- We model the TCM prescription generation problem as a graph representation problem in THIN, which is constituted by herbs, symptoms, and syndromes and their multiple relations extracted from clinical prescriptions.
- We propose a novel heterogeneous graph contrastive representation learning model, named HGCL, which combines the node- and semantic-level contrastive learning. To the best of our knowledge, this is the first attempt to take advantage of the heterogeneous graph contrastive learning for TCM prescription generation.
- Extensive experimental results have demonstrated that our proposed HGCL framework significantly outperforms seven state-of-the-art baselines, even though it is fully unsupervised.

2 Related Work

2.1 TCM Prescription Generation

TCM prescription generation has been a popular and challenging research issue in recent years. Wang et al. [23] identified the issue of detecting the relationship between symptoms and herbs as a machine translation problem and developed a transformer-based model to convert symptoms to herbs. Based on the idea of Transformer [18], Li et al. [11] presented a TCM knowledge enhanced Seq2Seq model to generate prescription. Although effective in prescription generation, Seq2Seq-based models have a weakness in dealing with short-text-like prescriptions, making it hard to capture the semantic information included in TCM prescriptions. Furthermore, due to lacking an explicit syndrome induction, most of the above methods do not follow TCM's philosophy of syndrome differentiation and treatment, which further limits their performance and applicability.

2.2 Graph Contrastive Learning

Lately, contrastive methods adopted for computer vision have also been adapted to graph domain and achieved great success. Velickovic et al. proposed DGI [20] which extended deep InfoMax [5] to graphs and contrasted node-local patches against global graph representations. Following this line of study, Sun et al. developed InfoGraph [17] which learned graph representations by maximizing the MI between the graph representations and sub-structural representations. For multiplex graph, Park et al. presented DMGI [13] which divided the original graph into several homogeneous ones and followed infomax objective of DGI for each relation graph. Inspired by SimCLR [1], MoCo [4] Zhu et al. presented GRACE [29] which generated two graph views by corruption and learned node representations by maximizing the agreement of node representations in these two views. Motivated by the above models, our proposed HGCL is tailored for THIN representation learning.

3 Preliminary

Definition 1. TCM Heterogeneous Information Network (THIN). As a HIN, THIN is defined as a heterogeneous graph $\mathcal{G} = (\mathcal{V}, \mathcal{E})$ where $\mathcal{V}$ and $\mathcal{E}$ represent the sets of nodes and edges respectively. A THIN is also associated with a node type mapping function $\phi(v) : \mathcal{V} \rightarrow \mathcal{A}, \forall v \in \mathcal{V}$ and a relation type mapping function $\varphi(e) : \mathcal{E} \rightarrow \mathcal{R}, \forall e \in \mathcal{E}$. $\mathcal{A}$ and $\mathcal{R}$ denote the sets of predefined node types and relation types. Specifically, Fig. 1(a) shows an example of THIN. In the THIN, we define three types of nodes corresponding to symptom, syndrome, herb, and two types of links representing various relationships between them. Symptom-Syndrome edges represent the generalization of syndrome to symptom in a prescription. Syndrome-Herb edges indicate the therapeutic or palliative effect of prescribed herbs on specific symptoms.

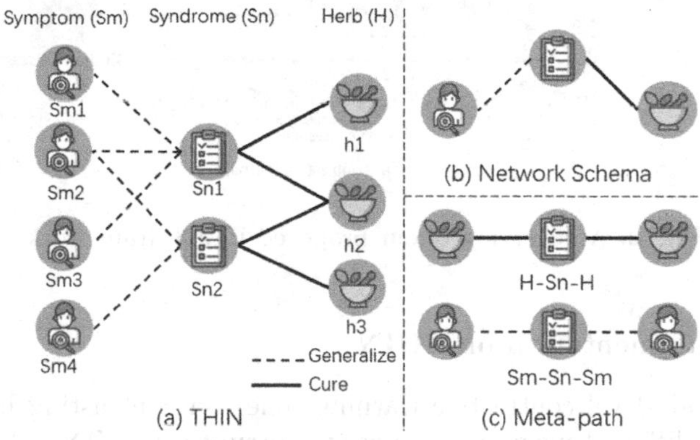

Fig. 1. A example of THIN and associated demonstration of network schema and meta-path.

Definition 2. TCM Meta-path. Given a THIN $\mathcal{G} = (\mathcal{V}, \mathcal{E})$, meta-path M is a path which is defined as $A_1 \xrightarrow{r_1} A_2 \xrightarrow{r_2} \cdots \xrightarrow{r_l} A_{l+1}$, where $r_i \in \mathcal{R}$, $A_i \in \mathcal{A}$. For the THIN $\mathcal{G}$, let $\mathcal{M} = \{M_1, M_2, \cdots, M_{|\mathcal{M}|}\}$. It is worth noting that a sequential nodes $m = \{v_1, v_2, \cdots, v_n\}$ conforming with the rule of meta-path M is a path instance of meta-path M. For example, Fig. 1(c) illustrates two meta-paths extracted from THIN in Fig. 1(a). Symptom-Syndrome-Symptom describes that a syndrome summarizes two interrelated symptoms, and Herb-Syndrome-Herb denotes that both herbs are effective for a specific syndrome.

4 Our Proposed Model: HGCL

Figure 2 illustrates the overall framework. To tackle the skewed data distribution problem, in Fig. 2(b), we design the node-level contrastive learning strategy, in which we first generate two augmented graph views by randomly corrupting the topology and feature of the THIN. Then, a novel node-level contrastive loss tailored for THIN is proposed to maximize the agreement of node embeddings in these two views. To capture high-order semantic information in THIN, in Fig. 2(c), we propose the semantic-level contrastive learning strategy based on meta-path instances. Finally, we jointly optimize the node- and semantic-level contrastive tasks to train the parameters of GNN.

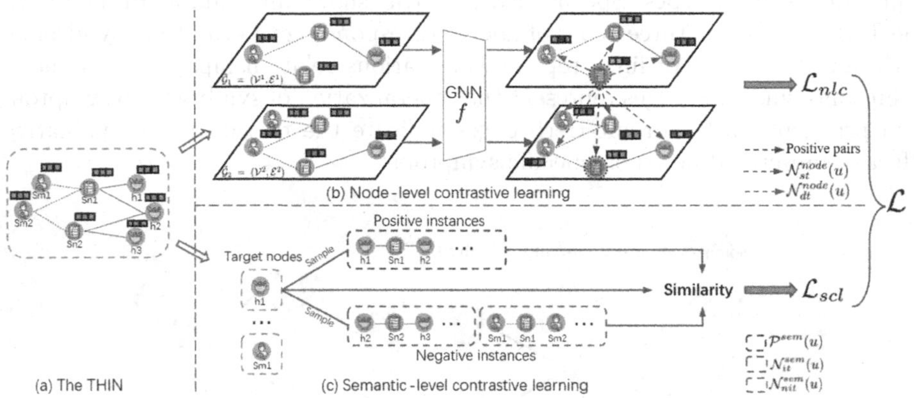

Fig. 2. An overview of our proposed HGCL framework.

4.1 Data Augmentation on THIN

Considering node-level contrastive learning relies on contrasting between node embeddings in different views, we propose to corrupt the THIN at both topology and attribute levels, thus constructing different node contexts for the model to be compared.

Node Dropping (ND) and Edge Remving (ER) randomly drop and remove a portion of nodes and edges in THIN. Formally, we sample two random vectors $\boldsymbol{N} \in \{0,1\}^{|\mathcal{V}|}$ and $\boldsymbol{E} \in \{0,1\}^{|\mathcal{E}|}$, where each element is sampled from a Bernoulli distribution $\boldsymbol{N}_i \sim Bernoulli(p_{nd})$, $\boldsymbol{E}_j \sim Bernoulli(p_{er})$ to determine whether to drop the i-th node and remove the j-th edge. Here p_{nd} and p_{er} are the probabilities for ND and ER. These operators are formulated as:

$$\mathcal{V}' = \mathcal{V} \odot \boldsymbol{N}, \tag{1}$$

$$\mathcal{E}' = \mathcal{E} \odot \boldsymbol{E}, \tag{2}$$

where $\odot$ denotes the Hadamard product (the same as below).

Feature Masking (FM) randomly masks a fraction of dimensions with zeros in node features. Formally, we first sample a random matrix $\boldsymbol{F} \in \{0,1\}^{|\mathcal{V}|\times d}$ where each element is sampled from a Bernoulli distribution $\widetilde{\boldsymbol{F}}_{ij} \sim Bernoulli(p_{fm})$ to determine whether to mask the feature matrix at position (i, j). Here p_{fm} is the masking rate for THIN features. The generated node features matrix $\widetilde{\boldsymbol{X}}$ can be computed as:

$$\widetilde{\boldsymbol{X}} = \boldsymbol{X} \odot \boldsymbol{F}. \tag{3}$$

By applying these augmentations on topology and feature in THIN $\mathcal{G}$, we generate two correlated graph views, denoted as $\tilde{\mathcal{G}}_1 = (\mathcal{V}^1, \mathcal{E}^1)$ and $\tilde{\mathcal{G}}_2 = (\mathcal{V}^2, \mathcal{E}^2)$ then the node-level contrastive learning will be conducted on these two views.

4.2 Node-level Contrastive Learning (NCL)

Having generated two augmented graphs for the THIN, as shown in Fig. 2(b), we consider the representations of the same node in two views as the positive pairs, and any different nodes in these two views as the negative pairs. In previous graph contrastive learning, however, the negative sampling is based only on homogeneous graph structures [28,29], which ignores the heterogeneity in the THIN. It is undesirable to graft it onto our scenario directly.

According to the alignment principle [22], similar samples have similar representations, and negative samples require more differences than positive ones. To make NCL exploit the semantics of node types in THIN, we need to characterize the differences between different types of negative samples. In specific, for a given anchor node u, we define two types of negative samples as:

$$\mathcal{N}_{st}^{node}(u) = \{v \mid \phi(u) = \phi(v), u \neq v, v \in \mathcal{V}^1 \cup \mathcal{V}^2\}, \tag{4}$$

$$\mathcal{N}_{dt}^{node}(u) = \{v \mid \phi(u) \neq \phi(v), v \in \mathcal{V}^1 \cup \mathcal{V}^2\}, \tag{5}$$

where $\mathcal{N}_{st}^{node}(u)$ and $\mathcal{N}_{dt}^{node}(u)$ represent the set of negative samples of the same and different type of the anchor node u respectively, as depicted by the purple and green dash lines in Fig. 2(b). Formally, we follow SimCLR [1]/MoCo [4] and utilize the normalized temperature-scaled cross entropy loss (NT-Xent) [12,25] to maximize the agreement of positive pairs and minimize it of negative pairs:

$$\begin{aligned}
\mathcal{L}_{nlc}^1(u) &= -\log \frac{\exp(s(h_u^1, h_u^2)/\tau)}{\Phi_1 + \Phi_2} \\
\Phi_1 &= \sum_{v \in \mathcal{N}_{dt}^{node}(u)} \exp(s(h_u^1, h_v)/\tau) \\
\Phi_2 &= \sum_{v \in \mathcal{N}_{st}^{node}(u)} \exp(s(h_u^1, h_v)/\tau)
\end{aligned} \tag{6}$$

where $s(\cdot,\cdot)$ denotes dot similarity and τ is a temperature parameter. Here, h_u^* indicates the representation of node u in the *-th view. Similarly, we can calculate the symmetrical loss $\mathcal{L}_{nlc}^2(u)$ for view 2.

Finally, by integrating above two losses, we obtain the final NCL as follows:

$$\mathcal{L}_{nlc} = \frac{1}{2|\mathcal{V}|} \sum_{u \in \mathcal{V}} (\mathcal{L}_{nlc}^1(u) + \mathcal{L}_{nlc}^2(u)). \tag{7}$$

4.3 Semantic-Level Contrastive Learning (SCL)

Meta-path is well used to explore the semantics and extract relations among nodes [16]. Consequently, to exploit the high-order semantic information on the THIN, we generate meta-path instances to generate the positive and negative samples, which capture the TCM semantic information on the THIN and are used to conduct SCL.

Sampling Positive Meta-path Instances. Given a meta-path $M \in \mathcal{M}$ and a target node u, we define a positive meta-path instance of u as a sequential nodes $m = \{v_1, v_2, \cdots, v_n\}$ conforming with the rule of meta-path M and including the target node u. For example, in Fig. 2(c), we have a meta-path instance as $m = \{h1, sn1, h2\}$. Formally, we generate the positive meta-path samples *w.r.t.* the target node u as

$$\mathcal{P}^{sem}(u) = \{m \mid m \in \Psi(M), u \in m, M \in \mathcal{M}\}, \tag{8}$$

where $\mathcal{M}$ is all of the pre-defined meta-paths, Ψ(M) denotes the set of all instances of M. Intuitively, sampling positive meta-path instances can capture not only local structural information, but also TCM semantic context.

Sampling Negative Meta-path Instances. To achieve fine-grained SCL and improve its semantic capturing capability, like NCL, we also define two types of negative meta-path instances of a target node u as:

$$\mathcal{N}_{it}^{sem}(u) = \{m \mid m \in \Psi(M), u \notin m, \phi(u) \in T(m), M \in \mathcal{M}\} \tag{9}$$

$$\mathcal{N}_{nit}^{sem}(u) = \{m \mid m \in \Psi(M), \phi(u) \notin T(m), M \in \mathcal{M}\} \tag{10}$$

where $T(m)$ denotes the set of all node types in the meta-path m, $\mathcal{N}_{it}^{sem}(u)$ represents the set of negative meta-path instances of the target node u, which contains the type of u, but not the u, $\mathcal{N}_{nit}^{sem}(u)$ denotes the set of meta-path instances that do not contain the u node type. These two types of negative instances are depicted by the purple and green dashed boxes in Fig. 2(c).

Given $\mathcal{N}_{it}^{sem}(u)$ and $\mathcal{N}_{nit}^{sem}(u)$, we then model the likelihood that the target node u is related to the positive samples while not being relevant to negative samples as follows:

$$\begin{aligned} \mathcal{L}_{scl} &= -\sum_{u \in \mathcal{V}} \sum_{I^+ \in \mathcal{P}^{sem}(u)} \log \frac{\exp(\mathbf{h}_u^\top f(I^+))}{\Phi_1 + \Phi_2} \\ \Phi_1 &= \sum_{I^- \in \mathcal{N}_{nit}^{sem}(u)} \exp(\mathbf{h}_u^\top f(I^-)) \\ \Phi_2 &= \sum_{I^- \in \mathcal{N}_{it}^{sem}(u)} \exp(\mathbf{h}_u^\top f(I^-)) \end{aligned} \tag{11}$$

where I^* represents a positive(+) or negative(-) meta-path instance to the target node u, $f(\cdot)$ is a mean pooling function which generates the representation of nodes in the meta-path instance I^*.

4.4 Model Training

We jointly optimize the both of the NCL and SCL contrastive losses (cf. Eq. (7) and Eq. (11)). Specifically, the final objective function is defined as:

$$\mathcal{L} = \mathcal{L}_{nlc} + \mathcal{L}_{scl}, \tag{12}$$

Our graph encoders f are 2-layer GCN and augmentation probabilities p_{nd}, p_{er}, p_{fm} are all set to be 0.5.

5 Experiments

In this section, we first describe our experimental settings, including datasets, baseline methods and detailed configuration, then extensive experiments are conducted to validate the effectiveness of the proposed framework.

5.1 Datasets

- **TCMRel** [21] is constructed based on the corpus of TCM literature, with herb, symptom, disease included.
- **ChP** [2] is built from the Pharmacopoeia of the People's Republic of China 2015 Edition, with formula, herb, symptom, and function included.
- **LuCa** is a real-world lung cancer clinical prescription dataset, collected from our cooperative hospital, which includes symptoms, syndromes, and herbs. We conduct the prescription generation task **on this dataset**.

5.2 Baseline Methods

We compare HGCL with two categories of baselines. For supervised methods, we select GCN [9], GAT [19], and HGT [6]. DGI [20], GRACE [29], and DMGI [13] are chosen as the self-supervised baselines.

5.3 Herb Classification and Similarity Search

For herb classification task, we implement a logistic regression model on the learned embeddings in the training set, and then evaluate the test set, 10 times repeat, 8:2 split rate, to get Micro-F1 and Macro-F1. For the similarity search task, we first calculate the cosine similarity scores of the learned embedding between all pairs of herbal nodes. For each node, we then rank the nodes based on the similarity score. Finally, we compute the percentage of nodes belonging to the same class among the top 5 nodes (Sim@5).

The results reported in Table 1 show that HGCL performs the best on LuCa and ChP, even compared with several supervised models. Furthermore, HGCL performs the second best on TCMRel in Macro F1, its performance is still very competitive with that of the best baseline HGT. For supervised methods, the method designed for heterogeneous graphs, HGT, obtains better results than

Table 1. Experiment results for the herbal classification and similarity search task.

Method	TCMRel			ChP			LuCa		
	MaF1	MiF1	Sim@5	MaF1	MiF1	Sim@5	MaF1	MiF1	Sim@5
GCN	0.1128	0.1304	0.0965	0.0488	0.1351	0.0885	0.0316	0.1321	0.0438
GAT	0.1128	0.1739	0.1246	0.02	0.1622	0.1027	**0.1238**	**0.2407**	0.2189
HGT	0.1818	0.2353	0.1069	0.0394	0.1538	0.0964	0.0314	0.1286	0.0957
DGI	0.0896	0.2877	0.1204	0.2	0.3415	0.1148	0.0194	0.1124	0.0713
GRACE	0.0514	0.2055	0.2459	0.0663	0.2033	0.1121	0.0069	0.1	0.22
DMGI	0.169	0.274	0.2633	0.07	0.187	0.1944	0.0258	0.1573	0.0582
HGCL	**0.1871**	**0.3132**	**0.2694**	**0.2169**	**0.4878**	**0.3124**	0.0408	0.1667	**0.339**

ones for homogeneous graphs, e.g., GCN and GAT. Through the above analysis, we can observe that our proposed node- and semantic-level contrastive learning on THIN can indeed explore the semantic information about the efficacy of herbs and be used in the downstream tasks of herb classification and similarity search.

5.4 Prescription Generation

For generating effective prescriptions, we start from the symptoms, first find the related syndromes by similarity search, then combine these syndromes with the corresponding syndromes, and finally get the target herbal collection.

This procedure highly conforms to the principle of syndrome differentiation and treatment. The precision@k and recall@k are employed as the evaluation metrics which denote the hit ratio of top-k herbs to true herbs and the coverage of true herbs in top-k herbs, respectively. The results are reported in Table 2.

Table 2. Performance of the prescription generation task on LuCa.

Method	p@10	p@20	r@10	r@20
GCN	0.2404	0.2969	0.1222	0.3017
GAT	0.0869	0.0434	0.0438	0.0438
HGT	0.0526	0.0611	0.0299	0.0322
DGI	0.0028	0.0202	0.0013	0.0197
GRACE	0.0485	0.0453	0.0250	0.0453
DMGI	0.0088	0.0368	0.0043	0.0359
HGCL	**0.3227**	**0.3485**	**0.1703**	**0.3372**

As shown in Table 2, our HGCL performs consistently much better than all baselines. For the dmgi, it splits the heterogeneous graph into muti-view network with the help of meta-path, where it loses the intermediate nodes of meta-path and a lot of semantics in it, so it does not perform well.

5.5 Ablation Study

To better understand our proposed HGCL model, we conduct experiments on TCMRel to answer the following two questions. ($Q1$) Is two-level contrastive learning superior to single-level comparative learning? ($Q2$) Can GCN, as an encoder of THIN, capture heterogeneous information? Here, we use HGCL_{ncl} and HGCL_{scl} to denote the ablated model with NCL loss $\mathcal{L}_{nlc}$ or SCL loss $\mathcal{L}_{scl}$ being masked. HGCL_{gat} and HGCL_{hgt} switch to adopting GAT and HGT as the encoder f to learn embeddings respectively.

Table 3. Ablation study on TCMRel dataset.

Method	Macro-F1	Micro-F1
HGCL_{ncl}	0.1111	0.3151
HGCL_{scl}	0.076	0.2877
HGCL_{gat}	0.1189	0.3699
HGCL_{hgt}	0.0222	0.2192
HGCL	**0.1871**	**0.4932**

For $Q1$, comparing HGCL with HGCL_{ncl} and HGCL_{scl}, we can see two-level contrastive learning, that benefits from capturing both local node and global semantic information, clearly contribute the superior performance over two single-level comparative learning. For $Q2$, the results of HGCL_{gat} and HGCL_{hgt} suggest that although GCN is used as encoder, the proposed model well captures the structural and semantic information of the heterogeneity in THIN via NCL and SCL (Table 3).

5.6 Parameters Study

Here we analyze the dimension of the final embedding H. We report herb classification (Macro F1 and Micro F1) on the TCMRel and ChP datasets in Fig. 3. We can find that herb classification performance increases with the growth of d', which shows that the high-dimensional representations successfully learn much semantic information of TCM formula. However, when d' reaches 32, the performance decreases. This may be caused by overfitting or additional redundancies. As $d' = 32$ shows relatively good performance, we set d' as 32 in the experiments.

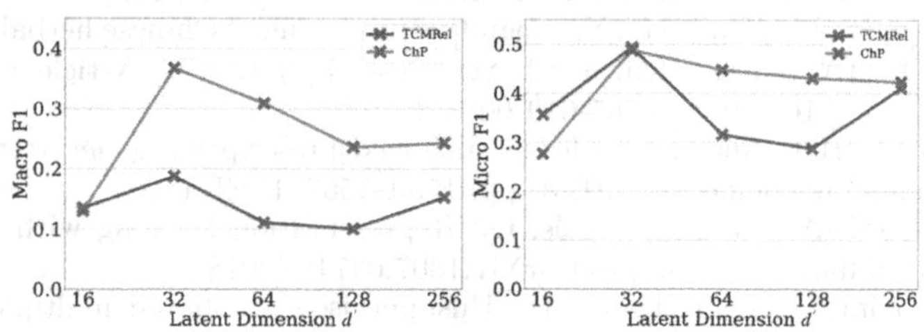

Fig. 3. Performance on various dimension of HGCL.

6 Conclusion

In this paper, we proposed a novel contrastive learning model, HGCL, to generate prescriptions following the philosophy of syndrome differentiation and treatment. For modeling rich semantics and complex relation in TCM literature and clinical prescription, we first model the TCM clinical prescriptions as a THIN, and then corrupt it at both topology and attribute aspect to support node-level contrastive learning. By sampling meta-path instances, we also implement semantic-level contrastive learning on THIN, so as to enhance the quality of node representations for several downstream tasks such as node classification, prescription generation, etc. In experiments, HGCL achieves state-of-the-art results on three real-world datasets in the node classification, similarity search, and prescription generation tasks. The ablation study also demonstrates the rationality of the design of the HGCL's components.

References

1. Chen, T., Kornblith, S., Norouzi, M., Hinton, G.: A simple framework for contrastive learning of visual representations. In: International Conference on Machine Learning, pp. 1597–1607. PMLR (2020)
2. Chen, X., Ruan, C., Zhang, Y., Chen, H.: Heterogeneous information network based clustering for categorizations of traditional Chinese medicine formula. In: BIBM, pp. 839–846. IEEE (2018)
3. Guo, L., Wang, Y.Y.: Study thoughts on complex phenomena in syndrome of Chinese medicine. Chin. J. Basic Med. Tradit. Chin. Med. **10**(2), 3–12 (2004)
4. He, K., Fan, H., Wu, Y., Xie, S., Girshick, R.: Momentum contrast for unsupervised visual representation learning. In: CVPR, pp. 9729–9738 (2020)
5. Hjelm, R.D., et al.: Learning deep representations by mutual information estimation and maximization. arXiv preprint arXiv:1808.06670 (2018)
6. Hu, Z., Dong, Y., Wang, K., Sun, Y.: Heterogeneous graph transformer. In: 2020 Proceedings of The Web Conference, pp. 2704–2710 (2020)
7. Jiang, M., et al.: Syndrome differentiation in modern research of traditional Chinese medicine. J. Ethnopharmacol. **140**(3), 634–642 (2012)
8. Jin, Y., Zhang, W., He, X., Wang, X., Wang, X.: Syndrome-aware herb recommendation with multi-graph convolution network. In: ICDE, pp. 145–156. IEEE (2020)
9. Kipf, T.N., Welling, M.: Semi-supervised classification with graph convolutional networks. In: 5th ICLR (2017). arXiv preprint arXiv:1609.02907
10. Lee, D., Xu, H., Liu, H., Miao, Y.: Cognitive modelling of Chinese herbal medicine's effect on breast cancer. Health Inf. Sci. Syst. **7**(1) (2019). Article number: 20. https://doi.org/10.1007/s13755-019-0083-3
11. Li, C., et al.: Herb-know: knowledge enhanced prescription generation for traditional Chinese medicine. In: BIBM, pp. 1560–1567. IEEE (2020)
12. van den Oord, A., Li, Y., Vinyals, O.: Representation learning with contrastive predictive coding. arXiv preprint arXiv:1807.03748 (2018)
13. Park, C., Kim, D., Han, J., Yu, H.: Unsupervised attributed multiplex network embedding. In: AAAI, vol. 34, pp. 5371–5378 (2020)
14. Ruan, C., Ma, J., Wang, Y., Zhang, Y., Yang, Y., Kraus, S.: Discovering regularities from traditional Chinese medicine prescriptions via bipartite embedding model. In: IJCAI, pp. 3346–3352 (2019)
15. Ruan, C., Wang, Y., Zhang, Y., Yang, Y.: Exploring regularity in traditional Chinese medicine clinical data using heterogeneous weighted networks embedding. In: Li, G., Yang, J., Gama, J., Natwichai, J., Tong, Y. (eds.) DASFAA 2019. LNCS, vol. 11448, pp. 310–313. Springer, Cham (2019). https://doi.org/10.1007/978-3-030-18590-9_35

16. Shi, C., Li, Y., Zhang, J., Sun, Y., Philip, S.Y.: A survey of heterogeneous information network analysis. IEEE Trans. Knowl. Data Eng. **29**(1), 17–37 (2016)
17. Sun, F.Y., Hoffmann, J., Verma, V., Tang, J.: InfoGraph: unsupervised and semi-supervised graph-level representation learning via mutual information maximization. arXiv preprint arXiv:1908.01000 (2019)
18. Vaswani, A., et al.: Attention is all you need. In: NeurIPS, pp. 5998–6008 (2017)
19. Veličković, P., Cucurull, G., Casanova, A., Romero, A., Lio, P., Bengio, Y.: Graph attention networks. arXiv preprint arXiv:1710.10903 (2017)
20. Velickovic, P., Fedus, W., Hamilton, W.L., Liò, P., Bengio, Y., Hjelm, R.D.: Deep graph infomax. In: ICLR (Poster) (2019)
21. Wan, H., et al.: Extracting relations from traditional Chinese medicine literature via heterogeneous entity networks. JAMIA **23**(2), 356–365 (2016)
22. Wang, T., Isola, P.: Understanding contrastive representation learning through alignment and uniformity on the hypersphere. In: ICML, pp. 9929–9939. PMLR (2020)
23. Wang, Z., Poon, J., Poon, S.: TCM translator: a sequence generation approach for prescribing herbal medicines. In: BIBM, pp. 2474–2480. IEEE (2019)
24. Wu, Y., et al.: A hybrid-scales graph contrastive learning framework for discovering regularities in traditional Chinese medicine formula. In: BIBM, pp. 1104–1111 (2021)
25. Wu, Z., et al.: Unsupervised feature learning via non-parametric instance discrimination. In: Proceedings of the IEEE Conference on Computer Vision and Pattern Recognition, pp. 3733–3742 (2018)
26. Yao, L., et al.: Discovering treatment pattern in traditional Chinese medicine clinical cases by exploiting supervised topic model and domain knowledge. J. Biomed. Inform. **58**, 260–267 (2015)
27. Yao, L., Zhang, Y., Wei, B., Zhang, W., Jin, Z.: A topic modeling approach for traditional Chinese medicine prescriptions. IEEE Trans. Knowl. Data Eng. **30**(6), 1007–1021 (2018)
28. Zhu, Y., Xu, Y., Liu, Q., Wu, S.: An empirical study of graph contrastive learning (2021). https://doi.org/10.48550/ARXIV.2109.01116, arXiv:2109.01116
29. Zhu, Y., Xu, Y., Yu, F., Liu, Q., Wu, S., Wang, L.: Deep graph contrastive representation learning. arXiv preprint arXiv:2006.04131 (2020)

Fractional Fourier Transform Aided Computerized Framework for Alcoholism Identification in EEG

Muhammad Tariq Sadiq[1(✉)], Hesam Akbari[2], Siuly Siuly[3], Yan Li[4], and Paul Wen[5]

[1] School of Architecture, Technology and Engineering, University of Brighton, Brighton BN2 4AT, UK
tariq_ee@hotmail.com
[2] Department of Biomedical Engineering, Islamic Azad University, 1584715414 Tehran, Iran
st_h.akbari@azad.ac.ir
[3] Institute for Sustainable Industries & Liveable Cities, Victoria University, Melbourne, VIC 3011, Australia
siuly.siuly@vu.edu.au
[4] School of Mathematics Physics and Computing, University of Southern Queensland, Toowoomba Campus, Toowoomba 4350, Australia
Yan.Li@usq.edu.au
[5] School of Engineering, University of Southern Queensland, Toowoomba Campus, Toowoomba 4350, Australia
Paul.Wen@usq.edu.au

Abstract. Alcoholism has a detrimental impact on brain functioning. Electroencephalogram (EEG) signals are commonly used by clinicians and researchers to quantify and document alcoholic brain activity. Despite widespread attention in these signals, the non-stationarity of physiological EEG signals has complications in alcoholism applications. Fourier Transform have been used to examine stationary signals in a straightforward manner. Non-stationary signal analysis, on the other hand, is unsatisfactory using such an approach because it cannot show the occurrence time of distinct frequency components. Furthermore, it is critical to capture both time and frequency characteristics. To overcome these aforementioned issues in alcoholism EEG signals, a computer-aided diagnosis (CAD) approach is proposed in this study to distinguish between normal and alcoholic subjects. The dataset is first split into multiple EEG signals, and the multiscale principal component analysis approach is used to remove noises. Second, as a novel and powerful feature extraction method for EEG signals, the Fractional Fourier Transform (FrFT) methodology with different coefficients is used. A generalization of the classical Fourier Transform, the FrFT, may reveal the fluctuating frequencies of non-stationary EEG signals. The t-test method is used to evaluate the FrFT derived coefficients as features. Finally, to categorize normal vs alcoholic signals, relevant features are tested on multiple machine learning classifiers accessible in the WEKA platform using a

A. Traina et al. (Eds.): HIS 2022, LNCS 13705, pp. 100–112, 2022.
https://doi.org/10.1007/978-3-031-20627-6_10

10-fold cross-validation technique. The obtained results effectively support the usefulness of FrFT coefficients as features.

Keywords: Electroencephalography · Computer-aided diagnosis · Alcoholism · Fractional Fourier Transform · Non-stationary · Classification

1 Introduction

Alcoholism is likely the most publicly acknowledged mental illness regarding widespread heinousness and fatality [1]. According to a World Health Organization (WHO) estimate from 2014, alcohol use accounts for about 3.3 million (5.9 percent) of total fatalities [2], making it the fifth major cause of mortality [3] and the leading risk factor for precipitate death and disability [4]. Alcoholism has a wide range of health effects on wellness, such as lung and kidney diseases, psychological disorders, some cancerous pustules, etcetera. Similarly, alcohol excess contributes to a variety of vandalism, including violent offences, car accidents, social troubles, and familial collapse [5,25]. Alcoholics experience a variety of mental problems, including neurocognitive deficits, difficulties with motor movements, and long-term behavioral changes that include restlessness and depression [6,7].

The electroencephalogram (EEG) is a vital diagnostic practice for assessing neurological events, competencies, and difficulties. EEG signals are measured electrical potential caused by the neuronal activity in various brain areas [8,27,44]. These captured EEG signals are quite complex in composition and add a plethora of information to consider. Visual evaluation is usually used by skilled doctors to determine changes in EEG signals between healthy or alcoholic people. Nevertheless, sometimes competent clinicians fail to perceive variations in signals ascribed to the effects of interference [9,45,46]. As a result of the increased need for adequate analysis and treatment of neurological irregularities, the rationale for this research is to foster an organized investigation framework for the accurate assessment of alcoholism. It can help to receive timely alerts of impending illnesses [26].

There are time-reliant, frequency-reliant, non-linear attributes, Auto-regressive (AR), and time-frequency techniques [22,23] reported in the literature for automatic detection of alcoholic and normal EEG signals. Since non-stationary EEG signals exhibit dynamic features, neither time nor spectral analysis approaches are acceptable for investigation; hence, time-frequency investigation is essential. AR and fast Fourier transform (FFT) strategies were used in literature to quantify power distribution of EEG signals for categorization [13]. Study [13] proposes an automated method that combines an AR model, a fuzzy-based adjustable methodology, and dimension reduction technique.

In articles [10–12] to discriminate normal and alcoholic EEG patterns, numerous non-linear characteristics like as approximate entropy (ApEn), largest Lyapunov exponent (LLE), sample entropy (SampEn), correlation dimension (CD),

Hurst exponent (H), and higher order spectral features are used. Time-frequency methods are implemented in studies [15] for discriminating between normal and alcoholic EEG data. In research [16] a spectral entropy-based method is implemented, suggesting the applicability of the gamma region to retrieve crucial results about alcoholism. Furthermore, a graph-based technique with non-linear features for identifying alcoholic subjects' signals was proposed. Although the substantial research in the area of alcoholism EEG, there is still a need to design a reliable automated system with a limited set of parameters that can deliver accurate recognition accuracy across a range of performance metrics.

A reliable computer-aided diagnosis approach is presented in the research design, according to the mentioned challenges, and it makes use of just one feature to produce high categorization results for various performance indicators. Most researchers in the area of alcoholism EEG focuses solely on classification accuracy and uses a number of different features to characterize EEG signals [34,35]. In the suggested computerised system, we first segment the EEG data for each group into a number of segments with an appropriate time frame, and then we use the Multiscale principal component analysis (MSPCA) technique to eliminate artifacts out of each segment. Every segment is treated as a separate signal. In order to investigate the nonlinearity and non-stationarity of the EEG signals, we implemented the fractional Fourier transform (FrFT) on each individual EEG signal. Thirdly, we use the absolute, angle, real, and imaginary components of the FrFT coefficients as features to aid in decision-making. Last but not least, k-nearest neighbour (KNN), k star, bagging, and random forest are handed the statistically important characteristics as input. The accuracy, sensitivity, specificity, precision, F-measure, area under the receiver operating curve (AUC), and Matthew's correlation coefficient (MCC) are some of the quality metrics used to validate the results from these classifiers.

2 Materials

The EEG alcoholism dataset was collected from the brains of alcoholic and non-alcoholic patients. This dataset is freely accessible for academic purposes at [21]. This dataset contains the 64 sensors recoding on the patients' scalps. The sensor locations corresponded to typical locations (American Electroencephalographic Association 1990). The frequency of the captured EEG signal being examined 256 Hz. There are two types of respondents: regular EEG and alcoholic EEG. There are 122 participants in the 2 groups, with each participant completing 120 preliminary exams. They divide EEG data into 32s. EEG record files are classified into three types: tiny sets, large data archives, and full records. The small database collection is used for experimentation reasons in this study [19, 20]. Figure 1 shows the visual representation of alcoholic and control EEG signal.

3 Methods

In this study, a Fractional Fourier Transform-based strategy for classifying normal and alcoholic EEG signals is introduced. The envisaged new framework

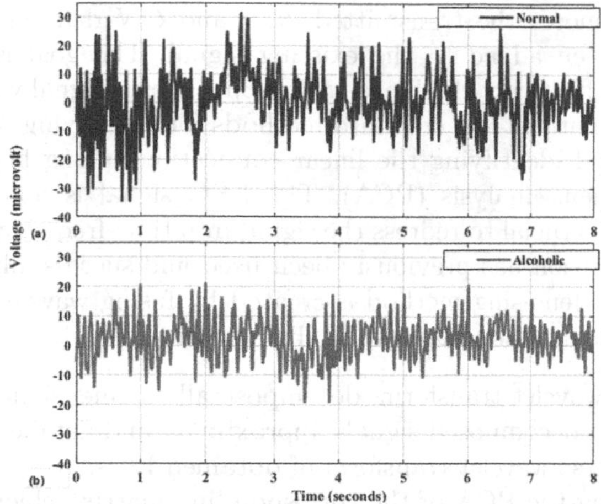

Fig. 1. Visual representation of alcoholic and control EEG signals

entire process is broken down into the following modules: pre-processing, fractional Fourier Transform as feature extraction, and classification, which is shown in Fig. 2. The above-noted components are explored further below.

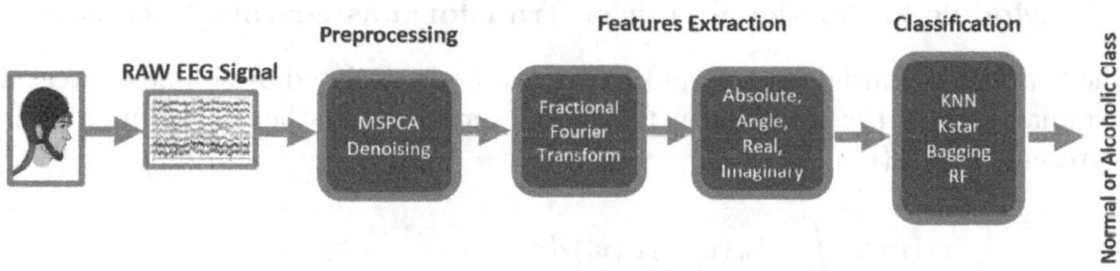

Fig. 2. Block diagram of the proposed Strategy

3.1 Module 1: Pre-processing

The dataset includes the recorded EEG signals 256 Hz sampling rate and 12-bit resolution for 32 s (about 16400 samples). In this study investigations are done utilizing smaller data sets where the baseline filter effectively removes artifacts such as blinking and muscle movements (>73.3 microv). The huge EEG recordings are divided into an eight-second window comprising 4 equal sections of 2048 samples for further investigation.

Any EEG signal acquired from the scalp of the subject is flimsy, vulnerable, and susceptible to a variety of interferences, including structured noise, electrical noise, eye movements signal noise, EMG noise, and others. This interference can be mathematical terms expressed in the form:

$$Q = Q_{EEG} + Q_N \tag{1}$$

where $QEEG$ denotes the transmitted data and QN denotes the artefact of noise that has been added to the existing signal. The goal is to simulate a scheme that can effectively eliminate noise from the raw signal without changing the $QEEG$ information. The standard methods for identifying correlated pieces of information and identifying the linear connection among both categories is principal component analysis (PCA). The EEG signal is non-stationary and non-linear, so it is crucial to redress the signal into time-frequency wavelets. The wavelet decomposition has previously been used and successfully demonstrated for this intent. A denoising method is created by fusing wavelet transform and PCA. The algorithm is summarised by the foregoing: [?]:

1. By executing wavelet transform, decompose all channel signals into n levels.
2. Apply PCA on decomposed signals approximate and detailed matrices.
3. Carry the inverse wavelet transform of obtained PC's.
4. Consider taking the PCA of the corresponding matrix achieved in the prior phase to yield a smoothed EEG signal sequence. Only a few PC's were chosen in the established system, in accordance with the Kaiser rule, for whom the eigenvalues were higher than the corresponding of all individual eigenvalues. Then, 5 levels of wavelets were chosen after numerous experiments. The detail and approximation signals were delivered by the Sym4 wavelet, and this function was selected empirical evidence.

3.2 Module 2: Fractional Fourier Transform as Feature Extraction

The Fractional Fourier Transform (FrFT) can be formulated by simplest integral formulation with the aid of linear transform kernel. Its mathematical function is represented as $e_b(v)$:

$$\begin{aligned} e_b(v) &\equiv \int_{-\infty}^{\infty} k_b\left(v, v'\right) e\left(v'\right) dv' \\ k_b\left(v, v'\right) &\equiv B_\beta \exp\left[i\pi\left(\cot\beta v^2 - 2csc\beta vv' + \cot\beta v'^2\right)\right] \\ B_\beta &\equiv \sqrt{1 - j\cot\beta}, \beta \equiv \frac{b\pi}{2} \end{aligned} \tag{2}$$

where in the aforementioned mathematical formulas, $kbleft(v, vprimeright)$ is the symmetric kernel and b is the amount of substitutions on the integrand $0leq|b|leq2$. The kernel has the following definition while $betaneq2pi$:

$$k_b\left(v, v'\right) = \sqrt{\frac{1 - j\cot\beta}{2}} \times e^{i\left(\frac{v^2}{2}\right)\cot\beta} e^{i\left(\frac{v'^2}{2}\right) - \cot\beta - ivv'\csc(\beta)} \tag{3}$$

The kernel has form $\delta\left(v - v'\right)$ when $\beta = 2n\pi$. On contrary, the kernel is $\delta\left(v + v'\right)$ while $\beta + \pi = 2n\pi$.

Despite the fact that the FrFT is a sequential canonical transmogrify, it also meets the commutative possessions and other characteristics of linear canonical transitions. According to the commutative criterion, $\left(e_{\beta1}e_{\beta2}\right)e_{\beta3} = e_{\beta1}\left(e_{\beta2}e_{\beta3}\right)$

[20]. Focusing on the commutative possessions and the inverse assets, it can be inferred that the inverse $(e_\beta)^{-1}$ of the β th order FrFT operator e_β is simply equal to the operator $f_{-\beta}$. In particular, the kernel of the inverse transform procured by substituting β with $-\beta$[20] demonstrates that FrFT is linear:

$$k_\beta^{-1}(v, v') = k_{-\beta}(v, v') = k_\beta^*(v, v') = k_\beta^*(v', v) = k_\beta^H(v, v')$$

After implementation of FrFT, its coefficients real, absolute, phase and imaginary components are considered as features and provide as an input to different classifiers.

3.3 Module 3: Classification

To segregate normal and alcoholic EEG signal features, we employed KNN, Kstar, Bagging and RF classifiers [28,29].

4 Results and Discussions

Table 1 tabulates the statistical power of features extracted from all trials (tr #). The probability (P) scores for all features are also very minimal, implying that the features are statistically significant. The envisaged framework's performance is measured using the performance indicators listed below [32,33]:

- Accuracy (ACC): Guesstimate tag to total tag percentage.
- True Positive Rate (TPR): The ability to precisely identify EEG signals caused by alcohol.
- True Negative Rate (TNR): The capacity to precisely recognise traditional EEG signals.
- Precision: The similarity of regular and alcoholic EEG signals.
- F-measure: A single number value estimate to investigate the sensitivity/precision trade-off.
- Matthews correlation coefficient (MCC): To evaluate the effectiveness of the categorization of regular and alcoholic EEG, true positive, true negative, false positive, and false negative are taken into account.
- Area Under the Receiver Operating Curve (AUC): AUC calculates a ranging between 0 and 1, with an amount close to 1 implying the validity of a classification model for recognising normal and alcoholic disoriented EEG signals.

The accuracy, TPR, TNR precision, and F-measure classification performance measures are displayed in Fig. 3. These findings pertain to features like the absolute, angle, real, and imaginary FrFT component parts. The conceptual approach produces benchmark scores for the KNN classifier's TPR, TNR, precision, and F-measure performance assessment. Angle, real, and imaginary FrFT coefficient attributes have recognition rate outcomes of 99.5%, 98.9%,

Table 1. Probability values of features

Trial #	P-value	Trial #	P-value	Trial #	P-value	Trial #	P-value
tr1	3.98E−25	tr31	1.28E−18	tr61	7.45E−39	tr91	2.21E−07
tr2	5.49E−18	tr32	4.61E−63	tr62	8.68E−93	tr92	5.03E−34
tr3	3.86E−36	tr33	4.08E−39	tr63	2.89E−134	tr93	8.29E−25
tr4	0.013157	tr34	6.70E−113	tr64	8.32E−35	tr94	3.14E−24
tr5	6.24E−77	tr35	1.89E−12	tr65	8.27E−07	tr95	1.70E−09
tr6	3.95E−49	tr36	1.15E−57	tr66	1.59E−11	tr96	3.71E−54
tr7	1.30E−64	tr37	1.13E−88	tr67	1.20E−18	tr97	1.75E−25
tr8	1.71E−36	tr38	0.20405	tr68	1.58E−09	tr98	1.36E−76
tr9	0.13081	tr39	0.71745	tr69	3.37E−34	tr99	4.31E−81
tr10	0.059152	tr40	1.06E−13	tr70	7.76E−102	tr100	3.44E−27
tr11	2.74E−61	tr41	9.38E−106	tr71	3.29E−46	tr101	7.56E−58
tr12	0.01719	tr42	2.66E−11	tr72	1.07E−27	tr102	7.57E−22
tr13	2.69E−34	tr43	4.75E−13	tr73	4.34E−95	tr103	1.47E−23
tr14	9.35E−08	tr44	0.0071636	tr74	5.61E−155	tr104	2.28E−63
tr15	0.33178	tr45	6.43E−22	tr75	1.89E−296	tr105	3.89E−68
tr16	6.26E−128	tr46	2.45E−58	tr76	1.40E−20	tr106	4.27E−41
tr17	1.05E−146	tr47	5.27E−62	tr77	3.91E−15	tr107	5.50E−07
tr18	1.22E−169	tr48	2.07E−126	tr78	2.56E−09	tr108	1.61E−20
tr19	2.68E−18	tr49	1.85E−34	tr79	5.57E−42	tr109	5.24E−262
tr20	1.56E−27	tr50	0.0070234	tr80	4.66E−13	tr110	7.24E−12
tr21	1.21E−62	tr51	4.47E−57	tr81	3.30E−09	tr111	6.36E−293
tr22	4.23E−66	tr52	5.29E−66	tr82	0.00029872	tr112	1.61E−203
tr23	1.31E−81	tr53	1.79E−33	tr83	0.88439	tr113	1.47E−128
tr24	9.23E−74	tr54	2.57E−73	tr84	1.08E−30	tr114	1.71E−101
tr25	1.89E−99	tr55	4.77E−14	tr85	0.39012	tr115	1.60E−135
tr26	3.69E−63	tr56	4.70E−90	tr86	1.64E−18	tr116	3.02E−47
tr27	8.16E−08	tr57	2.78E−126	tr87	0.10448	tr117	5.71E−36
tr28	1.77E−63	tr58	2.06E−42	tr88	1.76E−20	tr118	2.32E−48
tr29	0.011677	tr59	6.54E−114	tr89	0.0010761	tr119	6.13E−43
tr30	3.79E−41	tr60	1.52E−20	tr90	2.11E−09	tr120	8.02E−30

and 98.8%, respectively, and are ranked second, third, and last. It is important to note that the presented computerized guideline is nearly uniform because it can identify the normal and the alcoholic category with a detection rate variations of less than 1% only.

The MCC and AUC results provided by all features are shown in Fig. 4. As shown in Fig. 4 the absolute features received a value of 1 for both MCC

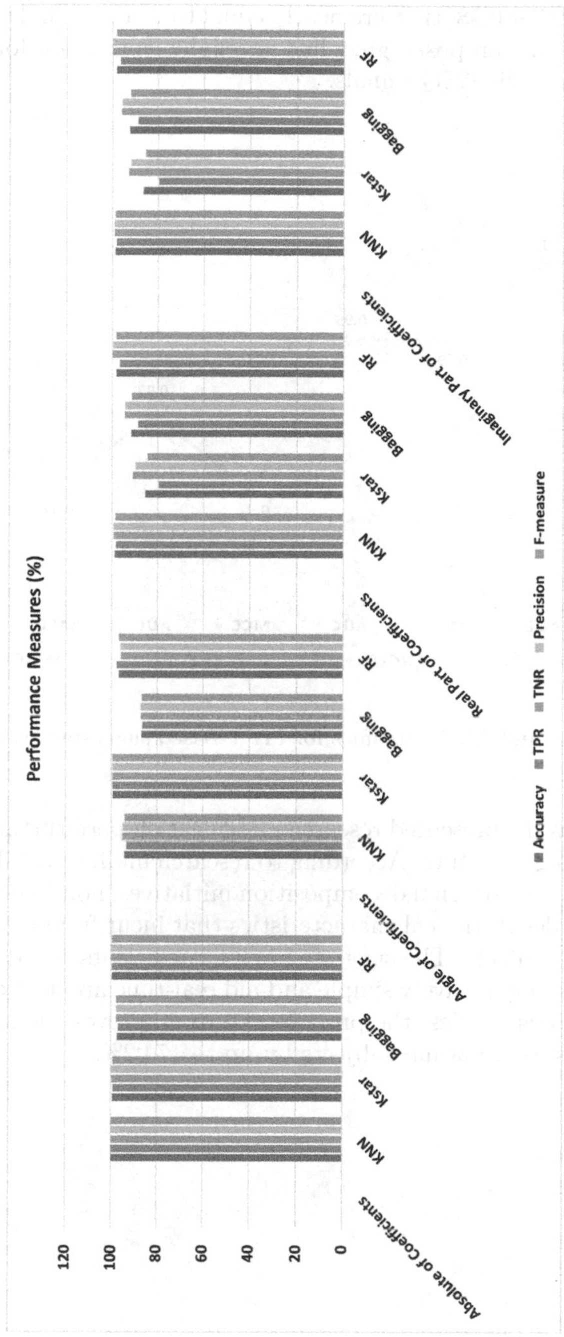

Fig. 3. Classification results obtained with proposed computerized framework

and AUC, indicating that it produces reliable results. Additionally, angle features contribute to the 0.99 value. Contrarily, real and imaginary functionalities produce values of 0.97 or 0.98, that are nearly equal to 1. These findings straightforwardly show that the proposed guideline is reliable and useful for classifying both normal and alcoholic EEG signals.

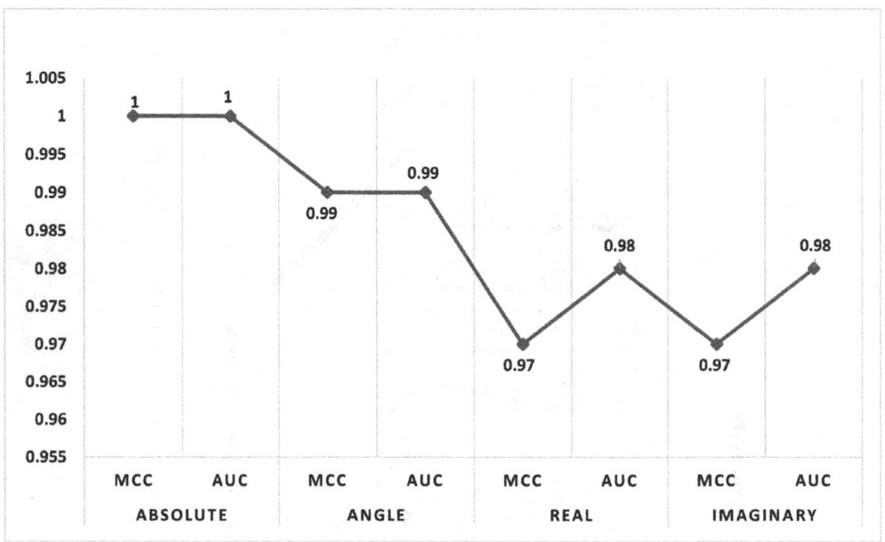

Fig. 4. MCC and AUC outcomes for FrFT-based suggested system

Table 2 compares the presented research classification performance outcomes towards other existing literature. According to research findings [12,36–43], all of these studies are related to signal decomposition initiatives, non-linear characteristics, and higher-order statistical characteristics that incur from mode mingling difficulty, and noise artifacts. The suggested FrFT coefficients-based features, on the other hand, are comparatively simple and aid real-time applications. In comparison to the previous studies, the proposed study improves the identification of alcoholic patients from normal subjects by up to 17.02%.

Table 2. Equating the conceptual methodology to previous works

Ref.	Author, Year	Method, Feature	FS	CV	Classifier	ACC (%)	SEN (%)	SPE (%)
[36]	Zhong and Ghosh (2002)	HMMs and Coupled HMMs	Not used	10-fold	NN	82.98	–	–
[12]	Acharya, Sree et al. (2012)	LLE, ApEn, SamEn and HOS Features	*p*-value	3-fold	SVM	91.7	90	93.33
[39]	Faust, Yu et al. (2013)	WPT, HOS	*p*-value	10-fold	KNN	95.8	95.8	95.8
[38]	Upadhyay, Padhy, et al. (2014)	CWT, Statistical Features	Not used	10-fold	SVM	94.29	–	–
[40]	Patidar, Pachori et al. (2017)	TQWT, Center Correntropy	PCA	10-fold	LS-SVM	97.02	96.53	97.5
[37]	Bae, Yoo et al. (2017)	Granger Causality	Not used	5-fold	SVM	90	95.3	82.4
[42]	Sharma, Sharma et al. (2018)	DTCWT, Two Entropies	*p*-value	10-fold	SVM	97.91	–	–
[41]	Sharma, Deb et al. (2018)	TBOWFB, Log-Energy Entropy	*p*-value	10-fold	LS-SVM	97.08	97.08	97.08
[43]	Mumtaz, Kamel et al. (2018)	Synchronization Likelihood	ROC	10-fold	SVM	98	99.9	95
This work	Sadiq et al. (2022)	Absolute of FrFT	Not used	10-fold	KNN	100	100	100

5 Conclusion

In the current study, a computerised method for classifying normal and alcoholic subjects is being developed. The developed scheme can segment, remove noise using a multivariate policy, use a strategy for heavily nonlinear time series signals, extract features, and classify data. Classification methods use fractional FT coefficient values as features to classify. The results indicate that using absolute FrFT coefficients as features provides benchmark classification accuracy results that outperform the state-of-the-art.

References

1. Enoch, M.-A., Goldman, D.: Problem drinking and alcoholism: diagnosis and treatment. Am. Fam. Physician **65**(3), 441 (2002)
2. World Health Organization: Global status report on alcohol and health 2018 (2019)
3. Lim, S.S., et al.: A comparative risk assessment of burden of disease and injury attributable to 67 risk factors and risk factor clusters in 21 regions, 1990–2010: a systematic analysis for the global burden of disease study 2010. Lancet **380**(9859), 2224–2260 (2012)
4. Rehm, J., et al.: Alcohol as a risk factor for global burden of disease. Eur. Addict. Res. **9**(4), 157–164 (2003)
5. MCOD Strategy: National drug strategy (2006)
6. Harper, C.: The neurotoxicity of alcohol. Hum. Exp. Toxicol. **26**(3), 251–257 (2007)
7. Brust, J.: Ethanol and cognition: indirect effects, neurotoxicity and neuroprotection: a review. Int. J. Environ. Res. Public Health **7**(4), 1540–1557 (2010)

8. Siuly, Li, Y., Wen, P.: EEG signal classification based on simple random sampling technique with least square support vector machine. Int. J. Biomed. Eng. Technol. **7**(4), 390–409 (2011)
9. Acharya, U.R., Bhat, S., Adeli, H., Adeli, A., et al.: Computer-aided diagnosis of alcoholism-related EEG signals. Epilepsy Behav. **41**, 257–263 (2014)
10. Ehlers, C., Havstad, J.: Characterization of drug effects on the EEG by power spectral band time series analysis. Psychopharmacol. Bull. **18**(3), 43–47 (1982)
11. Kannathal, N., Acharya, U.R., Lim, C.M., Sadasivan, P.: Characterization of EEG–a comparative study. Comput. Methods Programs Biomed. **80**(1), 17–23 (2005)
12. Acharya, U.R., Sree, S.V., Chattopadhyay, S., Suri, J.S.: Automated diagnosis of normal and alcoholic EEG signals. Int. J. Neural Syst. **22**(03), 1250011 (2012)
13. Faust, O., Acharya, R., Allen, A.R., Lin, C.: Analysis of EEG signals during epileptic and alcoholic states using AR modeling techniques. Irbm **29**(1), 44–52 (2008)
14. Yazdani, A., Ataee, P., Setarehdan, S.K., Araabi, B.N., Lucas, C.: Neural, fuzzy and neurofuzzy approach to classification of normal and alcoholic electroencephalograms. In: 2007 5th International Symposium on Image and Signal Processing and Analysis, pp. 102–106. IEEE (2007)
15. Sun, Y., Ye, N., Xu, X.: EEG analysis of alcoholics and controls based on feature extraction. In: 2006 8th International Conference on Signal Processing, vol. 1. IEEE (2006)
16. Akbari, H., Ghofrani, S., Zakalvand, P., Sadiq, M.T.: Schizophrenia recognition based on the phase space dynamic of EEG signals and graphical features. Biomed. Signal Process. Control **69**, 102917 (2021)
17. Snodgrass, J.G., Vanderwart, M.: A standardized set of 260 pictures: norms for name agreement, image agreement, familiarity, and visual complexity. J. Exp. Psychol. Hum. Learn. Mem. **6**(2), 174 (1980)
18. Acharya, J.N., Hani, A.J., Cheek, J., Thirumala, P., Tsuchida, T.N.: American clinical neurophysiology society guideline 2: guidelines for standard electrode position nomenclature. Neurodiagn. J. **56**(4), 245–252 (2016)
19. Asif, R.M., et al.: Design and analysis of robust fuzzy logic maximum power point tracking based isolated photovoltaic energy system. Eng. Rep. **2**(9), e12234 (2020)
20. Sadiq, M.T., Akbari, H., Siuly, S., Li, Y., Wen, P.: Alcoholic EEG signals recognition based on phase space dynamic and geometrical features. Chaos Solit. Fractals **158**, 112036 (2022)
21. Sadiq, M.T., Siuly, S., Ur Rehman, A., Wang, H.: Auto-correlation based feature extraction approach for EEG alcoholism identification. In: Siuly, S., Wang, H., Chen, L., Guo, Y., Xing, C. (eds.) HIS 2021. LNCS, vol. 13079, pp. 47–58. Springer, Cham (2021). https://doi.org/10.1007/978-3-030-90885-0_5
22. Sadiq, M.T., et al.: Motor imagery BCI classification based on multivariate variational mode decomposition. In: IEEE Transactions on Emerging Topics in Computational Intelligence, pp. 1–13 (2022)
23. Yu, X., Aziz, M.Z., Sadiq, M.T., Jia, K., Fan, Z., Xiao, G.: Computerized multidomain EEG classification system: a new paradigm. IEEE J. Biomed. Health Inform. (2022)
24. Semmlow, J.: Signals and Systems for Bioengineers: A MATLAB-Based Introduction, Academic Press (2011)
25. Akbari, H., et al.: Depression recognition based on the reconstruction of phase space of EEG signals and geometrical features. Appl. Acoust. **179**, 108078 (2021)
26. Hussain, W., Sadiq, M.T., Siuly, S., Rehman, A.U.: Epileptic seizure detection using 1 D-convolutional long short-term memory neural networks. Appl. Acoust. **177**, 107941 (2021)

27. Akbari, H., Sadiq, M.T., Rehman, A.U.: Classification of normal and depressed EEG signals based on centered correntropy of rhythms in empirical wavelet transform domain. Health Inf. Sci. Syst. **9**(1), 1–15 (2021). https://doi.org/10.1007/s13755-021-00139-7
28. Yu, X., Aziz, M.Z., Sadiq, M.T., Fan, Z., Xiao, G.: A new framework for automatic detection of motor and mental imagery EEG signals for robust BCI systems. IEEE Trans. Instrum. Meas. **70**, 1–12 (2021). https://doi.org/10.1109/TIM.2021.3069026
29. Sadiq, M.T., Yu, X., Yuan, Z., Aziz, M.Z., Siuly, S., Ding, W.: A matrix determinant feature extraction approach for decoding motor and mental imagery EEG in subject specific tasks. In: IEEE Transactions on Cognitive and Developmental Systems, p. 1 (2020). https://doi.org/10.1109/TCDS.2020.3040438
30. Akbari, H., Sadiq, M.T.: Detection of focal and non-focal EEG signals using non-linear features derived from empirical wavelet transform rhythms. Phys. Eng. Sci. Med. **44**(1), 157–171 (2021)
31. Fan, Z., Jamil, M., Sadiq, M.T., Huang, X., Yu, X.: Exploiting multiple optimizers with transfer learning techniques for the identification of COVID-19 patients. J. Healthc. Eng. **2020** (2020)
32. Akhter, M.P., Jiangbin, Z., Naqvi, I.R., Abdelmajeed, M., Sadiq, M.T.: Automatic detection of offensive language for Urdu and roman Urdu. IEEE Access **8**, 91213–91226 (2020)
33. Akhter, M.P., Jiangbin, Z., Naqvi, I.R., Abdelmajeed, M., Mehmood, A., Sadiq, M.T.: Document-level text classification using single-layer multisize filters convolutional neural network. IEEE Access **8**, 42689–42707 (2020)
34. Sadiq, M.T., et al.: Motor imagery EEG signals decoding by multivariate empirical wavelet transform-based framework for robust brain-computer interfaces. IEEE Access **7**, 171431–171451 (2019)
35. Sadiq, M.T., et al.: Motor imagery EEG signals classification based on mode amplitude and frequency components using empirical wavelet transform. IEEE Access **7**, 127678–127692 (2019)
36. Zhong, S., Ghosh, J.: HMMs and coupled HMMs for multi-channel EEG classification. In: Proceedings of the 2002 International Joint Conference on Neural Networks. IJCNN 2002 (Cat. No. 02CH37290), vol. 2, pp. 1154–1159. IEEE (2002)
37. Bae, Y., Yoo, B.W., Lee, J.C., Kim, H.C.: Automated network analysis to measure brain effective connectivity estimated from EEG data of patients with alcoholism. Physiol. Meas. **38**(5), 759 (2017)
38. Upadhyay, R., Padhy, P.K., Kankar, P.K.: Alcoholism diagnosis from EEG signals using continuous wavelet transform. In: 2014 Annual IEEE India Conference (INDICON), pp. 1–5. IEEE (2014)
39. Faust, O., Yu, W., Kadri, N.A.: Computer-based identification of normal and alcoholic EEG signals using wavelet packets and energy measures. J. Mech. Med. Biol. **13**(03), 1350033 (2013)
40. Patidar, S., Pachori, R.B., Upadhyay, A., Acharya, U.R.: An integrated alcoholic index using tunable-Q wavelet transform based features extracted from EEG signals for diagnosis of alcoholism. Appl. Soft Comput. **50**, 71–78 (2017)
41. Sharma, M., Deb, D., Acharya, U.R.: A novel three-band orthogonal wavelet filter bank method for an automated identification of alcoholic EEG signals. Appl. Intell. **48**(5), 1368–1378 (2018)
42. Sharma, M., Sharma, P., Pachori, R.B., Acharya, U.R.: Dual-tree complex wavelet transform-based features for automated alcoholism identification. Int. J. Fuzzy Syst. **20**(4), 1297–1308 (2018)

43. Mumtaz, W., Kamel, N., Ali, S.S.A., Malik, A.S., et al.: An EEG-based functional connectivity measure for automatic detection of alcohol use disorder. Artif. Intell. Med. **84**, 79–89 (2018)
44. Sadiq, M.T., Yu, X., Yuan, Z., Aziz, M.Z., Siuly, S., Ding, W.: Toward the development of versatile brain–computer interfaces. IEEE Trans. Artif. Intell. **2**(4), 314–328 (2021). https://doi.org/10.1109/TAI.2021.3097307
45. Khare, S.K., Bajaj, V.: Constrained based tunable q wavelet transform for efficient decomposition of EEG signals. Appl. Acoust. **163**, 107234 (2020)
46. Sadiq, M.T., et al.: Exploiting feature selection and neural network techniques for identification of focal and nonfocal EEG signals in TQWT domain. J. Healthc. Eng. **2021**, 24 (2021)

Learning Optimal Treatment Strategies for Sepsis Using Offline Reinforcement Learning in Continuous Space

Zeyu Wang[1](✉), Huiying Zhao[2](✉), Peng Ren[3], Yuxi Zhou[3], and Ming Sheng[3]

[1] Beijing Institute of Technology, Beijing 100081, China
wangzeyu@bit.edu.cn

[2] Peking University People's Hosipital, Beijing 100044, China
zhaohuiying109@sina.com

[3] BNRist, DCST, RIIT, Tsinghua University, Beijing 100084, China
{renpeng,yuxi,shengming}@tsinghua.edu.cn

Abstract. Sepsis is a leading cause of death in the ICU. It is a disease requiring complex interventions in a short period of time, but its optimal treatment strategy remains uncertain. Evidence suggests that the practices of currently used treatment strategies are problematic and may cause harm to patients. To address this decision problem, we propose a new medical decision model based on historical data to help clinicians recommend the best reference option for real-time treatment. Our model combines offline reinforcement learning and deep reinforcement learning to solve the problem of traditional reinforcement learning in the medical field due to the inability to interact with the environment, while enabling our model to make decisions in a continuous state-action space. We demonstrate that, on average, the treatments recommended by the model are more valuable and reliable than those recommended by clinicians. In a large validation dataset, we find out that the patients whose actual doses from clinicians matched the decisions made by AI has the lowest mortality rates. Our model provides personalized and clinically interpretable treatment decisions for sepsis to improve patient care.

Keywords: Sepsis · Optimal treatment strategies · Offline reinforcement learning · Continuous spaces

1 Introduction

Sepsis is a severe infection that can result in life-threatening acute organ dysfunction and is known as the leading cause of death in critically ill patients [1]. It affects more than 49 million people around the world each year, killing between one in six and one in three of those affected [2–4]. Early effective resuscitation and haemodynamic management are crucial for the stabilisation of sepsis-induced tissue hypoperfusion in sepsis and septic shock, and they are more important for the prognosis [5,6]. Although the Surviving Sepsis Campaign (SSC) guidelines

A. Traina et al. (Eds.): HIS 2022, LNCS 13705, pp. 113–124, 2022.
https://doi.org/10.1007/978-3-031-20627-6_11

2021 recommend an initial target mean arterial pressure (MAP) of 65 mmHg [5], the following questions are not answered: 1) what is the optimal dose of fluid and how should it be titrated? 2) what is the optimal approach to selection and dose titration for vasopressor therapy? 3) which patients should glucocorticoid therapy be initiated for? To resolve these concerns, it is essential to carry out personalized therapies in real time based on the individual characteristics and status of patients.

In previous study, high-granularity dataset and reinforcement learning approach were adopted to explore the sequential role of the therapy strategy [7,8]. However, its action and state are based on discrete space and there is a lack of more refined guidance for the treatment received by patients. Therefore, in our work, we propose a model to make medical decisions for sepsis patients based on historical data. We model in a continuous state-action space, representing the physiological state of a patient at a point in time as a continuous vector. LSTM mechanism is applied to capture the historical information of treatment received by the patient. In addition, offline deep reinforcement learning methods are used to determine the optimal treatment strategy. Finally, we conduct experiments to demonstrate that the strategy recommended by the model outperforms the clinician's strategy in terms of survival rate and safety rate. Also, we find out that the mortality rate of patients is the lowest when the clinician's treatment strategy is similar to the recommended strategy of the model.

Our contributions are as follows. We have introduced the offline reinforcement learning algorithms to better address the inability to interact with the environment in the medical field. The deep reinforcement learning models with continuous state-action spaces are implemented, and the optimal strategies are learned to improve patient outcomes and reduce patient mortality. We design experiments on the Medical Information Mart for Intensive Care version IV (MIMIC-IV) dataset to validate the model. The results show that the survival and safety rates of sepsis patients are significantly improved. At the same time, the analysis of the results reveals that the current method of drug use can be optimized, which is a guidance for the treatment of sepsis.

2 Related Work

Reinforcement learning approaches have been extensively explored in the treatment of patients with severe sepsis.

In discrete space, the Fitted-Q Iteration algorithm [9] was applied to learn treatment strategies for mechanical ventilation weaning from historical data [10]; Komorowski et al. [7] discretized the state and action space through k-means clustering, and then performed Q-learning [11] to generate the optimal strategy of managing intravenous fluids and vasopressors.

In continuous space, Raghu et al. [12] used Dueling Double-Deep Q Network [13,14] to learn medical treatment policies for sepsis. This approach used a vector representation of continuous states to extend the treatment of sepsis to a continuous space. Sun et al. [15] combined reinforcement learning and supervised learning, with the DDPG method adopted to develop strategies in a continuous value space.

In this work, we also focus on the treatment of sepsis, but aim to develop a model that does not interact with the environment in a continuous state-action space. In turn, it solves the performance problem of reinforcement learning in the medical field that it cannot do the exploration, while optimizing the treatment process. Additionally, more refined medical actions are taken.

3 Preliminaries

3.1 Reinforcement Learning

In reinforcement learning, time series data are often modeled with Markov Decision Processes (MDP) (S, A, p_M, r, γ), with state space S, action space A, and transition dynamics $p_M(s_0|s, a)$. At each discrete time step, the agent performs action a in the state s and arrives at the state s', while the agent receives a reward $r \in R$. The agent selects the action to maximize the expected discounted future reward, known as the return defined as $R_t = \sum_{t'=t}^{T} \gamma^{t'-t} r_{t'}$, where $\gamma \in (0, 1)$, represents the discount factor, capturing the tradeoff between immediate and future rewards and T refers to the terminal timestep. The agent selects action according to a policy $\pi : S \to A$. And each policy π has a Q function $Q^\pi(s, a) = \mathbb{E}_\pi[R_t|s, a]$. For a given policy, the Q function can be computed using the Bellman equation:

$$Q^\pi(s_t, a_t) = \mathbb{E}_{r_t, s_{t+1} \sim E}[r(s_t, a_t) + \gamma \mathbb{E}_{a_{t+1} \sim \pi}[Q^\pi(s_{t+1}, a_{t+1})]] \tag{1}$$

And if the target policy is deterministic, we use the policy directly:

$$Q^\pi(s_t, a_t) = \mathbb{E}_{r_t, s_{t+1} \sim E}[r(s_t, a_t) + \gamma Q^\pi(s_{t+1}, \pi(s_{t+1}))] \tag{2}$$

We consider continuous state-action space model-free RL and use historical data to find a good-quality policy π.

3.2 Extrapolation Error

As for reinforcement learning tasks in the medical field, it has to learn from historical data because of the high cost incurred by the interaction between agent and environment. This may lead to extrapolation errors. We define ϵ_{MDP} as the extrapolation error. This accounts for the difference between the value function $Q^\pi_{\mathcal{B}}$ computed with the history data and the value function Q^π computed with the environment:

$$\epsilon_{MDP}(s, a) = Q^\pi(s, a) - Q^\pi_{\mathcal{B}}(s, a) \tag{3}$$

Such errors will cause an even greater problem in continuous state space and multidimensional action space. Avoiding extrapolation errors plays a critical role in ensuring safe and effective patient care. Fujimoto et al. [16] relied on batch-constrained reinforcement learning to solve this problem well. Additionally, Fujimoto et al. [16] demonstrated that the extrapolation error can be eliminated and that BCQL can converge to the optimal policy on this MDP corresponding to dataset $\mathcal{B}$.

4 Datasets

Our experimental data are obtained from the Multiparametric Intelligent Monitoring in Intensive Care (MIMIC-IV) database. We focus on those patients who met sepsis-3 criteria [1] (6660 in total) within the first 24 h of admission to the hospital. Sepsis is defined as a suspected infection (prescription of antibiotics and sampling of bodily fluids for microbiological culture) combined with the evidence of organ dysfunction, as defined by a SOFA score ≥ 2 within 24 h of admission. In line with previous research, we assume a baseline SOFA of zero for all patients [6,17]. For each patient, we have the relevant physiological parameters, including demographics, comorbidities, vital signs, laboratory values, treatment interventions, intake/output events and 90 day mortality.

Since the first 24 h are extremely critical for the treatment of sepsis, we extract data within 24 h of patient onset. The data are aggregated into 2-hour windows. Besides, when there are several data points in a window, the average or sum (as appropriate) is recorded. This produces a 41×1 feature vector for each patient at each time period, which is the state s_t in the base MDP.

The physiological features used in our model are as follows:
Demographics: gender, age, ethnicity;
Comorbidities: elixhauser premorbid status;
Vital Signs: heart rate, mean arterial pressure (MAP), temperature, respiratory rate, peripheral capillary oxygen saturation (SpO2), glasgow coma scale (GCS);
Lab Values: white blood cell count (WBC), neutrophils, lymphocytes, platelets, hemoglobin, alanine aminotransferase (ALT), aspartate aminotransferase (AST), total bilirubin, blood urea nitrogen (BUN), creatinine, albumin, glucose, potassium, sodium, calcium, chloride, potential of hydrogen (PH), partial pressure of oxygen (PaO2), partial pressure of carbon dioxide (PaCO2), bicarbonate, PaO2/FiO2 ratio, lactate, prothrombin time (PT), activated partial thromboplastin time (APTT);
Organ Function Score: sequential organ failure assessment (SOFA) score;
Output Events: urine volume;
Treatment Interventions: 1) intravenous fluids volume; 2) the maximum dose of vasopressors: norepinephrine, phenylephrine, vasopressin, angiotensinii, epinephrine, dopamine, dobutamine; 3) whether hydrocortisone was used;

5 Model Architecture

Our model architecture consists of four main components: History capture model, Generative model, Perturbation model and Q-networks. By using this model, the offline reinforcement problem of optimal decision-making in continuous stateaction space is effectively solved.

5.1 History Capture Model

The goal of history capture model is to capture the change of states while incorporating the influence of the performed action over time. In the history capture model, the observation-action history is explicitly processed by an LSTM network and fed as input into other networks. For each moment of the patient's state, we use the historical treatment process ($\{o_1, a_1\}, ..., \{o_t, a_{t-1}\}$) as the input of the LSTM for calculation. Also, we will get an embedding representation s_t of the patient's current status by combining historical status and treatment information.

5.2 Generative Model

To avoid extrapolation error, a policy is supposed to induce a similar state-action visitation to the batch. The purpose of generative models as a model of imitative learning is to simulate the treatment strategies of clinicians by observing the state of the patient. By using this method, the model's strategies are distributed over the range of the dataset.

For the generative model, we use a conditional variational auto-encoder (VAE) [18]. The VAE G_ω is defined by two networks, an encoder $E_{\omega 1}(s, a)$ and decoder $D_{\omega 2}(s, z)$, where $\omega = \{\omega 1, \omega 2\}$. The encoder takes a state-action pair and outputs the mean μ and standard deviation σ of a Gaussian distribution $N(\mu, \sigma)$. The state s, along with a latent vector z as sampled from the Gaussian, is passed to the decoder $D_{\omega 2}(s, z)$ which outputs an action. The VAE is trained with respect to the mean squared error of the reconstruction along with a KL regularization term:

$$\mathcal{L}_{VAE} = \sum_{(s,a)\in\mathcal{B}} (D_{\omega 2}(s, z) - a)^2 + D_{KL}(\mathcal{N}(\mu, \sigma)||\mathcal{N}(0, 1)) \tag{4}$$

5.3 Perturbation Model

To enhance the diversity of actions, we introduce a perturbation model $\xi_\phi(s, a, \varphi)$. The perturbation model makes an adjustment based on action a which is generated from the generative model in the range $[-\varphi, \varphi]$. In this way, the output of the model is restricted to the scope of the dataset. This results in the policy π:

$$\pi(s) = \underset{a_i+\xi_\phi(s,a,\varphi)}{argmax} \; Q_\theta(s, a_i + \xi_\phi(s, a, \varphi)), a_i \sim G_\omega(s)_{i=1}^n \tag{5}$$

The perturbation model ξ_ϕ can be trained to maximize the $Q_\theta(s, a)$ through the deterministic policy gradient algorithm by sampling $a \sim G_\omega(s)$:

$$\phi \leftarrow \underset{\phi}{argmax} \sum_{(s,a)\in B} Q_\theta(s, a + \xi_\phi(s, a, \varphi)) \tag{6}$$

The choice of n and φ creates a trade-off between an imitation learning and reinforcement learning algorithm. If $\varphi = 0$ and $n = 1$, the model exhibits the characteristics of imitation learning, which imitates the clinician's strategy. And if φ is unconstrained and $n \to \infty$, the model approaches DDPG (Deep Deterministic Policy Gradient), an algorithm which searches the policy to greedily maximize the value function over the entire action space.

5.4 Q-Networks

Q-network is a method used to evaluate the value of a strategy with a neural network to approximate the value function. Deep Q-Network is an off-policy approach. Instead of using the real action of the next interaction for each learning, the target value function is updated by using the action currently considered to have the highest value. In this way, an overestimation of the Q value can occur. Clipped Double Q-learning estimates the value by taking the minimum between two Q-networks: $Q_{\theta 1}$ and $Q_{\theta 2}$. Also, taking the least operator also penalizes the high variance estimates in the uncertainty region and facilitates the action of strategy selection for the states contained in the dataset. In particular, we take a convex combination of the two values, with a higher weight on the minimum, to form a learning target which is used by both Q-networks:

$$r + \gamma \underset{a_i}{max}[\lambda \underset{j=1,2}{min} Q_{\theta'_j}(s', a) + (1 - \lambda) \underset{j=1,2}{max} Q_{\theta'_j}(s', a)] \quad (7)$$

Here is a summary of the model framework, which maintains four parametrized networks: a generative model $G_\omega(S)$, a perturbation model $\xi_\phi(s, a)$, and two Q-networks $Q_{\theta_1}, Q_{\theta_2}$. In the meantime, each of the perturbation and Q-networks has 1 target network. Similar to the DQN method, the parameters of the target network are updated after a certain period of time.

6 Experiment

This section describes the training details for our models.

6.1 Medical Action Selection

An immediate action for resolving hypotension should be taken as quickly as possible for those sepsis patients with hypoperfusion. Fluid resuscitation and vasopressor management are essential for the treatment of hypotension and hypoperfusion. Norepinephrine and vasopressin are the first-line and second-line vasopressor, respectively. Inotropes such as dobutamine and norepinephrine are recommended to the patients with septic shock and cardiac dysfunction with persistent hypoperfusion. Glucocorticoids (first choice is hydrocortisone) are also recommended for refractory septic shock. Therefore, in the experiment, for the choice of medical behaviors, we divide them into three parts of refinement. The first part is the fluid input for patients every two hours. The second part is the use of antihypertensive drugs, in which we classify norepinephrine and phenylephrine as the first type of vasopressors, vasopressin and angiotensin II as the second type of vasopressors, and epinephrine, dopamine and dobutamine as the third type of vasopressors, according to pharmacological characteristics. In turn, we optimize the three classes of antihypertensive drugs. The third part is the use of hydrocortisone, which is a discrete type of decision-making behavior. The above three parts are most critical to the treatment of sepsis and are of great importance to clinical application (Table 1).

Table 1. The selection of medical actions

Action	Content	Unit	Type[a]
liquid	Intravenous fluids	milliliter/2h	Continuous
vasopressor_1	Norepinephrine, phenylephrine	microgramme/kg.min	Continuous
vasopressor_2	Vasopressin, angiotensinii	U/min	continuous
vasopressor_3	Epinephrine, dopamine, dobutamine	microgramme/kg.min	Continuous
hydrocortisone	Hydrocortisone	–	Discrete

a: Continuous type of action implies that we decide the specific value of the action. Discrete type of action implies that we decide whether to adopt the action or not.

6.2 Reward Function

For the design of the patient reward function, we integrate the intermediate treatment process of the patient with the final outcome. Since our goal is to provide guidance for patients within 24 h after onset, we prefer to improve the change of patients' status within 24 h after onset. Therefore, for the change of patients in status, we consider a combination of two indicators, including the SOFA score and lactate level of patients. For the final outcome of the patient, we use the fact of whether the patient died while in the ICU as the final outcome.

Our reward function for intermediate timesteps is designed as follows:

$$r = C_0\, s_t^{SOFA} + C_1\,(s_{t+1}^{SOFA} - s_t^{SOFA}) + C_2\, tanh(s_{t+1}^{Lactate} - s_{t+1}^{Lactate}) \tag{8}$$

We conduct experiment with multiple parameters and opt to use $C_0 = -0.1$, $C_1 = -1$, $C_2 = -2$

At terminal timesteps, we set a reward of +25 if a patient survived their ICU stay, and a negative reward of −25 otherwise.

6.3 Training Process

For our training process, our pseudocode is shown below. The details about our specific implementation can be found in our project code https://github.com/taihandong-330/BCADRQN.

Algorithm 1. Batch-Constrained Action-specific Deep Recurrent Q-Network

Require: Records buffer $\mathcal{B}$ - observations O, actions A, reward function R;
Parameters - target network update rate τ, mini-batch size N, max perturbation φ, number of sampled actions n, minimum weighting λ, number of epochs M;

Randomly initialize LSTM data processing net L, with parameter ψ
Randomly initialize VAE $G_\omega = \{E_{\omega 1}, D_{\omega 2}\}$, with parameter ω
Randomly initialize main perturbation net ξ_ϕ, with parameter ϕ
Randomly initialize main Crisis net $Q_{\theta_1}, Q_{\theta_2}$, with parameter θ_1, θ_2
Target perturbation net ξ_ϕ: $\phi' \leftarrow \phi$
Target critic net $Q_{\theta_1'}, Q_{\theta_2'}$: $\theta_1' \leftarrow \theta_1, \theta_2' \leftarrow \theta_2$
for $m = 1 \rightarrow M$ **do**:
  Initialize the batch buffer $\mathcal{D}$
  for $i = 1 \rightarrow N$ **do**:
    Initialize the first action $a_0 = \textit{no operation}$
    Randomly select a patient at a time point t, sample a historical treatment episode $\langle(\{o_1, a_0\}, ...\{o_t, a_{t-1}\}, \{o_{t+1}, a_t\}), r_t\rangle$ from $\mathcal{B}$
    Store the historical treatment episode into $\mathcal{D}$
  end for
  $s = L(\{o_1, a_0\}, ...\{o_t, a_{t-1}\}), s' = L(\{o_1, a_0\}, ...\{o_{t+1}, a_t\}), a = a_t, r = t_t$
  $\mu, \sigma = E_{\omega_1}(s, a),\ \tilde{a} = D_{\omega_2}(s, z),\ z \sim \mathcal{N}(\mu, \sigma)$
  $\omega, \psi \leftarrow argmin_{\omega,\psi} \sum (a - \tilde{a})^2 + D_{KL}(\mathcal{N}(\mu, \sigma) || \mathcal{N}(0, 1))$
  Sample n actions:$\{a_i \sim G_\omega(s')\}$
  Perturb each action:$\{a_i = a_i + \xi_\phi(s', a_i, \varphi)\}_{i=1}^n$
  Set value target $y = r + \gamma \underset{a_i}{max}[\lambda \underset{j=1,2}{min} Q_{\theta_j'}(s', a) + (1 - \lambda) \underset{j=1,2}{max} Q_{\theta_j'}(s', a)]$
  $\theta \leftarrow argmin_\theta \sum (y - Q_\theta(s, a))^2$
  $\phi \leftarrow argmax_\phi \sum Q_{\theta_1}(s, a + \xi_\phi(s, a, \varphi)),\ a \sim G_\omega(s)$
  Soft update target networks: $\theta_i' \leftarrow \tau\theta + (1 - \tau)\theta_i'; \phi' \leftarrow \tau\phi + (1 - \tau)\phi'$
end for

7 Results

7.1 Result Analysis

For the results of the model training, we show the distribution of the model's output strategies relative to the clinician's original strategy. Figure 1 shows the difference between the model and the clinician's fluid input and the three classes of vasopressor within 24 h of patient onset.

After analysis we find out that for intravenous fluids, the model's strategy is approximately the same as that of the clinicians. However, the proportion of patients receiving vasopressors is only 10.7% and 11.8% for the first and second two hours after the onset of sepsis, but these would have been 14.1% and 13.7% if the recommendation made by AI Clinician was followed. There are also significant differences in the doses of the three classes of vasopressors. We find out that for the first and second classes of vasopressors, the model tends to select larger dosages. While for the third class of vasopressors, the model tends to select smaller dosages compared to the clinicians. In addition, we analyze the proportion of hydrocortisone use on the test set, discovering that the model use is essentially the same as the use by the clinician.

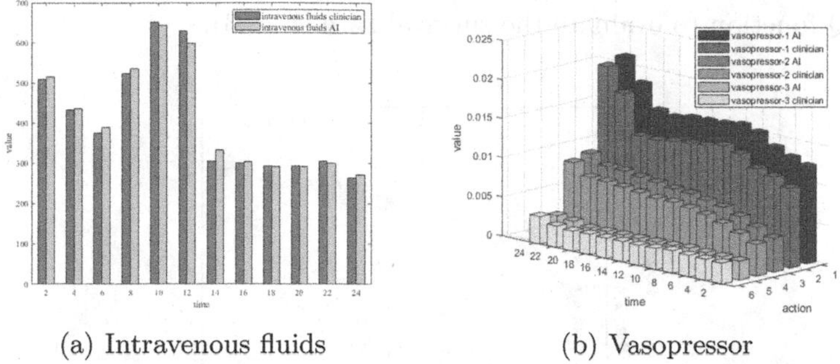

(a) Intravenous fluids (b) Vasopressor

Fig. 1. The distribution of clinicians and AI strategies is shown for every two hours. The value of the strategy represents the average measure of all patients at the corresponding moment in time.

We further analyze the change in patient mortality when there is a difference between the clinician's decisions and those of the model. We find out that, for the most part, patient mortality is lower when the clinician's strategy differs from the model's strategy insignificantly. Also, when the difference between the two is too large, the mortality rate of patients tends to increase substantially. This also demonstrates the validity of our model (Fig. 2).

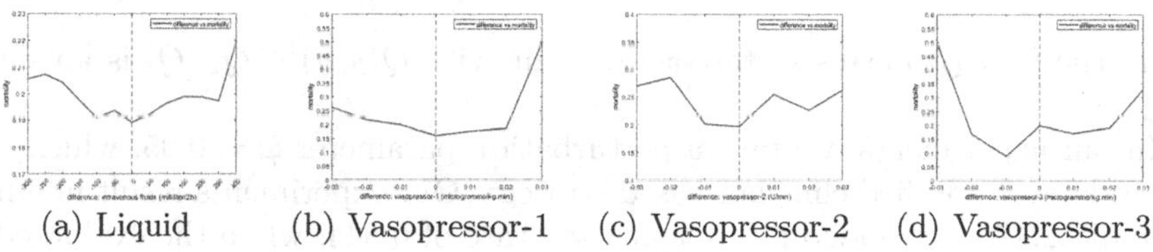

(a) Liquid (b) Vasopressor-1 (c) Vasopressor-2 (d) Vasopressor-3

Fig. 2. Compare how mortality varies with the difference between the dose recommended by the optimal policy and the dose used by the clinicians. When the difference is smaller, we see lower observed mortality rates, suggesting that patient survival can be improved when clinicians act on the learned policy in AI.

7.2 Evaluation Metric

Since offline reinforcement learning is more difficult to measure in continuous space, this experiment focuses on two metrics for evaluation and the result is analyzed on the test set.

Survival Rate. Improving patient mortality is particularly important in the healthcare process. Survival rate is an important metric for evaluating system performance. However, the offline reinforcement learning tasks in continuous space cannot interact with the environment to obtain rewards. Therefore, we use the Q function to evaluate the survival rate (Fig. 3).

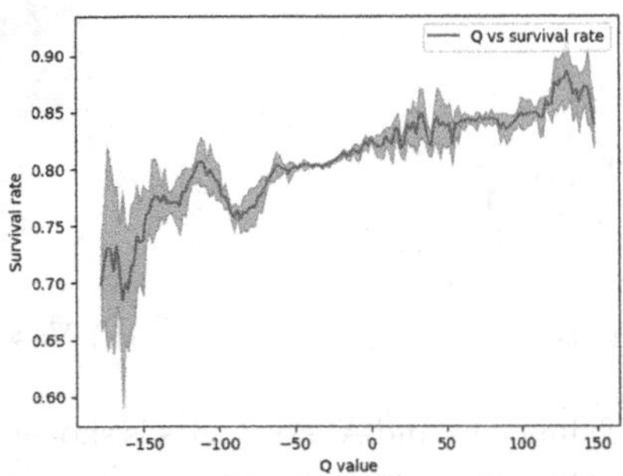

Fig. 3. The relationship between Q and survival rate. The shadows are the result range of 5-fold cross-validation and there is a positive correlation between Q and the survival rate. Thus, a reasonable Q evaluation mechanism can be used to measure the result of the strategy in the offline case.

Q vs. survival rate links expected returns Q to survival rates. The survival rate of a Q value is:

$$survival\_rate\,(Q) = \frac{\#of survival(s,a)_{Q_i}}{\#of(s,a)_{Q_i}} \tag{9}$$

where the $(s,a)_{Q_i}$ means a state-action pair with $Q(s,a) \in Q_i$. Q_i is an range of Q.

In our experiments, we take a perturbation parameter $\varphi = 0.05$, which corresponds to a modified clinician-based strategy. Our experiments result in our Q value of 52.47, corresponding to a survival rate of 0.844, while the evaluated Q value of the clinicians' strategy is 13.19, corresponding to a survival rate of 0.813. This indicates that our model is optimized based on the clinicians' strategy.

Safe Rate. Another evaluation metric under our consideration is the safety rate of the strategy. As for safety measures, we consider the AI-recommended drug doses in the range of 70%–130% of the clinician's strategy to be safe.

$$safe\_rate = \frac{1}{N}\sum_{i=0}^{N}\frac{1}{T}\sum_{t=0}^{T}\bigcap^{a_j}\mathbb{1}(0.7 < (\frac{V_{a_j}^{AI}}{V_{a_j}^{real}}) < 1.3) \tag{10}$$

The final result of the safety rate for our experiments is 0.902, which means the safety of the model results is guaranteed to a large extent. In addition, the data quality issue affects our safety rate calculation to some extent.

8 Conclusions

In this paper, we implement an effective decision optimization system for sepsis treatment in a continuous decision space. The experimental results show that the optimized medical decisions can effectively improve the survival and prognosis of patients. This work makes several key contributions.

At the algorithm level, on the one hand, our algorithm introduces an offline reinforcement learning method, which is an effective solution to the extrapolation error in the offline environment. On the other hand, we capture the patient's historical state, while extending the decision space to a continuous space, which is very important in reality.

At the medical level, our approach can well address the treatment of sepsis patients within 24 h, improving their prognosis. We also refines the action of three kinds of vasopressor, fluid input, and hydrocortisone, which has more practical implications for optimizing clinicians' decision.

Our analysis identifies that for intravenous fluids, the AI strategy is approximately the same as that of the clinician as well. Additionally, more fluid is required in the first 12 h after the onset of sepsis. We also find out that such vasopressors as norepinephrine and vasopressin need to be early initiated and administered in larger doses. However, such inotropes as dobutamine and norepinephrine may require lower doses in sepsis treatment because of increased sympathetic stress and oxygen consumption. Finally, we also discover that compared to the real strategy of clinicians, no more patients are needed to receive glucocorticoid therapy.

In our future work, we will focus on improving more robust clinical reward mechanisms and constructing interpretable deep learning models. At the same time, we will continue generalizing them to a wider range of medical scenarios.

Acknowledgements. This work was supported by National Key R&D Program of China (2020AAA0109603).

References

1. Singer, M., et al.: The third international consensus definitions for sepsis and septic shock (Sepsis-3). JAMA **315**(8), 801–810 (2016)
2. Rudd, K.E., et al.: Global, regional, and national sepsis incidence and mortality, 1990–2017: analysis for the global burden of disease study. Lancet **395**(10219), 200–211 (2020)
3. Fleischmann-Struzek, C., et al.: Incidence and mortality of hospital-and ICU-treated sepsis: results from an updated and expanded systematic review and meta-analysis. Intensive Care Med. **46**(8), 1552–1562 (2020)
4. Rhee, C., et al.: Incidence and trends of sepsis in us hospitals using clinical vs claims data, 2009–2014. JAMA **318**(13), 1241–1249 (2017)
5. Rhodes, A., et al.: Surviving sepsis campaign: international guidelines for management of sepsis and septic shock: 2016. Intensive Care Med. **43**(3), 304–377 (2017)

6. Lat, I., Coopersmith, C.M., De Backer, D.: The surviving sepsis campaign: fluid resuscitation and vasopressor therapy research priorities in adult patients. Intensive Care Med. Exp. **9**(1), 1–16 (2021)
7. Komorowski, M., Celi, L.A., Badawi, O., Gordon, A.C., Faisal, A.A.: The artificial intelligence clinician learns optimal treatment strategies for sepsis in intensive care. Nat. Med. **24**(11), 1716–1720 (2018)
8. Zhang, Y., et al.: HKGB: an inclusive, extensible, intelligent, semi-auto-constructed knowledge graph framework for healthcare with clinicians' expertise incorporated. Inf. Process. Manag. **57**(6), 102324 (2020)
9. Ernst, D., Geurts, P., Wehenkel, L.: Tree-based batch mode reinforcement learning. J. Mach. Learn. Res. **6**, 503–556 (2005)
10. Prasad, N., Cheng, L.F., Chivers, C., Draugelis, M., Engelhardt, B.E.: A reinforcement learning approach to weaning of mechanical ventilation in intensive care units. arXiv preprint arXiv:1704.06300 (2017)
11. Sutton, R.S., Barto, A.G.: Reinforcement Learning: An Introduction. MIT Press, Cambridge (2018)
12. Raghu, A., Komorowski, M., Ahmed, I., Celi, L., Szolovits, P., Ghassemi, M.: Deep reinforcement learning for sepsis treatment. arXiv preprint arXiv:1711.09602 (2017)
13. Wang, Z., Schaul, T., Hessel, M., Hasselt, H., Lanctot, M., Freitas, N.: Dueling network architectures for deep reinforcement learning. In: International Conference on Machine Learning, pp. 1995–2003. PMLR (2016)
14. Van Hasselt, H., Guez, A., Silver, D.: Deep reinforcement learning with double q-learning. In: Proceedings of the AAAI Conference on Artificial Intelligence, vol. 30 (2016)
15. Sun, C., Hong, S., Song, M., Shang, J., Li, H.: Personalized vital signs control based on continuous action-space reinforcement learning with supervised experience. Biomed. Signal Process. Control **69**, 102847 (2021)
16. Fujimoto, S., Meger, D., Precup, D.: Off-policy deep reinforcement learning without exploration. In: International Conference on Machine Learning, pp. 2052–2062. PMLR (2019)
17. Seymour, C.W., et al.: Assessment of clinical criteria for sepsis: for the third international consensus definitions for sepsis and septic shock (Sepsis-3). JAMA **315**(8), 762–774 (2016)
18. Kingma, D.P., Welling, M.: Auto-encoding variational bayes. arXiv preprint arXiv:1312.6114 (2013)

Health and Medical Data Processing

MHDML: Construction of a Medical Lakehouse for Multi-source Heterogeneous Data

Qi Xiao[1], Wenkui Zheng[1(✉)], Chenyu Mao[1], Wei Hou[1], Hao Lan[1], Daojun Han[1], Yang Duan[2], Peng Ren[3], and Ming Sheng[3]

[1] Henan University, Kaifeng 475004, China
{xiaoqi,houwei,hdj}@henu.edu.cn, zhengwenkui@126.com

[2] University of Illinois Urbana-Champaign, Illinois, USA
yangd4@illinois.edu

[3] BNRist, DCST, RIIT, Tsinghua University, Beijing 100084, China
{renpeng,shengming}@tsinghua.edu.cn

Abstract. In the medical field, the rapid growth of medical equipment produced a large amount of medical data which has a wide range of sources and complex structures. Besides, medical data contains essential information that contributes to data exploration. However, the existing platforms based on Data Warehouse or Data Lake cannot effectively integrate more comprehensive multi-source heterogeneous medical data and efficiently manage large-scale multi-modal medical data. This paper presents a **M**ulti-source **H**eterogeneous **D**ata of **M**edical **L**akehouse (MHDML), the platform that integrates multiple pieces of open-source software reasonably to integrate more comprehensive multi-source heterogeneous medical data. Multi-modal data fusion is an important method of the platform to improve multi-modal data management in the medical field. Finally, we customize Restful APIs for medical data exploration tasks. Based on the real data of sepsis and knee osteoarthritis, the platform realizes more comprehensive multi-source heterogeneous medical data acquisition and effective multi-modal medical data management, providing simple operations and visual data exploration functions for medical staff.

Keywords: Medical lakehouse · Multi-source heterogeneous data · Multi-modal data management · Data exploration

1 Introduction

Medical data processing is an important issue in current research [1]. There is no uniform storage standard for the information systems used by different medical institutions, which leads to differences in the structure of medical data. This data includes not only structured data, but semi-structured data (CSV, JSON, XML, etc.), and rapidly growing unstructured data (ECGs, CTs, MRIs, etc.) in the medical field. Facing massive multi-source heterogeneous data in the medical

A. Traina et al. (Eds.): HIS 2022, LNCS 13705, pp. 127–135, 2022.
https://doi.org/10.1007/978-3-031-20627-6_12

field, how to integrate, store and provide unified management methods become the key problems [2].

The Database is an important technology for early medical data management, and it can meet the needs of rapid insertion, deletion, and query of data in the case of less medical data. However, database technology is not well equipped to handle analysis tasks characterized by reading large amounts of data.

To solve this problem, the Data Warehouse has been applied in the medical field to provide data support for medical staff in data management analysis and treatment decision-making. However, as more and more high-precision medical technology devices are applied in the medical field, a large amount of unstructured data grows rapidly, making the data in the medical field complex and diverse. Data Warehouse cannot store multi-modal data effectively due to strict storage format requirements.

In order to solve the medical data storage challenges brought by the Data Warehouse, the researchers begin to pay close attention to the Data Lake technology for medical data management. The data storage system based on the Data Lake can store data in any format, solving the problems of multimodal medical data storage and facilitating data management by unifying data formats. However, due to the lack of effective data management, the Data Lake cannot effectively manage data. So researchers have been beginning to pay attention to the Lakehouse technology.

The Data Lakehouse is a new architecture, recently launched to overcome the problems existing in the Data Warehouse and the Data Lake [3]. With the introduction of the Data Lakehouse, medical data is presented in the form of structured queries and unstructured data analysis.

Contributions. The main contributions are summarized as follows:

1. We present the Medical Lakehouse to integrate more comprehensive multi-source heterogeneous medical data. With the support of open-source software, medical multi-source heterogeneous data is converted into one unified data storage. Our Lakehouse platform records the data sources and changes to ensure the traceability of the medcial data.
2. We customize Restful APIs for medical data exploration tasks. Meanwhile, we consider multi-modal data fusion to improve data management, thus providing more patient information to underpin doctors' rapid medical decision-making.

The rest of this paper is organized as follows. Section 2 introduces the related work. Section 3 gives the function architecture of medical Lakehouse. Section 4 shows the results of application and implementation. Section 5 summarizes the paper and points out future research direction.

2 Related Work

At present, the Data Warehouse system in the medical field is mainly used to solve the management of structured data. And unstructured data presents multi-modal characteristics in the medical field.

In order to solve the problem of multi-modal data storage of the Data Warehouse, the Data Lake architecture is adopted. The medical storage management system based on Data Lake can effectively solve the problem of multi-modal medical data storage. The existing Data Lake architecture solves the problem of data storage in arbitrary format, but there are still some deficiencies in the structured data query. Facing the problems in teh Data Warehouse and teh Data Lake, researchers focus on the Data Lakehouse technology.

As shown in Table 1, 1–4 are related studies of the Data Warehouse, 5–8 are the Data Lake related work, and the rest part of the Data Lakehouse related research.

However, the existing Lakehouse technology cannot integrate medical multi-modal data effectively, and it cannot effectively solve the problem of data traceability. Therefore, facing the problem of multi-modal data management in the medical field, we design the Medical Lakehouse to solve the problem of multi-modal data fusion and provide data traceability and data exploration functions.

Table 1. Comparison of related research.

	Author	Time	Multi-sources heterogeneous data of acquisition	Multi-sources heterogeneous data of storage	Multi-source heterogeneous data of management	Multi-modal data of fusion	Data source of trace	Unified APIs	Visual exploration
1	Nafees et al. [4]	2018	○	○	○	○	○	●	●
2	Ali et al. [5]	2020	○	○	○	○	○	○	●
3	Helmut et al. [6]	2020	○	○	○	○	○	○	●
4	Mohammad et al. [7]	2021	○	○	○	○	○	●	●
5	Ekta et al. [8]	2018	●	●	●	○	○	●	●
6	Joseph et al. [9]	2020	●	●	●	○	○	●	●
7	Iran A et al. [10]	2021	●	●	●	○	○	●	●
8	Peng et al. [11]	2021	●	●	●	●	-	●	●
9	Drazen et al. [12]	2021	●	●	●	○	○	●	●
10	Edmon et al. [13]	2021	●	●	●	○	○	●	●
11	**Ours et al.**	2021	●	●	●	●	●	●	●

Note: ● indicates that the table's feature is supported, and ○ is not

3 The Function Architecture of Medical Lakehouse

We design the Medical Lakehouse for integrating more comprehensive multi-source heterogeneous medical data, reducing the extra cost caused by data acquisition as much as possible. Considering the complexity of unstructured data in medical scenarios, our platform uses cluster computing power to fuse multi-modal data to generate high-quality data in a unified data format.

As shown in Fig. 1, the Lakehouse architecture is divided into six layers: Data Ingestion layer, Data Storage Layer, Data Management Layer, Data Scheduling Layer, Ecological Service Layer and Application layer.

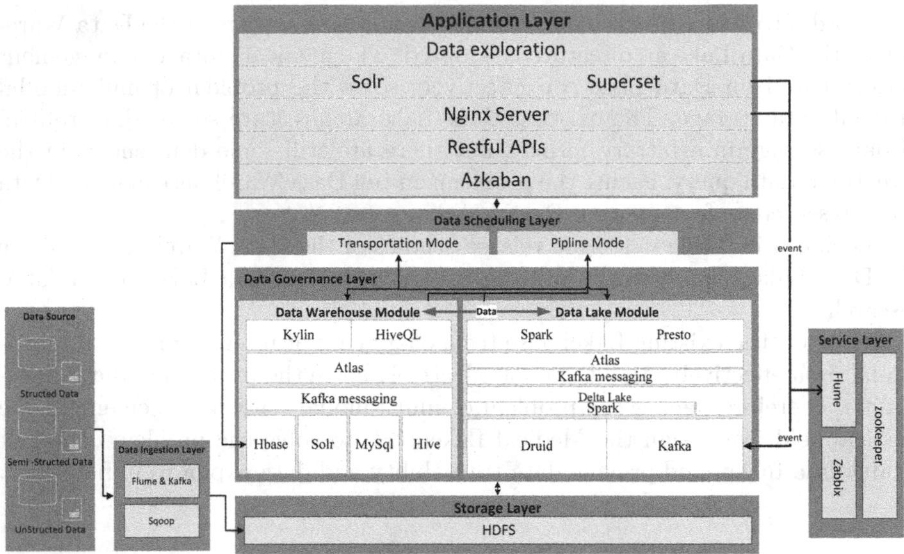

Fig. 1. The Lakehouse architecture.

3.1 Data Ingestion Layer

As there is no unified standard for the data storage format adopted by each medical institution, medical multi-source heterogeneous data needs to be converted into the storage structure of a unified platform for storage. Therefore, large-scale structured data and streaming data are quickly migrated to HDFS in this layer.

Using the Sqoop Import API, tables from relational databases can be stored in HDFS as individual records for each row. And we use Flume and Kafka to efficiently collect large-scale streaming data. So the Data Ingestion Layer offers a wide range of medical data for Data Management Layer.

3.2 Data Storage Layer

The Data Storage Layer must be able to store multi-modal data with different structures and the layer must have storage scalability and performance scalability. So HDFS is located at the bottom of the entire platform, it is the key link of data circulation between Data Warehouse and Data Lake.

3.3 Data Management Layer

Nowadays, medical institutions generate a large amount of data every day, and medical data is often unprocessed and fragmented, which cannot meet the requirements of data quality for downstream tasks. Through the Data Warehouse Module and the Data Lake Module, this layer performs different processing for different types of data, such as fragment fusion, metadata management and data format normalization.

Data Warehouse Module. Medical staff need to query the medical information of patients in large-scale data. Aiming at the efficiency data query, this module implements efficient data query function which can provide the required information for medical staff in a short time.

First, platform extract data from the Data Storage Layer to HBase, then platform use Hive to perform data ETL (Extract, Transform and Load) from HBase, and return the calculation results to HBase. Finally, platform use HiveQL to provide a data query function, and use Druid to help users query structured data.

For the medical information of patients, doctors need to know the reasons of data changes to provide reliable data support for medical decision-making. The Atlas component provides data traceability function, and information of each data change will be stored in HBase. And this module extracts the structural information describing the data schema.

Data Lake Module. For the Data Warehouse Module, it cannot efficiently store multi-modal medical data due to its strict storage format. The module uses DataFrame and DeltaTable to provide a unified data model for heterogeneous data, the platform can convert them into appropriate way of DataFrame to achieve persistent storage of multi-modal medical data.

Besides, through DeltaLake and Spark of this module, Spark provides the ability to accelerate computing and unify heterogeneous data into DeltaTable and DataFrame formats. DeltaTable and DataFrame can be converted to each other by using the provided DeltaMergeBuilder API, and DataFrame is used as the main format for subsequent tasks.

In the medical field, it is inevitable to query heterogeneous data. Medical staff not only need to query unstructured data but also need to query structured data at the same time. This module can be used through Presto to query multi-source data from Hive, Kafka and Druid.

Therefore, this module mainly processes multi-modal medical data to meet the requirements of the unified data format.

3.4 Data Scheduling Layer

After the ingestion phase, raw medical data is migrated to the Data Storage Layer, the platform divides data scheduling tasks into two modes for different users in different ways of using data.

Transmission Mode. This mode uses the SFTP protocol to upload data files to the reserved space of the data storage layer. During the uploading process, this mode will collect the metadata of the data file and store metadata in the HBase. The main purpose of this mode is to persistently store important medical data in the Data Storage Layer to ensure data security.

Pipeline Mode. The biggest difference between this mode and the Transmission Mode is that the platform does not save it in the Data Storage Layer and only stores the meta-information in the meta-information database when it is used. The main purpose of this mode is to provide memory usage, fusion, or query functions for uploaded medical data.

3.5 Ecological Service Layer

The main function of this layer is to ensure the normal operation of the cluster. As the core coordination component of the platform, Zookeeper is used to manage various components in the entire platform and coordinate the communication between components.

3.6 Application Layer

Through Restful APIs interface of the Application Layer, the data processing details are encapsulated into a visual module, and medical staff only need to submit the data to the platform without caring about how the data is processed.

According to the capabilities and requirements of medical personnel [14], they can use Restful APIs to call various functions of the platform, this layer provides a good interactive interface and provides visualization functions for data exploration.

4 Application and Implementation

We have applied multi-modal data fusion and query technology in some hospitals to assist medical experts in scientific research, involving multiple application scenarios. The treatment data of sepsis is illustrated below.

According to our Lakehouse platform, we can integrate more comprehensive types of multi-source heterogeneous medical data and effectively manage multi-modal medical data based on data fusion technology.

Under the sepsis treatment field, we gather a large number of data in the treatment process, including structured data 63.0 G, unstructured data 67.4 TB and most of the time-series data is produced after the patients received by hospitals. Our platform can unify multi-modal medical data formats and fuse the data for easy management.

Step 1: Through the Data Ingestion Layer, the data of any format is stored in the reserved space of HDFS. The platform adopts the combination of Flume and Kafka to improve the speed of streaming data ingestion, Table 2 norepinephrine injection log described the medical streaming data. As shown in Table 3, the streaming data is stored in the Data Management Layer.

Table 2. Example of injection data

03/19 18:20:01	INFO: Name:1001
03/19 18:20:05	INFO: Start:NaCl infusion
03/19 18:20:05	INFO: Main: rate:10 rateuom:ml/hr
03/19 18:25:20	INFO: Main: rate:20 rateuom:ml/hr
03/19 18:25:25	INFO: Start:NaCl infusion
03/19 18:25:25	INFO: Main: rate:20 rateuom:ml/hr
03/19 20:00:40	INFO: End:NaCl infusion

Table 3. Structure data of drug injection

Name	Item	START TIME	END TIME	RATE	RATEUOM
1042	Norepinephrine infusion	18:20	18:25	1	mcg/kg/min
1042	Norepinephrine infusion	18:25	20:00	2	mcg/kg/min

Step 2: According to the characteristics of a lot of unstructured data in the sepsis treatment scenario, our platform uses the Transmission Mode of the Data Scheduling Layer to persistently store data.

Step 3: For unstructured data, our platform uses ANNOY and NANOPQ methods to extract feature vectors of image data. As shown in Fig. 2, we converts time-series data, image data and structured data into a unified DataFrame format through Delata Lake of the Data Management Layer.

Step 4: Our platform converts DataFrame data into special tree and fuses the fragmented information of multi-modal data with the power of cluster computing, as shown in Fig. 3.

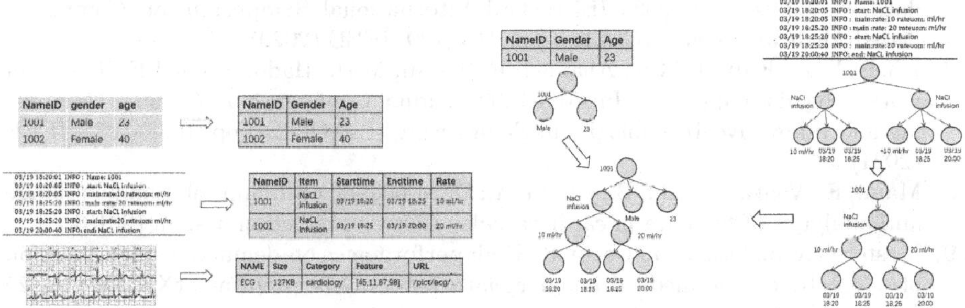

Fig. 2. Convert multi-type data to DataFrame

Fig. 3. Example of multi-modal data fusion

5 Conclusion and Future Work

In the medical field, the Lakehouse can be used as the basis of building the completely new platform. The Medical Lakehouse designed by us can integrate more extensive medical multi-source heterogeneous data and fuse multi-modal medical data with cluster computing power, so that the management of medical data have been improved. Our platform also provides doctors with easy-to-use data exploration functions through customized Restful APIs. In the future, we will use new features of Hudi to enhance the performance of the Medical Lakehouse.

Acknowledgements. This work was supported by National Key R&D Program of China (2020AAA0109603) and Foundation of University Young Key Teacher of Henan Province (2019GGJS040, 2020GGJS027).

References

1. He, J., Rong, J., Sun, L., Wang, H., Zhang, Y., Ma, J.: A framework for cardiac arrhythmia detection from IoT-based ECGs. World Wide Web **23**(5), 2835–2850 (2020). https://doi.org/10.1007/s11280-019-00776-9
2. Kalkman, S., Mostert, M., Udo-Beauvisage, N., Van Delden, J., Van Thiel, G.: Responsible data sharing in a big data-driven translational research platform: lessons learned. BMC Med. Inform. Decis. Mak. **19**(1), 1–7 (2019)
3. Armbrust, M., Ghodsi, A., Xin, R., Zaharia, M.: Lakehouse: a new generation of open platforms that unify data warehousing and advanced analytics. In: Proceedings of CIDR (2021)
4. Farooqui, N.A., Mehra, R.: Design of a data warehouse for medical information system using data mining techniques. In: 2018 Fifth International Conference on Parallel, Distributed and Grid Computing (PDGC), pp. 199–203. IEEE (2018)
5. Neamah, A.F.: Flexible data warehouse: towards building an integrated electronic health record architecture. In: 2020 International Conference on Smart Electronics and Communication (ICOSEC), pp. 1038–1042. IEEE (2020)
6. Spengler, H., Gatz, I., Kohlmayer, F., Kuhn, K.A., Prasser, F.: Improving data quality in medical research: a monitoring architecture for clinical and translational data warehouses. In: 2020 IEEE 33rd International Symposium on Computer-Based Medical Systems (CBMS), pp. 415–420. IEEE (2020)
7. Khan, M.Z., Kidwai, M.S., Ahamad, F., Khan, M.U.: Hadoop based EMH framework: a big data approach. In: 2021 International Conference on Advance Computing and Innovative Technologies in Engineering (ICACITE), pp. 1068–1070. IEEE (2021)
8. Maini, E., Venkateswarlu, B., Gupta, A.: Data lake-an optimum solution for storage and analytics of big data in cardiovascular disease prediction system (2018)
9. Mesterhazy, J., Olson, G., Datta, S.: High performance on-demand de-identification of a petabyte-scale medical imaging data lake. arXiv preprint arXiv:2008.01827 (2020)
10. Melchor-Uceda, I.A., Olivares-Rojas, J.C., Gutiérrez-Gnecchi, J.A., García-Ramírez, M.C., Reyes-Archundia, E., Téllez-Anguiano, A.C.: Data ingestion system for interoperability and integration of hospital data online and in real time. In: 2021 Mexican International Conference on Computer Science (ENC), pp. 1–5. IEEE (2021)
11. Ren, P., et al.: MHDP: an efficient data lake platform for medical multi-source heterogeneous data. In: Xing, C., Fu, X., Zhang, Y., Zhang, G., Borjigin, C. (eds.) WISA 2021. LNCS, vol. 12999, pp. 727–738. Springer, Cham (2021). https://doi.org/10.1007/978-3-030-87571-8_63
12. Oreščanin, D., Hlupić, T.: Data lakehouse - a novel step in analytics architecture. In: 2021 44th International Convention on Information, Communication and Electronic Technology (MIPRO), pp. 1242–1246. IEEE (2021)

13. Begoli, E., Goethert, I., Knight, K.: A lakehouse architecture for the management and analysis of heterogeneous data for biomedical research and mega-biobanks. In: 2021 IEEE International Conference on Big Data (Big Data), pp. 4643–4651. IEEE (2021)
14. Zhang, Y., et al.: HKGB: an inclusive, extensible, intelligent, semi-auto-constructed knowledge graph framework for healthcare with clinicians' expertise incorporated. Inf. Process. Manage. **57**(6), 102324 (2020)

A Hybrid Medical Causal Inference Platform Based on Data Lake

Peng Ren[1], Xingyue Liu[2(✉)], Shuxin Zheng[3], Lijun Liao[4], Xin Li[5], Ligong Lu[6], Xia Wang[7], Ruoyu Wang[2], and Ming Sheng[1]

[1] BNRist, DCST, RIIT, Tsinghua University, Beijing 100084, China
{renpeng,shengming}@tsinghua.edu.cn
[2] School of Mathematical Sciences, Beihang University, Beijing 102206, China
liuxingyue_buaa@163.com, zhangyong05@tsinghua.edu.cn
[3] School of Mathematics and Statistics, Beijing Jiaotong University, Beijing 100044, China
[4] Nanjing Nari Information and Communication Technology Co., Ltd., Nanjing, China
[5] Beijing Tsinghua Changgung Hospital, School of Clinical Medicine, Tsinghua University, Beijing 100084, China
[6] Zhuhai Institute of Translational Medicine Zhuhai People's Hospital Affiliated with Jinan University, Jinan University, Zhuhai 519000, Guangdong, China
[7] Institute for Intelligent Healthcare, Tsinghua University, Beijing 100084, China
wangxia_dt@tsinghua.edu.cn

Abstract. Causal inference platform is rather useful in the medical domain, and relies heavily on data quality and prior knowledge. Nowadays, the advancement of medical methods and the application of high-technology devices have brought a large amount of multi-source heterogeneous multi-modal data, which supports data-driven causal inference. In addition, when we need causal inference to assist medical research, it will be more reliable if we consider both data and prior knowledge. However, most of the current causal inference platforms only involve parts of the causal inference process, ranging from multi-modal data fusion, exploratory data analysis with doctor-in-loop, and causal inference based on data lake. A unified closed loop of causal inference that can be applied to most datasets and improve the reliability of research in the medical domain has not been established yet. Therefore, we propose a hybrid medical causal inference platform based on data lake, which is both data-driven and knowledge-driven. It can manage and fuse massive multi-heterogeneous data, interact well with doctors in data exploration process, and offer a convenient medical causal inference interface. This platform has been used on Knee Osteoarthritis disease, which proves the effectiveness of our work.

Keywords: Data lake · Heterogeneous medical data · Causal inference platform

A. Traina et al. (Eds.): HIS 2022, LNCS 13705, pp. 136–144, 2022.
https://doi.org/10.1007/978-3-031-20627-6_13

1 Introduction

The identification of the causal relationships among data is crucial to have a better understanding of making an accurate decision. In recent years, causal inference has attracted the interest of many researchers as an effective method to identify causal relationships. Scholars usually supplement the exploratory data analysis in the early stage of inference and also conduct cross-exploration with various fields such as medicine, psychology, sociology, etc.

Medical data is generated during the medical process, including structured data (MySQL, Oracle), semi-structured data (CSV, JSON), and unstructured data (CT, X-ray). With the advancement of the medical level and the application of various examining devices, medical data presents the characteristics of multi-source heterogeneity, large amounts, and redundancy in recent decades [1,2]. Therefore, when we do exploratory data analysis and causal inference in the medical domain, data should be combined and comprehensively considered. Besides, current medical data analysis is mostly rigid deletion and interpolation according to specific rules, which lacks feasibility in practical applications [3]. In this case, we consider that the participation of doctors is necessary and it can help the whole system obtain comprehensive and accurate prior knowledge [4].

Nowadays, causal inference has always been deeply connected with medical data analysis [5–7]. Currently, medical causal inference contributes to diverse medical methods [5]. The relationship between some pathological features is also unraveled with the help of causal inference [6]. Some medical models and data corrections also use causal inference [7]. Some of the above studies have proposed a new method for inference, others have discovered various new meanings of causal inference in a certain dataset, but how to realize a convenient medical causal inference platform on most datasets is still being explored.

Contributions. In this paper, we propose a platform based on data lake aiming to process causal inference in the medical domain. The main contributions are as follows:

1. We use data lake to store and integrate multi-source heterogeneous data. Different formats of structured and unstructured data are transformed into one unified format to store and fuse, eventually, summarize the whole information as a merged table.
2. We interact with doctors in the process of exploratory data analysis. Doctors are involved in loop and provide enormous prior knowledge to refine the entity selection and promote the quality of table merged in data lake.
3. We provide a platform for causal inference. Based on the merged table refined by doctors in exploratory data analysis, we execute causal inference in the platform, which allows most types of datasets to be processed uniformly and generally.

In the rest of this paper, we will provide the details. Section 2 introduces related work. Section 3 presents the overall system and the workflow of our platform. Section 4 discusses the fusion of multi-source heterogeneous data in data lake. Section 5 describes the process of medical exploratory data analysis with doctor-in-loop. Section 6 presents the steps of medical causal inference. The implementation and use case are introduced in Sect. 7. Section 8 concludes the paper.

2 Related Work

In order to highlight the great contribution of the causal inference platform in the medical domain, based on the underlying architecture of data lake, we hope to establish a complete closed loop in the research of causal inference, including data fusion, exploratory data analysis, causal inference, and verification. Moreover, the participation of doctors greatly improves the efficiency of the platform. Therefore, we started related work in the aspects of data lake, exploratory data analysis, and interaction with doctors [8–18].

Nowadays, many studies apply database and data warehouse technology to medical data management [8,9]. However, traditional methods limit the storage and management of data, as well as further analysis. Therefore, we manage various kinds of data based on the underlying architecture of the data lake and then realize multi-modal data storage, fusion, exploration, and causal inference [10].

The advantages of exploratory data analysis have been demonstrated in the medical domain. However, due to the lack of doctors' participation and the complexity of medical data [11,12], the conclusions are lacking in professionalism. In addition, the current data interaction platforms [13] still have the problem that the communication mode between doctors and exploratory data analysis professionals is not clear enough.

With the wide application of causal inference, many researchers consider applying it to the medical domain [14]. Due to the obvious advantages of causal inference in practical application, most studies carry out mathematical calculation and theoretical verification at the academic level [15]. However, there are few unified research methods for causal inference in application scenarios and many experiments used only a single data set to validate the model [16–18].

However, the recent causal inference systems mostly do not integrate various aspects of information. Besides, in most cases, there is no doctor participation in exploratory data analysis process. In addition, many studies aim at experimenting with a certain type of causal model, which is insufficient in generalization. Hence, a causal inference framework that can integrate comprehensive information, involve doctors in loop for exploratory data analysis, and be applied to most datasets has not been established.

3 Platform Design

In this section, We will describe the architecture and workflow of our platform in Sect. 3.1, analyze data-driven methods and knowledge-driven methods in Sect. 3.2, and then explain the advantages of our platform in Sect. 3.3.

3.1 Architecture and Workflow

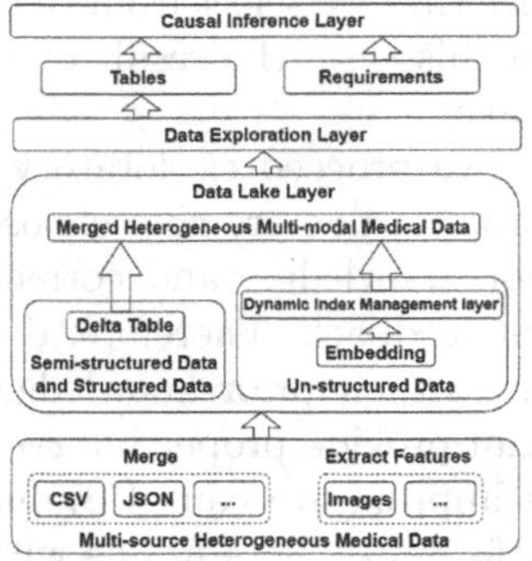

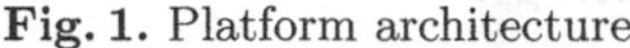

Fig. 1. Platform architecture

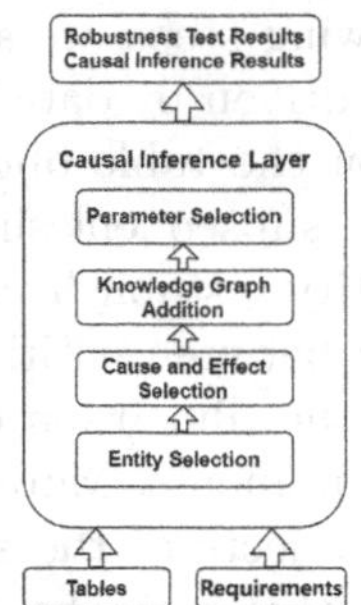

Fig. 2. Causal inference layer

Our platform is based on data lake and the whole process is divided into the following three parts: multi-source heterogeneous data fusion, exploratory data analysis with doctors in loop, and causal inference. The architecture of our platform is presented in Fig. 1. In the data lake layer, we process semi-structured data and structured data in one zone and unstructured data in the other zone, which enable us to integrate information using different methods. In the exploratory data analysis layer, we do exploratory data analysis under the guidance of doctors. After that, we obtain simplified tables, and these tables, as well as various extra requirements, are considered as input of the causal inference layer for final results. Our framework processes data with data-driven expansion in the data lake layer and knowledge-driven simplification in the exploratory data analysis layer, and eventually achieves causal inference and robustness test in causal inference layer. The workflow of causal inference layer is described in Fig. 2.

3.2 Data-Driven vs Knowledge-Driven Methods

On the one hand, data-driven methods can help obtain comprehensive information. However, relying on data-driven methods thoroughly may bring extra workload and affect the accuracy of causal inference. On the other hand, knowledge-driven methods can simplify the causal inference process. However, depending solely on knowledge-driven methods may produce empirical errors.

3.3 Integration of Data-Driven Expansion and Knowledge-Driven Simplification

Our platform combines data-driven and knowledge-driven methods, which can mitigate the problems mentioned above. With data lake and the participation of doctors, we can draw a more reliable conclusion that meets the needs of doctors.

In view of the characteristics of multi-source heterogeneous and multi-modal medical data, we use data lake to accomplish data storage, fusion and query.

Based on data lake, we can extract and synthesize diverse types of information from different formats of data, which finally get a comprehensive table. Due to the comprehensiveness of the table, specific entities that we select from the table in the following steps are also comprehensive. In this case, the result of causal inference is driven by data on the basis of data lake.

Based on the table obtained from data lake, we proceed exploratory data analysis and subsequent simplification. In this process, doctors help choose the suitable entity, establish causal graph with prior knowledge, and correct the relationship between entities according to instant feedback. Therefore, doctors can reduce the dimension of the table according to their prior knowledge and certain requirements. Moreover, doctor-in-loop can provide proper intervention and result objects of the study and help select appropriate causal evaluation methods. In this case, the final results of the platform are more in line with the actual needs of doctors, which is driven by knowledge.

4 Multi-source Heterogeneous Data Fusion

Data fusion is necessary to synthesize all aspects of information about medical data. The basis of data fusion is data lake. In data lake, we use a unified concept for representation and adopt a new management mode for structured data and unstructured data. We consider that each of files contains items with identified keys and various attached features. To specify, for structured data, we regard it as a tree and the nodes of each tree are the features and keys. There will be three situations: if keys and all the sub-trees are identical, we regard them as the same tree; if keys are the same while sub-trees are different, we regard them as partly same trees; if keys are different, we regard them as different trees. In the process of fusion, we reserved only one of the same tree and both of the different trees. Meanwhile, we fuse partly same trees according to the same features. For unstructured data, we also regard it as a tree. In this case, the nodes store not only features and keys, but also some unstructured aspects, including feature vector, path information, and other underlying information. The fusion of unstructured data is similar to the process of structured data mentioned above, which means that we also match the nodes of each tree. Moreover, it is worth noting that the fusion can happen not only between the same data type from various sources, but also between different data types.

5 Exploratory Data Analysis

After the fusion based on data lake, we will get a table that integrates the information of multi-modal medical data. However, some of the features in this table are useless for further study, which increases workload and decreases efficiency. Moreover, some irrelevant features may reduce the significance of those vital ones. Thus, we still need to conduct exploratory data analysis to reduce dimensions and simplify the table. Our exploratory data analysis process is designed according to the need of doctors and aimed at assisting doctors in scientific research. Doctors can click any part of the table according to their needs to merge, delete or interpolate any column or row in the table. Besides, the table can be visualized as bar chart, histogram, line graph or pie chart and any part of the visualized graph can be selected by clicking on the graph. Eventually, the simplified form serves in the platform as a new input for subsequent causal inference. The final form preserves the comprehensiveness of the data fusion and eliminates unnecessary information to focus on individual requirements.

6 Causal Inference

Causal inference is divided into four steps: Entity selection, Cause and Effect selection, Constraint Creation, and Parameter Selection.

Entity Selection: In this step, we select all entities which will be used later. The default is set to select all entities and we can click the box to deselect unnecessary ones. In Fig. 3, we can see the blue options are the selected entities that will present as nodes in the cause-and-effect graph.

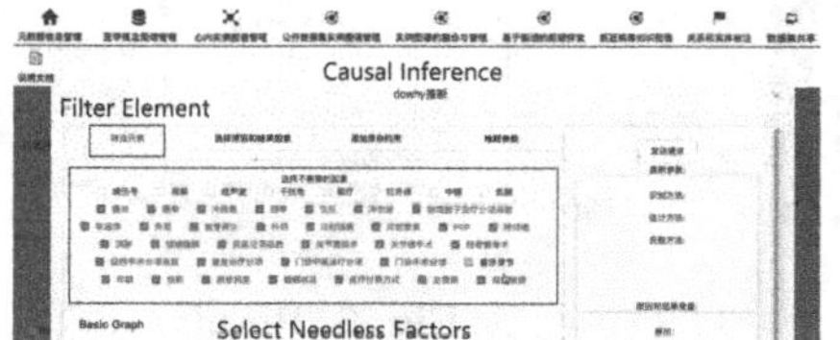

Fig. 3. Entity selection

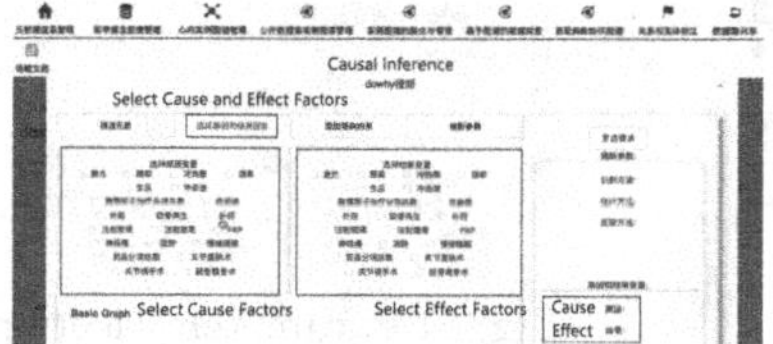

Fig. 4. Cause and effect selection

Cause and Effect Selection: In this step, we select the cause and effect variables, which we want to prove whether there exists a causal relationship, as Treatment and Outcome. At the same time, the name of the selected variable is shown on the right side for checking. The process is shown as Fig. 4.

Constraint Creation: In this step, we add the diverse constraints that the entities selected in the first step needs to meet. In Fig. 4, we can see that cause variables and result variables are on the left of the screen. Every time we select one cause variable and one result variable and click "Add Factor" button, a set of constraints is added to the prior knowledge graph as a red edge, which will also be displayed at the corresponding position on the right side of the screen. Finally, the graph of prior knowledge is completed and displayed.

Parameter Selection: In this step, identification method, estimation method and refutation method should be selected:

1. Identification criteria: Back-door criterion, Front-door criterion, Instrumental Variables, and Mediation (Direct and indirect effect identification).

2. Estimation methods: Propensity Score Matching, Regression discontinuity, Inverse Propensity Weighting, Linear Regression, Generalized Linear Models, and Binary Instrument.
3. Refutation methods: Add Random Common Cause, Placebo Treatment, Data Subsets Validation, and Bootstrap Validation.

We choose one parameter from each item. For example, as we can see in Fig. 5, we choose *Back-door Criterion*, *Linear Regression* and *Add Random Common Cause*. Then, the platform calculates the estimation result and the robustness test result, which is demonstrated as Fig. 6. The minus sign indicates a negative correlation between the cause variable and the effect variable. The value indicates the degree of the correlation and the result passes the robustness test.

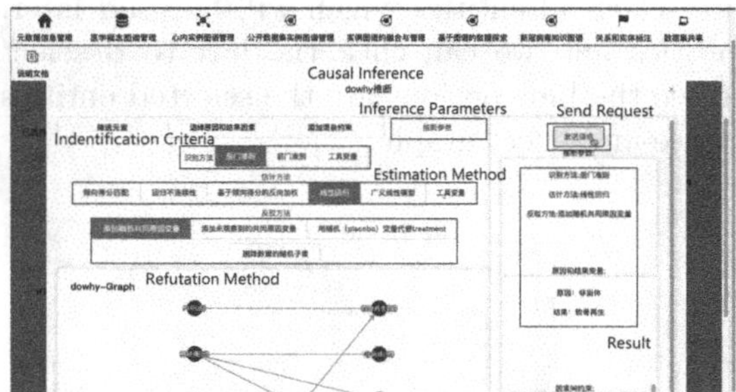

Fig. 5. Parameter selection

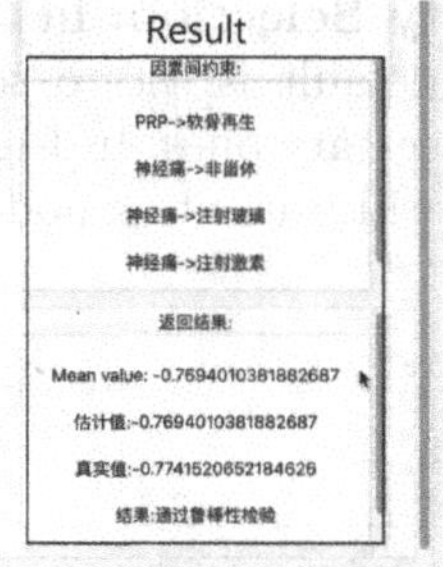
Result
PRP->软骨再生
Mean value: -0.7694010381882687
估计值:-0.7694010381882687
真实值:-0.7741520652184626

Fig. 6. Result

7 Implementation and Use Case

The implementation of our platform is summarized as follows: Our platform is based on Delta Lake[1]. Massive multi-source heterogeneous data is input to manage and fuse in data lake, in which the information is extracted and stored in the merged table. After obtaining the table, we conduct exploratory data analysis to refine the table under the guidance of doctors, including merging some rows or columns, and deleting some features according to individual requirements. The refined table is regarded as a sub-table of the original table and input it into causal inference process. Then, the sub-table starts causal analysis by four steps: selecting entity elements, determining cause and effect factors, adding confounding constraints, and choosing inference parameters. The final output includes whether there is a causal relationship, whether it is positive if the causal relationship exists, and whether the result passes the robustness test.

An example dataset came from all electronic medical records of tertiary hospitals patients diagnosed with Knee Osteoarthritis from 2014 to 2020. This dataset includes 6000 patients and 16000 medical records, which contains 10 tables about

[1] https://delta.io.

personal information, basic information, medical cost, ultrasound examination, imaging diagnosis, auxiliary examination, doctor's advice, and other related information. There are 35 kinds of medical influencing factors including drugs, physical factors, rehabilitation treatment and surgery, and more than 2500 kinds of medical advice in the dataset, which is used for various statistical research.

8 Conclusion

This paper proposes a causal inference platform based on data lake to achieve the fusion of multi-source heterogeneous medical data, perform exploratory data analysis with doctor-in-loop, and conduct causal inference and robust tests. To increase the accuracy and reliability of causal inference, we combine data-driven and knowledge-driven methods. Based on Data Lake, we accomplish the integration of information. After that, we adopt a new exploratory data analysis method with the participation of doctors. This platform has been used on Knee Osteoarthritis disease, which proves the effectiveness of our work.

Acknowledgement. This work was supported by National Key R&D Program of China (2020AAA0109603).

References

1. Zhang, Y., Sheng, M., et al.: HKGB: an inclusive, extensible, intelligent, semi-auto-constructed knowledge graph framework for healthcare with clinicians' expertise incorporated. Inf. Process. Manage. **57**(6), 102324 (2020)
2. Du, J., Michalska, S., Subramani, S., Wang, H., Zhang, Y.: Neural attention with character embeddings for hay fever detection from twitter. Health Inf. Sci. Syst. **7**(1), 1–7 (2019). https://doi.org/10.1007/s13755-019-0084-2
3. Jasu, J., Tolonen, T., et al.: Combined longitudinal clinical and autopsy phenomic assessment in lethal metastatic prostate cancer: recommendations for advancing precision medicine. Eur. Urol. Open Sci. **30**, 47–62 (2021)
4. Wartner, S., Girardi, D., Wiesinger-Widi, M., Trenkler, J., Kleiser, R., Holzinger, A.: Ontology-guided principal component analysis: reaching the limits of the doctor-in-the-loop. In: Renda, M.E., Bursa, M., Holzinger, A., Khuri, S. (eds.) ITBAM 2016. LNCS, vol. 9832, pp. 22–33. Springer, Cham (2016). https://doi.org/10.1007/978-3-319-43949-5_2
5. Castro, D.C., Walker, I., Glocker, B.: Causality matters in medical imaging. Nat. Commun. **11**(1), 1–10 (2020)
6. Qi, Z., Yaping, W., et al.: Research on influencing factors of prognosis treatment for lung cancer patients based on causality. Comput. Technol. Dev. **31**(08), 145–149 (2021)
7. Decruyenaere, A., Steen, J., et al.: The obesity paradox in critically ill patients: a causal learning approach to a casual finding. Crit. Care **24**(1), 1–11 (2020)
8. Mitchell, J., Naddaf, R., Davenport, S.: A medical microcomputer database management system. Methods Inf. Med. **24**(2), 73–78 (1985)
9. Sebaa, A., Chikh, F., Nouicer, A., Tari, A.K.: Medical big data warehouse: architecture and system design, a case study: improving healthcare resources distribution. J. Med. Syst. **42**(4), 1–16 (2018). https://doi.org/10.1007/s10916-018-0894-9

10. Ren, P., et al.: MHDP: an efficient data lake platform for medical multi-source heterogeneous data. In: Xing, C., Fu, X., Zhang, Y., Zhang, G., Borjigin, C. (eds.) WISA 2021. LNCS, vol. 12999, pp. 727–738. Springer, Cham (2021). https://doi.org/10.1007/978-3-030-87571-8_63
11. Cominetti, O., et al.: Identification of a novel clinical phenotype of severe malaria using a network-based clustering approach. Sci. Rep. **8**(1), 1–10 (2018)
12. Pareekutty, N.M., Kadam, S., Ankalkoti, B., Balasubramanian, S., Anilkumar, B.: Gastrectomy with D2 lymphadenectomy for carcinoma of the stomach in a standalone cancer centre in rural India. Indian J. Surg. Oncol. **11**(2), 256–262 (2020). https://doi.org/10.1007/s13193-020-01059-w
13. Sauver, J.L.S., et al.: Peer reviewed: Rochester epidemiology project data exploration portal. Prev. Chronic Dis. **15** (2018)
14. Wu, J.Q., et al.: Automated causal inference in application to randomized controlled clinical trials. Nat. Mach. Intell. **4**(5), 436–444 (2022)
15. Whata, A., Chimedza, C.: Evaluating uses of deep learning methods for causal inference. IEEE Access **10**, 2813–2827 (2022)
16. Wang, X., Xu, X., Tong, W., Roberts, R., Liu, Z.: InferBERT: a transformer-based causal inference framework for enhancing pharmacovigilance. Front. Artif. Intell. **4**, 659622 (2021)
17. Pandey, D., Wang, H., et al.: Automatic breast lesion segmentation in phase preserved DCE-MRIs. Health Inf. Sci. Syst. **10**(1), 1–19 (2022). https://doi.org/10.1007/s13755-022-00176-w
18. Sarki, R., Ahmed, K., Wang, H., Zhang, Y.: Automated detection of mild and multi-class diabetic eye diseases using deep learning. Health Inf. Sci. Syst. **8**(1), 1–9 (2020). https://doi.org/10.1007/s13755-020-00125-5

Data Exploration Optimization for Medical Big Data

Shuang Ding[1,2], Chenyu Mao[1,2], Wenkui Zheng[3](✉), Qi Xiao[3], and Yitao Wu[4]

[1] School of Software, Henan University, Kaifeng 475004, China
ds@vip.henu.edu.cn
[2] Henan International Joint Laboratory of Intelligent Network Theory and Key Technology, Kaifeng 475004, China
[3] Henan University, Kaifeng 475004, China
zwk@vip.henu.edu.cn, xiaoqi@henu.edu.cn
[4] International College, Beijing University of Posts and Telecommunications, Beijing 100876, China

Abstract. In medical domain, huge amounts of data are generated at all times. Data exploration is very important to help physicians or medical researchers to find the required datasets. However, the storage and computation of large-scale data surpass the performance limits of traditional relational databases, which are prone to performance bottlenecks, and it is difficult to expand the storage capacity and computational power. To solve the above problems, this paper studies the distributed migration storage and computing methods of medical data, and proposes a distributed computing and storage strategy of medical data to achieve efficient medical data exploration. We use the open source tools to migrate the MIMIC-IV medical database and optimize the sepsis data exploration. The experimental results show that compared with the traditional single node method, our optimization method based on Hive-ORC and its indexes, partition table reduces the storage space by 85% and the query time by 86%. This mechanism has higher efficiency in data management in the medical field. In addition, with the increase of data volume and cluster nodes, the strategy can achieve better optimization results.

Keywords: Hadoop · Hive · Medical big data · Data exploration

1 Introduction

With the progress of information technology, most hospitals and other medical institutions have achieved large-scale informationization. However, the early work of hospital information system (HIS) used traditional relational database [1,2], which can only meet the needs of fast insertion, deletion and query when medical data is relatively small. Until recently, these data have been difficult to obtain, especially large amounts of data, often lacking a useful organization, and therefore are generally underutilized in clinical studies. If

A. Traina et al. (Eds.): HIS 2022, LNCS 13705, pp. 145–156, 2022.
https://doi.org/10.1007/978-3-031-20627-6_14

used effectively, these data may better predict patient outcomes, personalized medication treatment, and more targeted interventions.

Sepsis is a major problem and challenge facing the medical field at present. With the rapid development of modern medicine, the research and exploration of sepsis in various fields has become more and more in-depth measures, but the morbidity and mortality of sepsis remain high. If the electronic case information is used for sepsis-related data exploration in clinical research, it can not only provide a comprehensive diagnosis and treatment reference for clinicians, but also provide a reliable diagnosis and treatment basis for reducing the development of sepsis in infected patients.

Facing the challenges of database management in massive medical data management, Data Warehouse technology is applied to medical data management [3,4]. It can migrate data to Hive data warehouse, query and filter data. By default, data is stored in a text file format. Although this method is more efficient than traditional databases, it still has the possibility of further optimization. Therefore, the method of storing the data in Hive as ORC file format then using the Row Group Index and Bloom Filter Index, and partition the table in Hive to further optimize the query of big data was proposed in this paper. This method will import a public intensive care medical database (mimic-IV) into the relational database MySQL. It uses ordinary PC organizations to build Hadoop distributed clusters, fully migrates data from relational databases to clustered hive data warehouses through Sqoop, and optimizes the exploration of mimic-iv data in Hive.

The rest of this paper is organized as follows. Section 2 presents related work. Section 3 covers data migration and storage. Section 4 introduces the optimization scheme for medical big data exploration. Section 5 presents the experiments performed to evaluate the method and analyzes the experimental results. Section 6 summarizes the paper and points out future research direction.

2 Related Work

In recent years, with the rapid development of computer technology and its wide application in the medical field, the amount of medical data has increased rapidly. Y. Tu et al. [5] has proposed a Spark-based distributed medical big data platform architecture design, which is specially designed for large-scale health data. G. Song et al. [6] introduced a medical service system BDMSP based on big data technology, designed a patient-centered service model, and realized the rational allocation and sharing of medical resources. D. Li et al. [7] proposed a platform named Data Mid-Platform (DMP) to solve the problems of missing information, data dispersion, information islands, and redundancy in most hospitals, and to serve other big data projects as well as scientific.

B. Du et al. [8] designed and implemented a distributed large-scale time series processing analysis system based on Spark platform. In order to improve the analysis efficiency of massive monitoring data of air quality monitoring system, B. Peng et al. [9] proposed a method of storing data in ORC file format based on Hive data warehouse, and then creating Row Group Index and Bloom Filter Index. Optimize the query of the air quality monitoring system. M. Kvet et al. [10] designed experiments using Hadoop, Spark, and Hive transformation tools that transform data from MySQL relational databases to non-relational MongoDB databases, conducting experiments on distributed data in relational and non-relational databases Transformations and queries were compared for performance.

C. M. D. Ranade et al. [11] used the MIMIC-IV database to conduct an exploratory analysis of the disease characteristics and demographic data of neonatal patients. The analysis of the MIMIC-IV database will help researchers gain insight into the characteristics of neonatal diseases and their mortality. Z. Nowroozilaki et al. [12] performed real-time mortality prediction through a comparative analysis of ICU data in MIMIC-IV.

Zhang, Y et al. [13] proposed Health Knowledge Graph Builder (HKGB), an end-to-end platform which could be used to construct disease-specific and extensible health knowledge graphs from multiple sources. Sarki, R et al. [14] established an automatic classification system using deep learning (DL) to classify mild and multi class diseases between healthy or diseased retinas. A. Opaliński et al. [15] integrated data from patients with obstructive sleep apnea (OSA) and proposed a medical data exploration based on an aggregation system of heterogeneous data sources.

Using artificial intelligence to predict sepsis from clinical data, R. M. Demirer et al. [16] developed an AI-based early warning and treatment decision-making system to reduce sepsis-related hospital mortality. N. Shanthi et al. [17] proposed a novel machine learning approach for early prediction of sepsis. A dataset of patients is identified and validated using algorithms with different models to predict performance metrics.

3 Data Storage and Migration

The storage system of the big data platform is mainly composed of HDFS distributed file system and NoSQL non-relational database. The HDFS distributed file system is the underlying storage support of the system. At the end of the day, both structured and unstructured data are stored in the HDFS distributed file system. The NoSQL non-relational database is deployed on the basis of the HDFS distributed file system. The non-relational database used in this article is mainly Hive database. For data migrated to the big data platform, operations such as adding, deleting, modifying, and querying data are also included.

3.1 Data Migration Process

The MIMIC-IV database mainly contains four types of information, namely, the basic information and transfer information of the patient, the relevant information of the patient's hospital outpatient treatment, and the relevant information and auxiliary information of the patient's treatment in the ICU. Almost all mining and analysis of MIMIC-IV database are carried out in traditional relational database. However, in the face of massive data in MIMIC-IV database, traditional relational database cannot efficiently and quickly process the exploration of such data.

First download the original data of the MIMIC-IV database to the nodes of the cluster, configure the software environment in the server cluster, create the corresponding MIMIC-IV database and table in the Mysql database, and import the data into each table through the load command. Structured storage of MIMIC-IV data. Then install the Sqoop plug-in, access each data table through Sqoop, obtain the MIMIC-IV database stored in Mysql and migrate it to the Hive data table. The process of migrating the MIMIC-IV database through Sqoop is shown in Fig. 1.

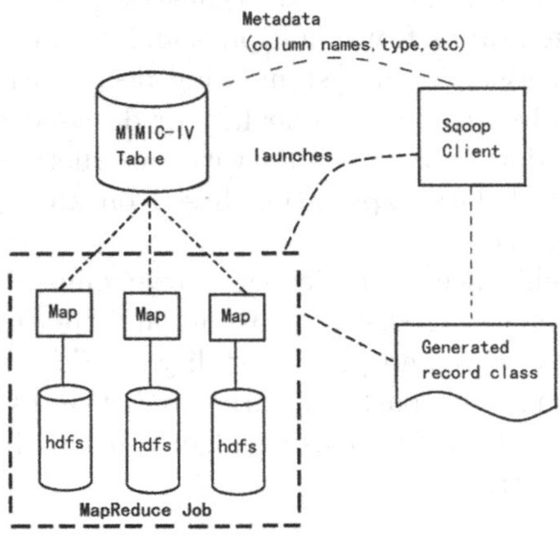

Fig. 1. Data import process.

3.2 Implementation of Data Migration

During the data migration process, there are not only data tables in the database, but also views designed to facilitate our joint query. Therefore, views need to be migrated to Hive along with data tables. The process is shown in Fig. 2.

4 Optimization Method for Medical Big Data

If the possibility of sepsis can be predicted from the characteristics of the population, the pathogen and site of infection, and the severity of the disease in the early stage of infection, an effective clinical scoring system can be used to evaluate patients, and more active measures are taken for patients with high risk of

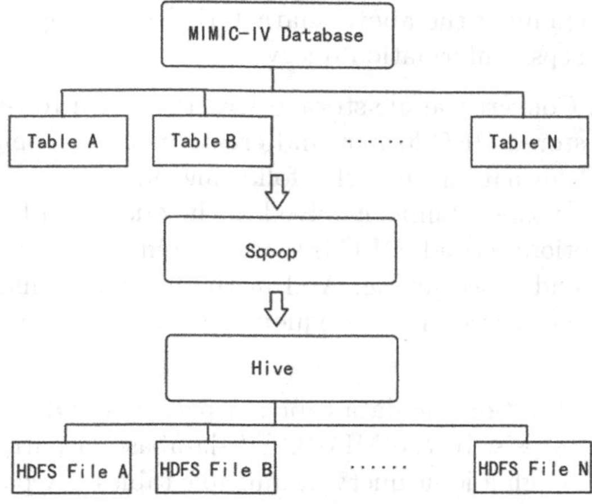

Fig. 2. MIMIC-IV data migration process.

sepsis. Therefore, it is particularly important to efficiently perform sepsis-related data exploration on clinical data.

After the structured medical data is cloned into the Hive data warehouse through Sqoop, the medical structured data is stored in the storage layer in the form of text files. When Hive's filtering query involves some data in the data table, the MapReduce task needs to load the HDFS text file corresponding to the patient information table, and then filter out the data that meets the conditions. Therefore, effectively organizing the file structure of the data table and avoiding full loading or full reading of the file can reduce the time for loading data and the consumption of query calculation.

4.1 MIMIC-IV Data Exploration and Optimization Scheme

In the currently adopted international guidelines for sepsis Sepsis 3.0, infection + SOFA score ≥ 2 is used as the diagnostic criteria for sepsis. In this paper, the data exploration and optimization of MIMIC-IV database is mainly divided into hot query and sepsis information query. It is known from the hospital research that the hot query includes querying the patient's blood chemical indexes and querying the items related to blood gas in the patient's perspective. The sepsis information query is the value measured for the first time after the patient enters the ICU. The above two parts of the query are both linked table queries on the MIMIC-IV database.

By analyzing the MIMIC-IV data table, we can find that the table with a large amount of data has two characteristics: First, the number of columns is fixed, but the number of rows is much larger than the number of columns. For example, the number of columns in a patient information table is only 6, but the number of rows is hundreds of thousands; secondly, a table with a large amount of data has hundreds of millions of rows, but the value of a column is hundreds of fixed values. Combining the above characteristics, two optimization schemes for hot query and sepsis information query are proposed:

Optimization 1: Convert the file storage structure from row-stored TXT text format to column-stored ORC format and create indexes. Compared with TXT text format, ORC format file has the following advantages: First, ORC is a column store, so only the columns involved in the query can be read, which can reduce IO consumption; second, ORC is stored in binary mode, which has higher compression ratio and space saving. And in the hot query, indexes are created for the fields that are queried more frequently to reduce the time consuming of the hot query.

Optimization 2: Partition the data table. A patient's SOFA score is the diagnostic criterion for sepsis. In the MIMIC-IV database, a patient's SOFA score can be obtained through a joint query of multiple tables. By partitioning sepsis-related tables, load consumption can be reduced. For example, the chartevents table has more than 300 million rows of data, but the itemid value of a column of patients is only 2226. The table is partitioned based on the itemid column. Hive can select read table partitions based on filter conditions to reduce load consumption. For the same reason, the labevents table is also partitioned on the itemid column to optimize sepsis-related data exploration.

4.2 Importing Data into ORC Table and Creating Views

After the table is created, the data from the TextFile table needs to be imported into it. Because of the rowgroup index, when importing data, the data must be sorted by the index column. Also put the partition field itemid at the end and insert it into the ORC table.

After storing the MIMIC-IV database in hive, we need to create multiple views to efficiently complete the hot query and data exploration of sepsis to quickly query age, height, weight, complications, experiments within 24 h of entering the ICU Room indicators, vital signs, sofa, sapsii score, ventilation, medication and other information. The concept of views created in Hive is the same as that of views created in RDBMS. When a query references a view, Hive combines the view's definition with the query. We implements joint query of multiple tables by creating views on MySQL and Hive, and records the execution time of the query for analogy. Finally, the query performance is plotted and displayed on a graph.

5 Experiment and Analysis

To evaluate the performance of the method proposed in this paper, an experiment was designed to compare the efficiency of hot query and sepsis data exploration in the MIMIC-IV database. On Hive, compare the execution time of five view queries between the method of default storage as textfile and the method of creating ORC partition table and indexing proposed in this paper. Each query is executed three times, and the average is taken as the experimental result.

5.1 Experimental Environment

The hardware environment of the cluster is shown in Table 1, and the host is used to build a cluster with a master-slave structure.

Table 1. System configuration.

Manufacturer	Lenevo
Processor	11th Gen IntelR coreT i7-11700F@ 2.50 GHz ×16
Installed memory	16.00 GB (15.4 GB usable)
System type	Ubuntu 18.04.6 LTS 64-bit Operating system

The software environment of the cluster is shown in Table 2. Hadoop, Hive, and Sqoop are all programs written in the Java language. Firstly, we need to install the operating system and the Java software development kit.

Table 2. System configuration.

Name	Version	Remarks
JDK	1.8.0	JAVA Software development kit
Hadoop	2.7.2	Distributed architecture (with MapReduce)
Hive	2.3.6	WareHouse
Sqoop	1.4.6	ETL Tools
Tez	0.9.1	Hive engine
MySQL	8.0.28	Relational database

5.2 Experimental Data and Scheme

There are 27 tables in the MIMIC-IV database, including the emar_detail table, the labevents table, and the chartevents table. The chartevents table has 329499789 rows of data. When stored in textfile format, the size is 32G. However, when stored as Orc file format, its size is 4.13G. It can be seen that the orc format file reduces the storage space required by the chartevents table by 87%. This is because the orc file uses the compressed storage method and the data is compressed according to the specified format. Like the chartevents table, the storage space required for the labevents table and emar_detail is reduced by 82% and 93%, respectively, when stored in the Orc file format. The data set information is shown in Table 3.

Experiments for query comparison of hot queries and sepsis-related information were performed by querying five views in the MIMIC-IV database in

Table 3. Detail of the experiment data sets.

Table	Size of TextFile	Size of ORC	Reduction of size
chartevents	32G	4.13G	87%
labevents	15G	2.63G	82%
emar_detail	10G	0.63G	93%

MySQL and hive, respectively. The first chemistry view is designed to query and aggregate blood chemistry indicators as the center, and the second bg view is designed to query the entries related to blood gas. It is known from the hospital study that these two views are hot query, and the above two views are used in most data query process. The following three views provide the indicators of the patient's first day of admission to the ICU. The third view provides the minimum, maximum and average values of the vital signs measured on the first day, and the fourth view provides the minimum and maximum values of the laboratory parameters measured on the first day. Based on these two views, Information about sepsis in ICU patients can be queried and extracted in the fifth view. Table 4 gives the list of query statements for MySQL and Hive:

Table 4. List of executed queries.

Query No.	Query	Query description
Q1	Select * from chemistry;	This query pivots laboratory indicators and aggregates them
Q2	Select * from bg;	The aim of this query is to pivot entries related to blood gases
Q3	Select * from first_day_vitalsign	This query pivots vital signs and aggregates them
Q4	Select * from first_day_lab;	Minimum and maximum measured value of the first day in the laboratory
Q5	Select * from first_day_sofa;	This query extracts the sequential organ failure assessment

Default methods and Proposed optimization methods are used for queries in hive, and tez is used for execution engines in hive. Each of the above five views is queried three times and tested on multiple clusters. Finally, the average execution time is calculated as the experimental result.

5.3 Experimental Results and Analysis

The queries are executed on five different views, each query is executed three times, and the Q3, Q4, Q5 queries are compared in a cluster of 3 to 8 nodes.

Finally, the average execution time is calculated as the experimental result. The final test time is shown in Table 5, Table 6 and Fig. 3. The comparison results between the two optimization methods and hive's default method are shown in Fig. 4. As the number of nodes in the cluster increases, the time-consuming comparison of Q3, Q4, Q5 queries is shown in Fig. 5.

Table 5. Execution time (min) using different methods.

Query No.	MySQL	Hive on Tez	Hive-ORC	Hive partition	Hive-orc and partition
Q1	8	2.2	1.9	1.6	1.4
Q2	15	9.6	5.8	3.3	1.5
Q3	19	9.2	5.1	3.9	2.7
Q4	40	10.3	7.1	5.8	4.6
Q5	116	61.4	48.3	18.9	16.1

Table 6. Execution time (min) using different nodes.

Number of nodes	3	4	5	6	7
Q3	2.7	2.3	1.9	1.6	1.4
Q4	4.6	4.1	3.7	3.3	2.9
Q5	16.1	14.2	11.9	10.6	9.7

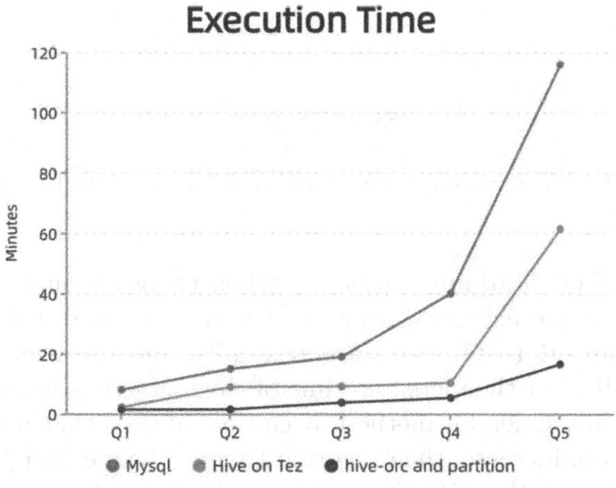

Fig. 3. Time consuming comparison of query statements.

As we can see from Table 5, when using MySQL, the average execution time of Q5 is 116 min. When using Hive and Tez as the computing engine, the average

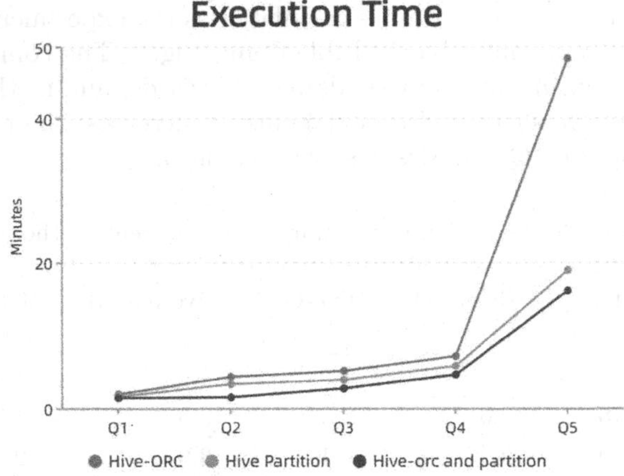

Fig. 4. Time consuming comparison of different methods in Hive.

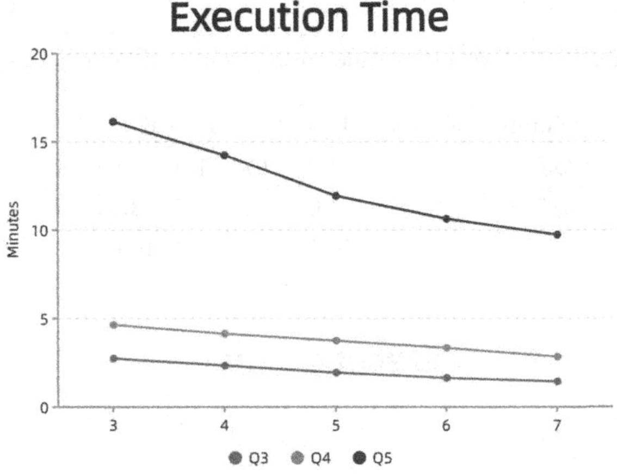

Fig. 5. Time consuming comparison of different nodes in a cluster.

execution time of Q5 is 61 min. However, when using the method proposed in this paper, its average execution time is 16 min. The total amount of data to be processed from Q1 to Q5 increases gradually, and the execution time also increases gradually, but the increased time of the method proposed in this paper is less than that of the default method. It can be inferred that when the amount of data continues to increase, the execution time of the method proposed in this paper will still be less than Hive's default method, and the optimization effect of the method proposed in this paper will be better.

5.4 Analysis

Since Hive is deployed on a cluster and can use MapReduce for parallel computing, it can support large-scale data. Therefore, using tez computing engine in hive takes less time than mysql. Optimized hot queries and sepsis queries took less time. On the one hand, after the table is changed from the text file storage structure to the orc column storage structure, the column data database scans the data in a column by column manner. Therefore, when the amount of data is large, the column data has better scanning efficiency and effectively reduces the time-consuming of hot query. On the other hand, the sepsis related tables are partitioned to reduce the data set, so as to avoid full table scanning, improve query speed and performance.

6 Conclusion and Future Work

There are a lot of structured data in medical data. The traditional business relational database is limited by poor scalability and high cost. Combined with MapReduce architecture in big data technology, this paper migrates the data in mimic-iv medical database from relational database MySQL to Hadoop cluster through sqoop, carries out distributed storage and query of medical structure in NoSQL database Hive, and optimizes the query speed. In the future, we will focus on the storage and fusion of medical multi-source heterogeneous data. We not only convert medical multi-source heterogeneous data into a unified data model to store data efficiently and permanently, but also fuse and effectively centralize the scattered data after medical data storage.

Acknowledgements. This work was supported in part by the China Postdoctoral Science Foundation under Grant 2020M672217, and in part by the Science and Technology Research Key Project of Henan Province Science and Technology Department under Grant 222102210133.

References

1. Joyce, A.M., Naddaf-Dezfbli, A., Davenport, S.L.: A medical microcomputer database management system. Methods Inf. Med. **24**(02), 73–78 (1985)
2. Mohamad, B., d'Orazio, L., Gruenwald, L.: Towards a hybrid row-column database for a cloud-based medical data management system. In: Proceedings of the 1st International Workshop on Cloud Intelligence, pp. 1–4 (2012)
3. Sebaa, A., Chikh, F., Nouicer, A., Tari, A.: Medical big data warehouse: architecture and system design, a case study: improving healthcare resources distribution. J. Med. Syst. **42**(4), 1–16 (2018)
4. Farooqui, N.A., Mehra, R.: Design of a data warehouse for medical information system using data mining techniques. In: 2018 Fifth International Conference on Parallel, Distributed and Grid Computing (PDGC), pp. 199–203. IEEE (2018)
5. Tu, Y., Lu, Y., Chen, G., Zhao, J., Yi, F.: Architecture design of distributed medical big data platform based on spark. In: 2019 IEEE 8th Joint International Information Technology and Artificial Intelligence Conference (ITAIC), pp. 682–685. IEEE (2019)

6. Song, G., Wen, Y., Jia, Y., Liu, H.: Research on medical service system based on big data technology. In: 2019 International Conference on Intelligent Transportation, Big Data & Smart City (ICITBS), pp. 302–304. IEEE (2019)
7. Li, D., Ye, Z., Li, L., Wei, X., Qin, B., Li, Y.: Practical data mid-platform design and implementation for medical big data. In: 2019 IEEE 4th Advanced Information Technology, Electronic and Automation Control Conference (IAEAC), vol. 1, pp. 1042–1045. IEEE (2019)
8. Du, B.: Distributed large-scale time-series data processing and analysis system based on spark platform. In: 2021 International Conference on Big Data Analysis and Computer Science (BDACS), pp. 105–110. IEEE (2021)
9. Peng, B., Liu, L.: Query optimization for air quality big data based on hive-orc. In: 2020 5th International Conference on Control, Robotics and Cybernetics (CRC), pp. 19–23. IEEE (2020)
10. Čerešňák, R., Kvet, M.: Comparison of distributed data transformation and comparing query performance in relational and non-relational database. In: 2019 17th International Conference on Emerging eLearning Technologies and Applications (ICETA), pp. 108–114. IEEE (2019)
11. Ranade, M.D., Deshpande, A.: Exploratory analysis of disease characteristics and demographic data of neonatal patients using MIMIC-IV database. In: 2021 International Conference on Communication Information and Computing Technology (ICCICT), pp. 1–6. IEEE (2021)
12. Nowroozilarki, Z., Pakbin, A., Royalty, J., Lee, D.K., Mortazavi, B.J.: Real-time mortality prediction using MIMIC-IV ICU data via boosted nonparametric hazards. In: 2021 IEEE EMBS International Conference on Biomedical and Health Informatics (BHI), pp. 1–4. IEEE (2021)
13. Zhang, Y., et al.: HKGB: an inclusive, extensible, intelligent, semi-auto-constructed knowledge graph framework for healthcare with clinicians' expertise incorporated. Inf. Process. Manage. **57**(6), 102324 (2020)
14. Sarki, R., Ahmed, K., Wang, H., Zhang, Y.: Automated detection of mild and multi-class diabetic eye diseases using deep learning. Health Inf. Sci. Syst. **8**(1), 1–9 (2020)
15. Opaliński, A., et al.: Medical data exploration based on the heterogeneous data sources aggregation system. In: 2019 Federated Conference on Computer Science and Information Systems (FedCSIS), pp. 591–597. IEEE (2019)
16. Demirer, R.M., Demirer, O.: Early prediction of sepsis from clinical data using artificial intelligence. In: 2019 Scientific Meeting on Electrical-Electronics & Biomedical Engineering and Computer Science (EBBT), pp. 1–4. IEEE (2019)
17. Shanthi, N., et al.: A novel machine learning approach to predict sepsis at an early stage. In: 2022 International Conference on Computer Communication and Informatics (ICCCI), pp. 1–7. IEEE (2022)

Improving Data Analytic Performance in Health Information System with Big Data Technology

Hung Ba Ngo[1](✉) and Nguyen Chi Tran[2]

[1] Can Tho University, Can Tho, Vietnam
nbhung@cit.ctu.edu.vn
[2] VNPT Ca Mau, Ca Mau, Vietnam

Abstract. For many years, the Health Information System (HIS) has been an integral part of the day-to-day operations of healthcare organizations such as clinical centers and hospitals. HIS collects, stores and manages healthcare data from different sources related to patients' electronic medical record and other daily operational activities of healthcare organizations. HIS analyzes its database to create reports that help healthcare organizations improve patient outcomes, quality of services, treatment cost efficiency and support healthcare policy decisions. Over time, the HIS data has grown enormously and that makes the HIS's data analytic module become overloaded, affecting the overall system performance of HIS and resulting in a denial of service from HIS. This paper presents a case study of applying big data technology to improve the performance of data analytic modules in a traditional HIS.

Keywords: Health information system · HIS · Business intelligence · BI · Big data · Performance · Hadoop · Analysis

1 Introduction

Hospital Information System (HIS) is an integrated information system that collects, stores and processes healthcare data from different sources to support a hospital's operational activities in all aspects, such as administrative, financial and clinical work. HIS is used to digitize business processes such as patient admission, therapeutic actions, medication orders and diagnostics, accounting, pharmacy, and warehouse in a healthcare organization [1]. HIS can help an organization avoid duplication data created and tasks done between units, integrate patient's data created from different sources into patients' electronic medical records that are quickly and efficiently exchanged between staff so that staff efficiency and quality of healthcare outcome are improved. In addition, many analysis reports related to different aspects such as patient's diagnosis, financial report, staff performance, facility, pharmacy need to be submitted by a healthcare organization to different stakeholders for different purposes at different times and periods. For instance, a typical public hospital of a city or province in Vietnam has to create 67 annual reports for the City Health Department, 8 monthly, quarterly and annual reports

A. Traina et al. (Eds.): HIS 2022, LNCS 13705, pp. 157–164, 2022.
https://doi.org/10.1007/978-3-031-20627-6_15

for Health insurance agencies, 5 monthly, quarterly and annual reports for social insurance agencies and dozens of daily reports for the purpose of internal management. These kinds of reports are so-called operational reports. The main goal of operational reports is to ensure effective operation of health organizations. They are generated by an analytic module of HIS, a kind of descriptive analytic to tell administrative staff what was happening in a health organization. In a traditional HIS, analytic module explores relational databases from different modules of HIS to generate operational reports, typically using SQL to aggregate and statistically analyze. Through time, HIS data volume is increasing, making the analytic module of HIS consume much calculating resources. In some cases, when the analytic module is activated, the performance of the whole HIS system becomes very poor; the other modules of HIS are stalled. In this paper, a popular used HIS in Vietnam, so-called VN-HIS, is taken as a case study. VN-HIS was deployed as a cloud service and is being used by 6,500 commune health stations, 270 district health centers and 200 provincial specialized hospitals in Vietnam. Usually there is one VN-HIS instance serving for commune health stations and district health centers of a province and one instance for each provincial specialized hospital. For instance, in the province where this research took place, there is one VN-HIS instance serving 101 commune health stations and 8 district health centers and 3 instances for 3 provincial specialized hospitals. In 30 months, from January 2017 to June 2020, four VN-HIS instances in the province generated around 250 Gbytes of data in their relational databases and around 13 Terabytes of data in whole Vietnam. As being designed a long time ago, based entirely on relational database techniques, recently, when performing the functions of creating reports, VN-HIS in the studied province and many other provinces operated very slowly, even stalled, denying the use of other functions. This paper presents the results of a case study in applying big data technology to improve the performance of data analytic modules in the process of creating analysis reports of a traditional HIS, such as VN-HIS. The next section presents more details about technical aspects used by VN-HIS and big data technologies related to the proposed solution. The third section will introduce a new big data technology-based data analytic module proposed for VN-HIS to improve its performance. The implementation and testing results will be discussed in the fourth section. The conclusion and future work will be presented in the last section.

2 Related Works

VN-HIS provides functions that cover 10 general aspects related to healthcare organizations in Vietnam such as outpatient treatment management, inpatient treatment management, hospital's fee, medical and biomedical equipment management, health insurance settlement, diagnostic imaging, laboratory management, medical procedures and surgery, and operational analysis reporting. VN-HIS represents a typical HIS designed as a web-based application without using big data technology, developed based on Java Spring MVC framework and using Oracle 12.c as database management system. To enhance performance and throughput, VN-HIS is deployed into two layers. The first layer is a cluster of application servers orchestrated by a load balancing server supporting horizontal scaling. The second layer is a high performance database server using vertical scaling. Nine of ten modules of VN-HIS respond well to workloads in almost every use case using this deployment model but the data analytic module. A test case at the studied hospital where VN-HIS was deployed on a cluster of 4 application servers (CPU 32 cores, 36 GB RAM), and a database server (CPU 48 cores, 96 GB RAM). The real data of the hospital from January 2017 to June 2020 was used. It showed that it took from six to nine minutes to create several analysis reports related to the data created from January 2020 to June 2020. Moreover, while the reports were being generated the other modules were almost out of service. The whole system was considered to be in stall. The analysis showed that the data analytic module needed to access data from 67 tables with the data in six months around 225 Gbytes and 209 million rows. In 9 min of creating reports, 100% of the CPU is occupied and used by the operational report module. Data warehouse technology can be used to improve data analysis and report creation in information systems [19]. Data warehouse is a subject oriented, nonvolatile, integrated, time variant collection of data in support of management decisions [18]. Data warehouse is the core component of Business Intelligence (BI) solutions [2, 15] that support descriptive analytics [10]. A solution transforming a traditional online transactional processing (OLTP) system in healthcare towards building an online analytical processing (OLAP) solution based on relational database is proposed by [3] so that HIS can focus more on data analytics to provide healthcare organization with new business solutions and more insight of the organization. Recently, Big data technology with the capacity to handle large amounts of data that is unmanageable using traditional software and relational databases can enhance the BI solution in HIS with new capabilities to not only provide analysis reports but also data interpretation in supporting decision making [11]. With the nature of big data that can handle data in different formats such as structured data, semi structured data and unstructured data, BI in healthcare can be enhanced with smarter and cost-effective descriptive, diagnostic, predictive, prescriptive analysis reports [12, 20]. Many existing big data tools and technologies that are ready for healthcare in management, analysis and future prospects are identified in [12]. The next section will propose a solution that is applying big data technology to improve data analysis performance of traditional health information systems.

3 Applying Big Data Technology to Improve Data Analytic Performance in Traditional Health Information Systems

This section uses VN-HIS as a traditional health information system that implements OLAP to provide operational reports and has a big problem in performance when its related database increases in volume. A new data analytic module using big data technology will be integrated into VN-HIS to provide the same previous operational reports with improved performance. When the new data analytic module is running to generate required reports, it must not affect the performance of the other modules of VN-HIS.

3.1 Conceptual Model of Proposed Data Analytic Module for HIS

The conceptual model for the new data analytic module, so-called HIS-BI is presented in Fig. 1 with seven components.

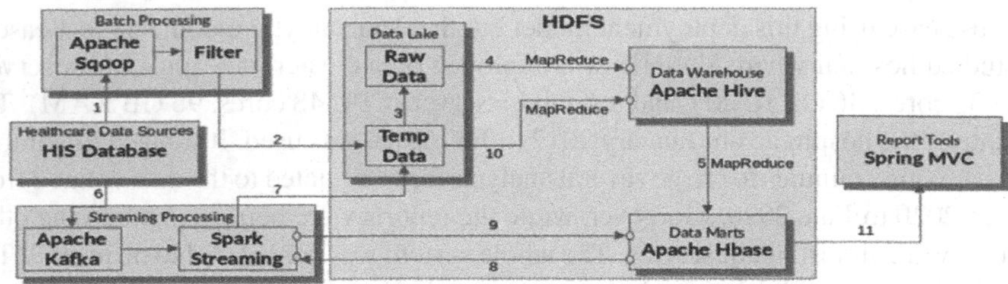

Fig. 1. A big data technology-based conceptual model of data analytic module for HIS.

Healthcare Data Sources: This component represents data sources related to healthcare that can be collected for a later analysis process. It may be structured data in HIS databases and other semi structured and unstructured data created by file systems or medical devices from the past to a determined point of time.
Batch Processing: This component is responsible for transforming related data existing in HIS database into text format to be stored in Data Lake.
Streaming Processing: This component is responsible for collecting data created and modified in HIS databases after the transformation point of time determined in Batch processing, transforming them into text format to be stored in Data Lake and Data Marts.
Data Lake [14]: This component stores the whole HIS data in the form of text, which is divided into a raw pool and a temp pool. The raw pool contains whole data collected from the Batch Processing and Streaming Process, which is the principal data used to create a Data Warehouse. The temp pool is used to store data collected by Streaming Processing, usually with small size for necessary processing before inserting them to the Data Warehouse without accessing data in the big size raw pool.
Data Warehouse: This component receives data from the Data Lake after normalizing and filtering unnecessary data for generating reports. This data is analyzed later by big data technology such as Mapreduce to create the results in the form of text files that will be stored in appropriate data marts.
Data Marts with small size and subject-oriented data make analysis processing more efficient in terms of time.
Report Tools: This component provides a user interface to access reports generated from data stored in Data Marts.

3.2 Implementation Model of HIS-BI

The HIS-BI solution is implemented using big data technology and tools as described in Fig. 2. Apache Sqoop [9] is used to transfer all data in the relational database of VN-HIS into text format and effectively store it in the big data file system HDFS [16].

Each row in a table will be converted into a line (1). Only tables necessary for report generation will be taken into account by Sqoop. The filter will eliminate duplicate data from being collected and stored in the Temp Data pool of HDFS (2). Periodically, data from Temp Data pool will be moved to Raw Data pool (3). A Hadoop MapReduce [4, 13] process will read data from the Raw Data pool (4) to create multidimensional and time series data for the Data Warehouse component implemented by Apache Hive [6].

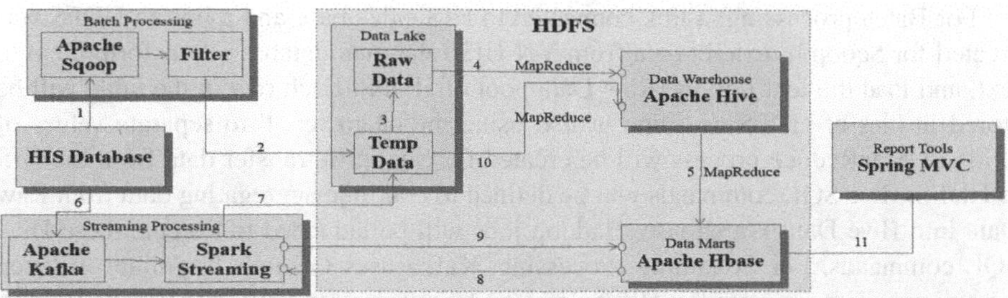

Fig. 2. A big data technology-based implementation model of data analytic module for HIS.

Several MapReduce processes are used to create data marts for specific subjects that contain data ready for analysis to generate specific groups of reports (5). In the case study, 4 data marts were created for specific subjects for HIS reports. Hbase [5] is used to store Data Marts. The workflow from (1) to (5), so-called Batch Processing workflow, is usually executed one time to feed the Data Warehouse with the HIS's data from the past until a determined point of time. Next, the Streaming Processing workflow will be executed periodically to update the Data Warehouse and the Data Marts with the new income data in HIS's database. In the Streaming Processing workflow, new income data in HIS's database (6) will be buffed in Kafka [7] and processed by Spark [8] to create text data having the same format as step (2) and stored in Temp Data pool (7) which is periodically processed by a MapReduce process (10) to update Data Warehouse then moved to Raw Data pool (3). To quickly update reports with this new incoming data, Spark will calculate and update Data Marts with new incoming data (8), (9). Report Tools is a web-based application using data from Data Marts to create operational reports.

4 Experiment and Results

The proposed solution HIS-BI was deployed onto an experimental cluster of one master node and seven slave nodes with big data tools installed as illustrated in Fig. 3. On HDFS, 4 predefined directories (/temp, /raw-his, /hive and /hbase) were reserved for storing data of Temp Data pool, Raw Data pool, Hive database and Hbase database. In Hive Data Warehouse, objects/entities related to the operational reports for HIS were created. In Hbase Data Marts, one or more tables that contained data for each type of report were created.

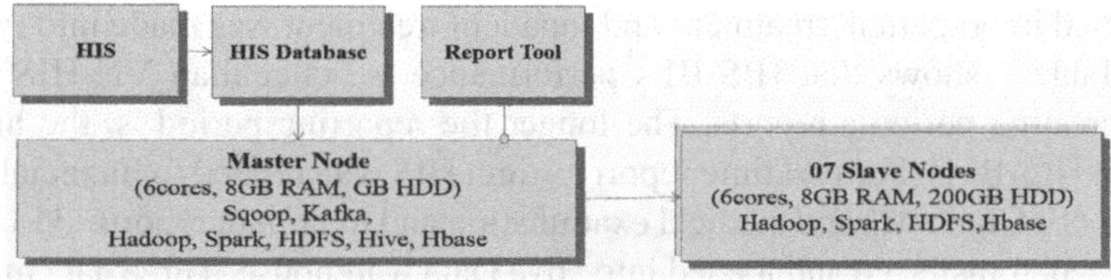

Fig. 3. Experiment model of proposed data analytic module for HIS.

For Batch processing, a link connected to HIS's database and a link to HDFS was created for Sqoop to extract data from VN-HIS relational database, transform them to text, and load the text into the Raw Data pool of HDFS. Each row in the table will be stored in files of HDFS as a line of text using the character '|' to separate values of fields. A MapReduce process will be created for Sqoop to transfer data from the HIS to HDFS. Hive SQL commands will be defined to continue aggregating data from Raw Data into Hive Data Warehouse. Hadoop jobs will be launched to execute these Hive SQL commands. For Streaming Processing, Kafka uses Oracle's Logminer to listen for any new data generated in HIS's data and feed them into Spark for processing. An application needs to be developed using Spark API to process new data and load it to Temp Data, to update Raw Data, Data Warehouse and Data Marts. Report Tool is a web-based application deployed on a laptop getting data from Data smart to present different kinds of operation analysis reports for users.

Table 1. Time generating reports of VN-HIS report module and HIS-BI module.

Report types	VN-HIS (second)	HIS-BI (second)
Monthly reports	6	0.12
Quarterly-reports	10	0.13
Half year reports	13	0.14
Annual reports	30	0.64
Two years report	10	1.40
Three years report	200	2.00
Online reports	5	0.12

The experiment used real data from VN-HIS deployed in the cloud to serve 101 commune health stations, 8 district health centers, and 3 provincial specialized hospitals in the studied province of Vietnam. The database contained data from January 2017 to October 2020. Time for generating each type of report by the VN-HIS module and by the new HIS-BI was measured. Each type of report was repeated 5 times with 15 min of delay between two successive times to ensure that the data were not cached by Oracle server.

First, 14 Gbytes data of inpatient treatment and 16 Gbytes data of outpatient treatment were loaded into Data Warehouse and Data Marts by Batch processing workflow consuming 572 s to complete. Next, a test for creating a periodical report related to medicine used in outpatient treatment and inpatient treatment was made into two report modules. Table 1 shows that HIS-BI's performance is better than VN-HIS's performance in creating periodic reports. The longer the reporting period is, the higher the time gain of HIS-BI is. For real time report testing, HIS data related to financial supervision reports (17 Gigabyte) and medical examination and treatment reports (31 Gigabyte) were extracted, transferred and loaded into Hive Data warehouse. Three data marts were created for online reports related to medical examination, subclinical, and hospital fees. The average time for generating online reports by the VN-HIS module and by the new

HIS-BI was measured in the last line of Table 1. It shows that the new HIS-BI has more performance than the traditional VN-HIS module. So in both of the cases, the new HIS-BI module using big data technologies and tools demonstrates better performance in creating healthcare reports than does the traditional HIS based on OLAP model with related databases.

5 Conclusions and Future Work

The data analytic module in an HIS analyzes its databases to create reports that can help healthcare organizations improve patient outcomes, quality of services, treatment cost efficiency and support healthcare policy decisions. When HIS data increases in volume, using OLAP models on related databases to create operational reports can cause HIS's performance to slow down, even stop other HIS modules. This paper proposes to integrate into traditional HIS a new data analytic module based on big data technology and tools to improve performance of HIS's data analysis. The Batch Processing workflow transfers all data in relational databases of HIS into text format and stores them in a Data Lake where the data are ready to be extracted, transformed into subject, multidimensional and time serial data to load into a Data Warehouse. For each type of required reports, a data mart is defined to extract from the Data Warehouse the data that is only required for the corresponding report. The size of data marts is too small in comparison to a data warehouse's size. That explains why the creation time of reports from data marts is very short. For the updated data in HIS's database, after Batch Processing has finished, Streaming Processing Workflow will collect these new incoming data, process them and update Data Lake, Data Warehouse and Data marts correspondingly. The proposed solution chose the most efficient tools in the domain such as HDFS file system, Hive database, and Hbase database for big data storage, and Hadoop and Spark for big data processing. Experiments were established with real data from VN-HIS deployed and used by healthcare organizations in the provinces of Vietnam. The testing results show that the new HIS-BI module based on big data technology gives good performance in creating operational reports required by VN-HIS. For future work, the proposed solution can be extended to store HIS's semi-structured data and unstructured data such as healthcare documents, scanning images in HDFS so that they can be ready to be analyzed using data mining techniques and tools. Analyzing these semi structured data and unstructured data can give healthcare professionals more insight and better decision making for their organizations.

References

1. Aghazadeh, S., Aliyev, A., Ebrahimnezhad, M.: Review the role of hospital information systems in medical services development. Int. J. Comput. Theory Eng. **4**(6), 866–870 (2012)
2. Alhyasat, E.B., Al-Dalahmeh, M.: Data warehouse success and strategic oriented business intelligence. A theoretical framework. J. Manag. Res. **5**(3) (2013)
3. Ali-Ozkan, O., Nassif, A., Capretz, L.: Business intelligence solutions in healthcare a case study: transforming OLTP system to BI solution. In: The 3rd International Conference on Communications and Information Technology, pp. 209–214. IEEE, Lebanon (2013)

4. Apache Hadoop. https://hadoop.apache.org
5. Apache Hbase. https://hbase.apache.org
6. Apache Hive. https://hive.apache.org
7. Apache Kafka. https://kafka.apache.org
8. Apache Spark. https://spark.apache.org
9. Apache Sqoop. https://attic.apache.org/projects/sqoop.html
10. Bayrak, T.: A review of business analytics: a business enabler or another passing fad. Proc. – Soc. Behav. Sci. **195**, 230–239 (2015)
11. Chen, K.L., Lee, H.: The impact of big data on the healthcare information systems. In: Transactions of the International Conference on Health Information Technology Advancement, p. 25. WMU (2013). https://scholarworks.wmich.edu/ichita_transactions/25
12. Dash, S., Shakyawar, S.K., Sharma, M., et al.: Big data in healthcare: management, analysis and future prospects. J. Big Data **6**, 54 (2019)
13. Dean, J., Ghemawat, S.: MapReduce: simplified data processing on large clusters. In: The 6th conference on Symposium on Operating Systems Design & Implementation, vol. 6, pp. 137–150. USENIX, US (2004)
14. Fang, H.: Managing data lakes in big data era: what's a data lake and why has it became popular in data management ecosystem. In: 2015 IEEE International Conference on Cyber Technology in Automation, Control, and Intelligent Systems (CYBER), pp 820–824. IEEE, China (2015)
15. Gad-Elrab, A.A.A.: Chapter 8 modern business intelligence: big data analytics and artificial intelligence for creating the data-driven value. In: E-Business - Higher Education and Intelligence Applications, 19 May 2021. https://doi.org/10.5772/intechopen.97374. ISBN 978-1-78984-685-0
16. HDFS Architecture Guide. https://hadoop.apache.org/docs/r1.2.1/hdfs_design.html
17. IBM Cloud Learn Hub. https://www.ibm.com/cloud/learn/data-mart
18. Inmon, W.H.: What is a data warehouse? Prism Solutions, Inc. (1995). www.cait.wustl.edu/cait/papers/prism/vol1_no1/
19. Sharma, S., Jain, R.: Enhancing business intelligence using data warehousing: a multi case analysis. Int. J. Adv. Res. Comput. Sci. Manag. Stud. **1**(7), 40–56 (2013)
20. Sun, Z., Zou, H., Strang, K.: Big data analytics as a service for business intelligence. In: Janssen, M., et al. (eds.) I3E 2015. LNCS, vol. 9373, pp. 200–211. Springer, Cham (2015). https://doi.org/10.1007/978-3-319-25013-7_16

HoloCleanX: A Multi-source Heterogeneous Data Cleaning Solution Based on Lakehouse

Qin Cui[1], Wenkui Zheng[1(✉)], Wei Hou[1], Ming Sheng[2], Peng Ren[2], Wang Chang[1], and XiangYang Li[3]

[1] Henan University, Kaifeng 475004, China
zwk@vip.henu.edu.cn
[2] BNRist, DCST, RIIT, Tsinghua University, Beijing 100084, China
{shengming,renpeng}@tsinghua.edu.cn
[3] Beijing SGITG-Accenture Information Technology Co., Ltd., Beijing 100031, China

Abstract. The storage of multi-source heterogeneous data has been solved effectively by using Lakehouse, but there are no universal and effective solutions for cleaning in existing systems. Based on Lakehouse MHDP, this paper proposes a cleaning scheme with interactivity based on DCs (Denial Constraints) for cleaning multi-source heterogeneous data. Firstly, we optimize Holoclean to achieve better results on small datasets, which improves F1 by at least 5%. Furthermore, we propose algorithms to parse various types of data, which can effectively reconstruct data. Secondly, we implement an interactive system with real-time feedback which extracts and visualizes the basic metadata and allows users to participate in cleaning work by building DCs. Finally, the cleaned data is saved in the original data format without removing the original data. The experiment results prove that our solution can effectively clean multi-source heterogeneous data with both high accuracy and easy usability.

Keywords: Multi-source heterogeneous data · Data cleaning · MHDP · Holoclean · Lakehouse

1 Introduction

With the rapid advancement of Big Data technology in numerous industries, data from a single source is no longer sufficient for large-scale data analysis [1–4]. For example, multi-source data with the same concept, such as user information, must be combined for integrated analysis. Structured tables, semi-structured files, and unstructured images are all common data structures in multi-source data. The fusion and storage problems of multi-source heterogeneous data have been well solved, as evidenced by research for elevator data [5], a framework for Multi-Source Data Fusion [6], and MHDP [7] for medical data, etc. However, there are no general and effective cleaning solutions, and data cleaning solutions typically focus on specific data contents [8, 9].

Challenge. The fusion effect of multi-source heterogeneous data can be affected by the quality of the original data [10], and data cleaning usually occurs before and after the

A. Traina et al. (Eds.): HIS 2022, LNCS 13705, pp. 165–176, 2022.
https://doi.org/10.1007/978-3-031-20627-6_16

data fusion, which is optional, so a fixed cleaning procedure is not flexible to cope with this process. Consequently, there are three challenges as follows:

1. Independence: Data cleaning should be performed at any time and does not affect other data processing tasks such as data storage or data analysis
2. Effectiveness: It should be able to handle data of all sizes, and produce high-quality cleansed data.
3. Generality: It should be able to deal with different kinds of data from different sources.

Contribution. This paper introduces HoloCleanX, an extension of HoloClean [11] for multi-source heterogeneous data based on the MHDP. To address the three challenges mentioned above, we contributed to three aspects as follows:

1. We propose the HoloCleanX framework, based on the Lakehouse MHDP, for cleaning structured data with ER relationships, such as SQL, or semi-structured data, such as nested JSONs, to No SQL data in Key-Value stores, such as HBase.
2. We design a new algorithm to better handle multi-source data, which has better results in processing small data.
3. We design a visible interactive interface with real-time feedback to make data cleaning an independent systematic task, allowing professionals to contribute DCs and providing tailored cleaning solutions.

In this paper, Sect. 2 will contain references to related work. Section 3 will cover the HoloCleanX framework. The Framework's specified layers will be described in depth. Section 4 contains the input layer, Sect. 5 contains the data cleaning and data export layers, Sect. 6 contains the implementation and specifics of the real-time feedback interactivity, and Sect. 7 contains the conclusion and future development. Furthermore, the contribution of these three elements above is contained in Sects. 4, 5, and 6.

2 Related Work

This section presents three parts of our research: cleaning methods in multi-source heterogeneous data processing platforms, cleaning methods that have been proposed for multi-source heterogeneous data, and effective methods for general dataset cleaning.

The study of cleaning methods in multi-source heterogeneous data processing platforms. The process of multi-source heterogeneous data processing or professional platform does not have a common data cleaning scheme or no cleaning [5, 12]. H Li et al. proposed establishing constraints based on the dataset itself to detect and correct anonymous data before fusing multi-source heterogeneous power system log data [13]. A Gledson et al. decoupled the data cleaning of multi-source data and encapsulated it into an interface for user selection [14]. C Wang et al. performed simple processing of multi-source heterogeneous data from elevators [6]. Q Yuan et al. standardized the data from each source before data fusion for grid data [15], etc. We deploy cleaning work on MHDP, a high arithmetic platform, to improve cleaning performance.

The study of cleaning methods for multi-source heterogeneous data. There is no both open-source and general repair tool for multi-source heterogeneous data repair work. The cleaning work is typically done for specific data sets, such as the cleaning of smart grid big data based on SVM [16], building Tan network for cleaning of multi-source heterogeneous grid data [17], the data cleaning by content replacement based on the similarity of character sequences for medical big data [18], constructing PSL neural networks by extracting fuzzy rules of multi-source data for renewable energy data detection and repair work [9]. The tools for automated cleaning of multi-source heterogeneous data based on advanced repair methods, such as these [19, 20] have a good performance on multi-source datasets but are not open source.

The study of various methods for data cleaning. Data cleaning is the process of eliminating erroneous and inconsistent data and requires solving the problem of outliers and tuple duplication [10]. Research works have been experimentally demonstrated to automate and perform quite well on datasets with ER properties, such as HoloClean [11], HoloDetect [21], AlphaClean [22], Raha [23], Pclean [24], etc. And HoloClean, the first data cleaning system to integrate integrity restrictions, external data, and quantitative statistics, has grown to be one of the most popular and relatively successful cleaning frameworks [21, 22]. Previous works were more used to improve HoloClean in terms of detection [23] and correctness [24] but did not make it compatible with multi-source heterogeneous data. We improve Holoclean so that it can help effectively solve the problem of cleaning multi-source heterogeneous data.

3 Architecture of HoloCleanX

The proposed HoloCleanX's architecture is shown in Fig. 1.

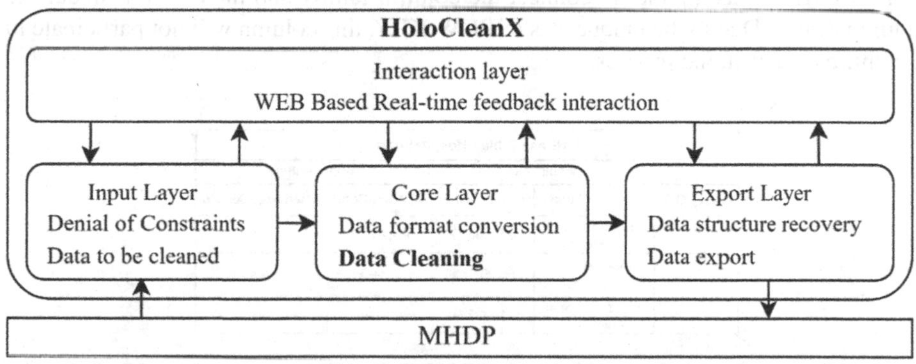

Fig. 1. HoloCleanX's platform architecture

The architecture is divided into four layers, including the Input Layer, Core Layer, Export Layer, and Interaction Layer.

Interaction Layer: It is an interactive platform for users to participate in data cleaning work and evaluate the effect of data cleaning instantly.

Input Layer: It can obtain the data source and DCs selected by the user (The abstract DCs will be transformed and recognizable by the program).

Core Layer: The key of data cleaning work includes the most critical parts of data cleaning work, such as the detection of abnormal data, the training of inferred models, the model correction of abnormal data, etc.

Export Layer: The restored data is saved in the same path as the input data, and users can perform subsequent operations on the cleaned data.

4 Heterogeneous Data Fusion

The solution is based on MHDP architecture and aims to improve the HoloClean engine for data cleaning. The Processing Layer of MHDP is primarily responsible for data processing and management, including data cleaning.

HoloCleanX is capable of handling datasets from multiple data sources with multiple standards, thus uniform data standardization is required before formal data cleaning efforts. We select the Python DataFrame as our standardized data structure. We employ the pre-processing algorithm of MHDP which parses each type of data into Spark DataFrame. To restore the structured data to the original data structure, we retain the name of the parent node in the naming of column names, that is, ":" as a connection symbol to connect the names of columns at all levels.

In addition to structured data from data sources such as SQL Server or semi-structured data such as JSON, No SQL data is also considered an important data source. We take the column family database HBase as an example, as shown in Fig. 2. To rebuild a structured table, we use ":" as a joiner to connect the column family and the columns under the column family. Due to the uniqueness of ROW KEY, this column will not participate in the entire data cleaning process.

HBase Table: Hospital(part)				
	HospitalInfo		TreatmentInfo	
ROW_KEY	HospitalName	PhoneNumber	MeasureCode	EmergencyService
1	callahan eye foundation	2053258100	scip-inf-1	yes
10	helen keller memorial hospital	2563864556	ami-3	yes
100	mizell memorial hospital	3344933541	ami-8a	no

Structured Table(part)				
ROW_KEY	HospitalInfo:HospitalName	HospitalInfo:PhoneNumber	TreatmentInfo:MeasureCode	TreatmentInfo:EmergencyServic
1	callahan eye foundation hospital	2053258100	scip-inf-1	yes
10	helen keller memorial hospital	2563864556	ami-3	yes
100	mizell memorial hospital	3344933541	ami-8a	no

Fig. 2. No SQL type data parsing (HBase as an example)

5 Data Cleaning

This section will introduce the critical components of data cleaning in HoloCleanX and the improvements of HoloCleanX compared to the HoloClean cleaning engine.

5.1 Interactive Cleaning Procedure

The relationship and technical dependencies of the various modules of the interactive data cleaning work are shown in Fig. 3, where the bolded parts represent improvements of HoloCleanX over other cleaning tools or HoloClean.

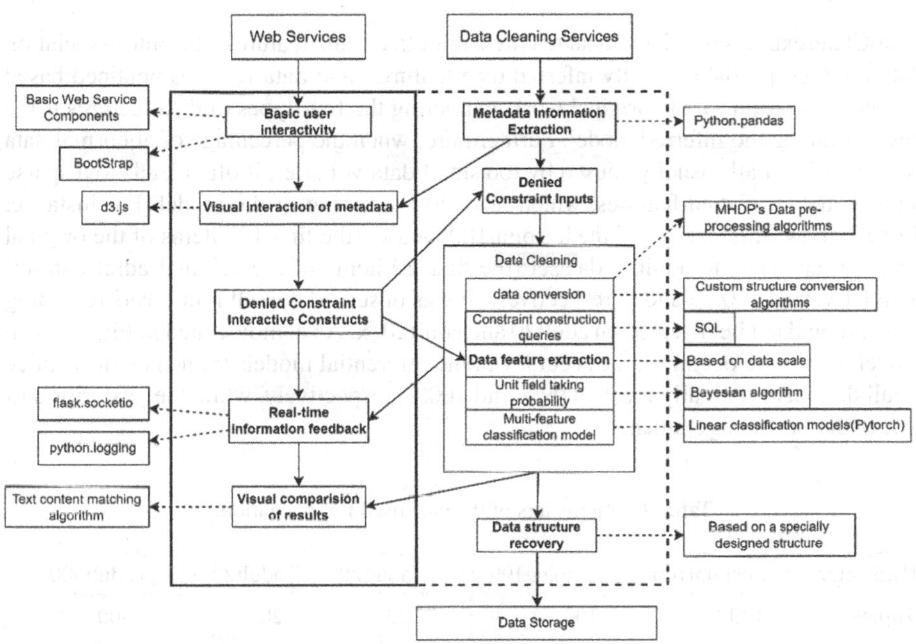

Fig. 3. Procedure of data cleaning

HoloCleanX interacts with MHDP in the form of HTTP API service for data interaction, decoupling from the platform functions and encapsulating the key methods of MHDP data processing part as an open interface for HoloCleanX to access.

Web Services: HoloCleanX is developed based on WEB services to achieve user interaction functions. To achieve real-time feedback on crucial information functions, HoloCleanX is based on Socketio to achieve real-time bidirectional communication between the server and the client after formally entering the data cleaning work. To provide real-time feedback to the user, HoloCleanX redirects all the log information to the log file on the server-side, based on the logging library, and sets a file listener to listen to the changes in the log file. When the data cleaning work of a client is completed, the real-time communication established between the client and the server is terminated.

Data Cleaning Service: except for the processing of part of the multi-source heterogeneous data, which will request MHDP open pre-processing interface, HoloCleanX will complete the Main Modules of data cleaning on the independent service side. The main modules of data cleaning include connection and manipulation of the SQL engine, various statistical calculations, and linear weight sharing based on PyTorch. These modules enable lightweight PyTorch-based classification models. HoloCleanX's data cleaning services are built on top of the Flask framework to provide better API services for open access to MHDP's web platform.

5.2 Improved Inference Model

HoloClean extracts four basic data features: initialized data features, attribute association data features, probabilistically inferred data features, and data features obtained based on DCs extraction. In the original work, extracting the four types of data features is the key to training the inferred model. Furthermore, when the percentage of abnormal data is extremely small (usually caused by too small data volume), it often leads to a sparse feature matrix of data features, which leads to overfitting of the model. For instance, Table 1 shows the features of the hospital100 dataset (the first 100 items of the original hospital dataset) and adult20 dataset (the first 20 items of the original adult dataset) with F1 values of 0.73 and 0, respectively. It was observed that all four errors regarding gender could not be detected on adult20 and adult20_x. As demonstrated in Fig. 4, when model overfitting occurred, the accuracy of the inferential models trained on these three small datasets eventually reached 99% and 100%, respectively, while the posterior cost values did not change much.

Table 1. Parameters of the data used for evaluation.

Parameter	hospital100	hospital100_x	adult20	adult20_x	adult500
Tuples	100	100	20	20	500
Attributes	19	15	11	4	11
Violations	59	59	4	4	6
ICs	9DCs	9DCs	2DCs	2DCs	2DCs
Parameter	hospital100	hospital100_x	adult20	adult20_x	adult500

The extracted data features were found to have the characteristic of One-hot, with most of the elements having the value of 0 and the effective features ranging from 0 to 1. Due to the highly logical and related in HoloClean's every part, HoloCleanX does not pursue the dimensionality reduction of the extracted data features but focuses its efforts on the reasonable selection of the extracted data features. As discussed in the previous section, HoloClean builds data sets to train inferential models, relying on four basic data feature extractors, which are not always helpful for experimental results. As for the initialized data features, if too few types of detection attributes are selected in the negation constraint or too little data for outliers, the feature matrix will become a sparse matrix with overwhelmingly zero values. The correlated data features of attribute pairs require a strong value correlation between each attribute of the dataset, based on the Bayesian algorithm to calculate the connection between the values taken by each attribute pair. If there is no correlation between the attribute pairs in the dataset, the extracted feature matrix will also become a sparse matrix. The latter two data feature extractors, on the other hand, are the most critical parts of the feature extractor. One is the probabilistic inferred data feature, which works by calculating the value with the highest probability among all possible fetched values identified in the cell being detected. The other is the negation constraint data feature, which works by detecting the data feature of outliers based on the input negation constraint. We do not make changes to the process of data feature extraction, but open the potential attributes of the dataset as metadata access to the user, thus providing flexibility in selecting the first two data features.

Because its role is mostly represented in the type of attributes that negate the constraint selection, the initialized feature extractor is analyzed in conjunction with the number of DCs and the number of associated Attributes in the DCs. The attribute pair feature extractors are related to whether or not the participating attribute pairs are associated, and the correlations are calculated based on Bayesian and quantified as the extracted data features. The comparison of the extracted results after choosing different feature extractors is shown in Fig. 4. After using the optimization method, the individual datasets gradually stabilized in terms of the loss values of the trained models (a, b of Fig. 4), and the accuracy of the trained models were not concentrated above 90% (c, d of Fig. 4). This shows that our strategy successfully prevented the occurrence of overfitting.

Due to the inconsistency of attribute features in different datasets, it is difficult to find a uniform method to select feature extractors. Therefore, HoloCleanX encourages users to manually select feature extractors on small datasets and compare the effect of model cleaning. Since the feature size will become very small on small datasets (valid data size < 100), it is difficult to provide enough valid features to train the inferred model, and we hope to further improve it by referring to augmented datasets or generated datasets [21] in the future.

5.3 Data Restoration and Storage

HoloCleanX, as a functionally independent cleaning tool, attempts to restore the data to its original structure for subsequent work, regardless of whether the data being processed is before or after the fusion work. At the beginning of the cleaning work, HoloCleanX will record the channel of the category to which the source data belongs, mainly including SQL/CSV/JSON/HBase/XML/Pandas.DF/Spark.DF. After the data cleaning is finished, the recorded metadata information will be recorded, including the storage path of the data, the file name of the data, the data type of each layer, etc.

SQL/CSV. Structured data requires no further processing, and various tools based on the pandas' library can convert DataFrames into the corresponding data types.

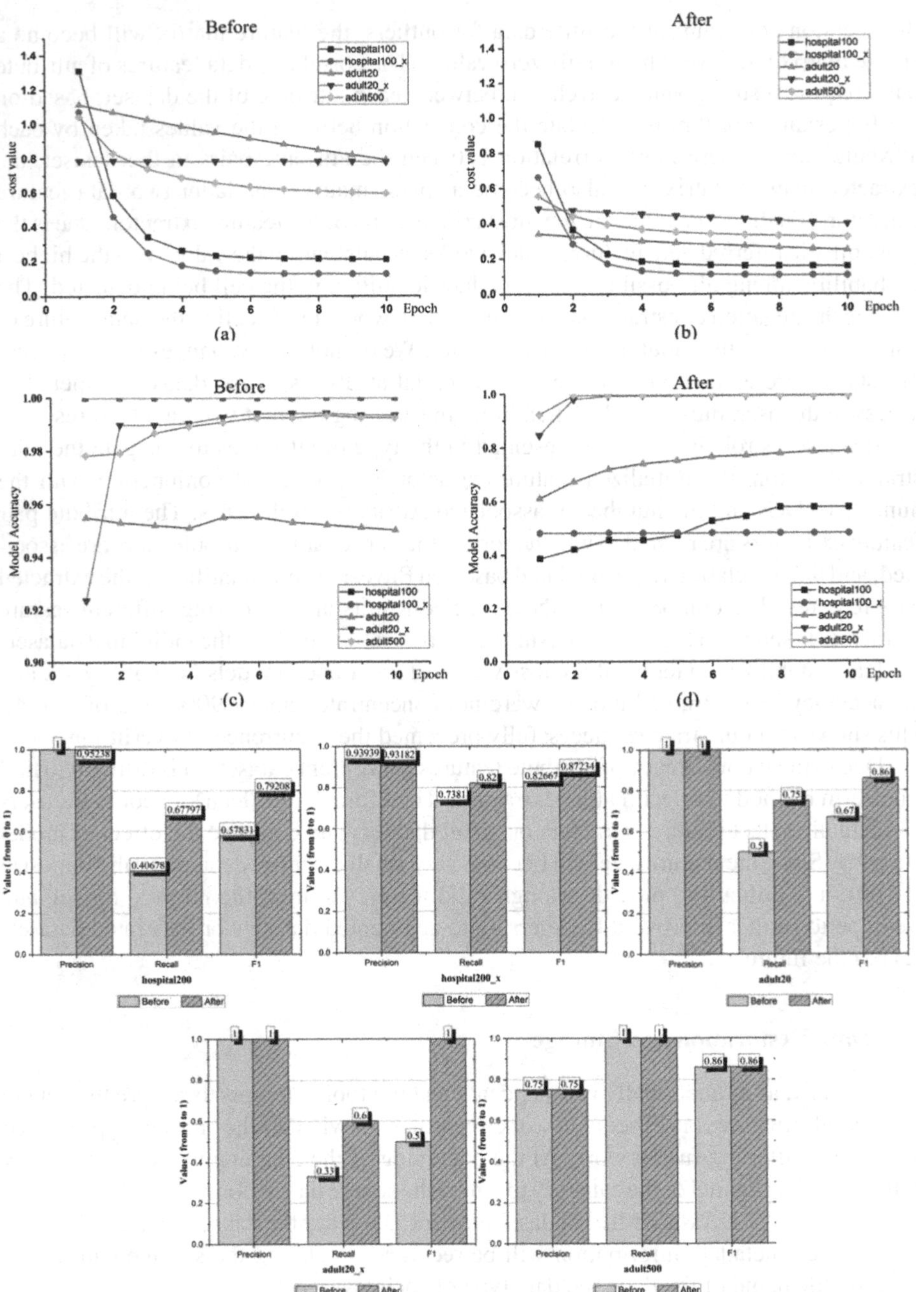

Fig. 4. Comparison of HoloCleanX and HoloClean cleaning results on small datasets

***-DF (DataFrame).** When accepting such data, we unify the various DataFrames into Pandas-DF to facilitate subsequent data format conversion in PyTorch. When returning data, the data format is converted based on the tools already available in the pandas' library.

JSON/HBase/XML. This type of data is generally nested data, and we already process the original data by parsing multiple layers of nesting into a single layer. When recovering, we split the ":" to recursively construct a tree structure, as in Fig. 5. Structured data we build can be directly converted and put into HBase based on methods in Python-happybase. And the parse string tool in Python-XML can reduce the nested data we parsed into XML format.

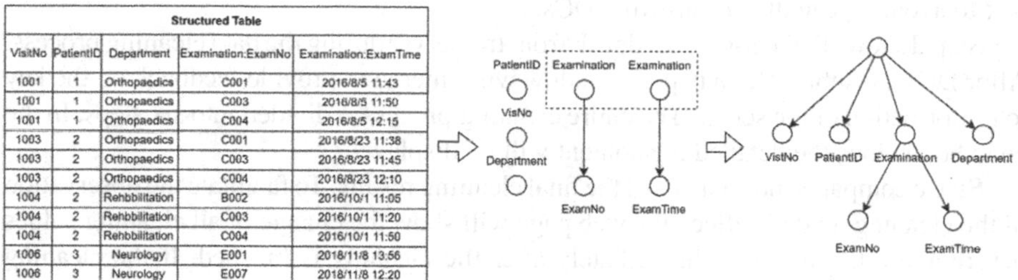

Structured Table				
VisitNo	PatientID	Department	Examination:ExamNo	Examination:ExamTime
1001	1	Orthopaedics	C001	2016/8/5 11:43
1001	1	Orthopaedics	C003	2016/8/5 11:50
1001	1	Orthopaedics	C004	2016/8/5 12:15
1003	2	Orthopaedics	C001	2016/8/23 11:38
1003	2	Orthopaedics	C003	2016/8/23 11:45
1003	2	Orthopaedics	C004	2016/8/23 12:10
1004	2	Rehbbilitation	B002	2016/10/1 11:05
1004	2	Rehbbilitation	C003	2016/10/1 11:20
1004	2	Rehbbilitation	C004	2016/10/1 11:50
1006	3	Neurology	E001	2018/11/8 13:56
1006	3	Neurology	E007	2018/11/8 12:20

Fig. 5. Structured data recovery

6 System Implementation and Usage

This section will introduce the tools we used and the implementation of the system visualization interaction.

6.1 Implementation

The implementation is dependent on Java (1.8.0_291) and Python (3.8). The main components of the LakeHouse for data storage mainly include Hadoop (3.2.1), Spark (2.4.6), and Hbase (2.3.7). We use Postgresql (14.1) as our data query engine and train the inference model based on the torch (1.10.0+cu113). For the implementation of the interactive system, we use Bootstrap (3.4.1), D3 (3.0), and flask (2.0.3) which includes flask-socketio (3.0.2).

6.2 Usage

To facilitate testing the cleaning effect, we use the hospital dataset with the nested structure as our baseline dataset without changing the exact data content. Steps from a to e are key stages in the cleaning process.

Step a shows the metadata extraction and visualization interface. The visual interface gives the user a tree structure to show the hierarchical relationship of the data. In addition, it displays the data features (null ratio, duplicate ratio, and sample values) of each leaf node through a table or mouse hover node. These functions facilitate the user to analyze whether each column is valuable for cleaning and to perform automatic feature extraction based on the effective tuple length of the data.

Step b demonstrates how users construct a DC. After determining the properties of the data to be cleaned, the data will enter the constraint entry interface. When initializing a constraint relationship, the user is required to select the number of tuples (optional values are 1 and 2).

Step c depicts the user interface for summarising, checking, and submitting DCs. When the DCs are submitted, all the DCs that have been entered so far will be displayed in a pop-up window. Users can also directly paste the already written DCs to the input box to avoid repeatedly constructing DCs.

Step d shows the real-time feedback from the server during the data cleaning process. After DCs are submitted, a pop-up window will emerge to provide feedback on the key log information of the server. The entire cleaning process is divided into six steps. In the code box below, the detailed log content will be displayed.

Step e compares the contents of the final cleaning results. To facilitate the observation of the cleaning model's effect, the web page will show the change of all cleaning values before and after in a table immediately after the cleaning is finished. If the cleaning effect is not satisfactory, the process can begin anew. The hospital dataset can be tested on the original HoloClean tool, and the fixes within each attribute are consistent with HoloCleanX, including 456 valid fixes.

7 Conclusion and Future Work

In this paper, we propose HoloCleanX, a data cleaning tool to clean multi-source heterogeneous data based on LakeHouse. Unlike common approaches to clean multi-source heterogeneous data, HoloCleanX is a multi-source heterogeneous data cleaning solution that enables separate services. Furthermore, it is built on a high computational platform. We improve the data feature extraction process and design an interactive interface with real-time feedback, which not only increases data cleaning capabilities for big data sets but also improves usability.

In the future, we will improve our work in two aspects: first, we will add visual charts to illustrate more details; second, we will migrate the query engine to Spark SQL under Spark Platform to further speed up data cleaning.

Acknowledgement. This work was supported by National Key R&D Program of China (2020AAA0109603).

References

1. Zhang, Y., et al.: Hkgb: an inclusive, extensible, intelligent, semi-auto-constructed knowledge graph framework for healthcare with clinicians' expertise incorporated. Inf. Process. Manage. **57**(6), 102324 (2020)

2. Du, J., Michalska, S., Subramani, S., Wang, H., Zhang, Y.: Neural attention with character embeddings for hay fever detection from Twitter. Health Inf. Sci. Syst. **7**(1), 1–7 (2019). https://doi.org/10.1007/s13755-019-0084-2
3. Supriya, S., Siuly, S., Wang, H., Zhang, Y.: Automated epilepsy detection techniques from electroencephalogram signals: a review study. Health Inf. Sci. Syst. **8**(1), 1–15 (2020). https://doi.org/10.1007/s13755-020-00129-1
4. Sarki, R., Ahmed, K., Wang, H., Zhang, Y.: Automated detection of mild and multi-class diabetic eye diseases using deep learning. Health Inf. Sci. Syst. **8**(1), 1–9 (2020). https://doi.org/10.1007/s13755-020-00125-5
5. Wang, C., Feng, S.: Research on the collection and preprocessing of multisource heterogeneous elevator data. In: 2020 IEEE International Conference on Power, Intelligent Computing and Systems (ICPICS), pp. 490–493. IEEE (2020)
6. Liu, W., Zhang, C., Yu, B., Li, Y.: A general multi-source data fusion framework. In: Proceedings of the 2019 11th International Conference on Machine Learning and Computing, pp. 285–289 (2019)
7. Ren, P., et al.: Mhdp: an efficient data lake platform for medical multi-source heterogeneous data. In: Xing, C., Fu, X., Zhang, Y., Zhang, G., Borjigin, C. (eds.) WISA 2021. LNCS, vol. 12999, pp. 727–738. Springer, Cham (2021). https://doi.org/10.1007/978-3-030-87571-8_63
8. Chen, C.S., Hu, H.R., Fang, L.L., Xiang, Y.X.: Research on equipment situation display based on multi-source data fusion. In: 2020 International Conference on Computer Engineering and Intelligent Control (ICCEIC), pp. 207–211. IEEE (2020)
9. Sun, R., et al.: Research on multi-source heterogeneous data cleaning technology based on integrating neural network with fuzzy rules for renewable energy accommodation. In: 2020 IEEE 4th Conference on Energy Internet and Energy System Integration (EI2), pp. 3024–3027. IEEE (2020)
10. Rahm, E., Do, H.H.: Data cleaning: problems and current approaches. IEEE Data Eng. Bull. **23**(4), 3–13 (2000)
11. Rekatsinas, T., Chu, X., Ilyas, I.F., Ré, C.: Holoclean: Holistic data repairs with probabilistic inference. arXiv preprint arXiv:1702.00820 (2017)
12. Jiming, H., Wei, S.: An object-centric multi-source heterogeneous data fusion scheme. In: 2021 IEEE International Conference on Information Communication and Software Engineering (ICICSE), pp. 24–29. IEEE (2021)
13. Li, H., Zhou, G., Zhou, S., Chen, S., Mao, S., Jin, T.: Multi-source heterogeneous log fusion technology of power information system based on big data and imprecise reasoning theory. In: 2020 IEEE 20th International Conference on Communication Technology (ICCT), pp. 1609–1614. IEEE (2020)
14. Gledson, A., Dhafari, T.B., Paton, N., Keane, J.: A smart city dashboard for combining and analysing multi-source data streams. In: 2018 IEEE 20th International Conference on High Performance Computing and Communications; IEEE 16th International Conference on Smart City; IEEE 4th International Conference on Data Science and Systems (HPCC/SmartCity/DSS), pp. 1366–1373. IEEE (2018)
15. Yuan, Q., Pi, Y., Kou, L., Zhang, F., Li, Y., Zhang, Z.: Multi-source data processing and fusion method for power distribution internet of things based on edge intelligence. arXiv preprint arXiv:2203.17230 (2022)
16. Lv, Z., Deng, W., Zhang, Z., Guo, N., Yan, G.: A data fusion and data cleaning system for smart grids big data. In: 2019 IEEE Intl Conference on Parallel & Distributed Processing with Applications, Big Data & Cloud Computing, Sustainable Computing & Communications, Social Computing & Networking (ISPA/BDCloud/SocialCom/SustainCom), pp. 802–807. IEEE (2019)

17. Ying, Z., Huang, Y., Chen, K., Yu, T.: Big data cleaning model of multi-source heterogeneous power grid based on machine learning classification algorithm. In: Journal of Physics: Conference Series, vol. 2087, p. 012095. IOP Publishing (2021)
18. Deshpande, P., Rasin, A., Tchoua, R., Furst, J., Raicu, D., Antani, S.: Enhancing recall using data cleaning for biomedical big data. In: 2020 IEEE 33rd International Symposium on Computer-Based Medical Systems (CBMS), pp. 265–270. IEEE (2020)
19. Ye, C., Li, Q., Zhang, H., Wang, H., Gao, J., Li, J.: AutoRepair: an automatic repairing approach over multi-source data. Knowl. Inf. Syst. **61**(1), 227–257 (2019)
20. Ye, C., Wang, H., Zheng, K., Gao, J., Li, J.: Multi-source data repairing powered by integrity constraints and source reliability. Inf. Sci. **507**, 386–403 (2020)
21. Heidari, A., McGrath, J., Ilyas, I.F., Rekatsinas, T.: HoloDetect: few-shot learning for error detection. In: Proceedings of the 2019 International Conference on Management of Data, pp. 829–846 (2019)
22. Krishnan, S., Wu, E.: AlphaClean: automatic generation of data cleaning pipelines. arXiv preprint arXiv:1904.11827 (2019)
23. Mahdavi, M., et al.: Raha: a configuration-free error detection system. In: Proceedings of the 2019 International Conference on Management of Data, pp. 865–882 (2019)
24. Lew, A., Agrawal, M., Sontag, D., Mansinghka, V.: PClean: Bayesian data cleaning at scale with domain-specific probabilistic programming. In: International Conference on Artificial Intelligence and Statistics, pp. 1927–1935. PMLR (2021)

The Construction and Validation of an Automatic Crisis Balance Analysis Model

Long Yin Guo[1], Lin Xia[1], Xin Yi Huang[1], Yu Xin Fu[1], Xin Yi Li[1], Si Chen Zhou[1], Chao Zhao[2], and Bing Xiang Yang[1(✉)]

[1] School of Nursing, Wuhan University, Wuhan, China
00009312@whu.edu.cn
[2] Faculty of Science, Leiden University, Leiden, The Netherlands

Abstract. *Background*: With the development of Internet, many people with suicide risk tend to express their thoughts on social media platforms. AI-based model can early identify social media users with suicide risk and analyze their cognitive and interpersonal characteristics. Then we can do early intervention to help them.

Objective: To build an automatic crisis balance analysis model based on artificial intelligence which can perform automatic early suicide identification, suicide risk classification and analyze cognitive distortion and interpersonal relationship of users. Then to validate the predictive efficiency of model.

Method: Firstly, based on the suicide knowledge graph, free annotation data set was generated and then Bert-based model was built. Secondly, the data set was refined by psychology students and experts to build fine-tuning model and Psychology+ model. The Psychology+ model was used as final suicide risk assessment model. We enriched and quantified the variables of cognitive and interpersonal characteristics and built the cognitive distortion and interpersonal relationship analysis model. Using F1 score, precision, recall and accuracy to evaluate the model performance and the consistence of model results with expert judgment and scales results to evaluate the model prediction ability.

Results: For the suicide risk assessment model, the F1 score, precision, recall rate and accuracy rate of the model are 77.98%, 80.75%, 75.41% and 78.68% respectively. For the cognitive distortion and interpersonal relationship analysis model, the F1 score, accuracy and recall rate of the model are 77.26%, 78.22% and 76.33% respectively. Comparing the results with the results of the scale by chi square test, there was no significant difference in cognitive distortion($P = 0.521$) and interpersonal relationship($P = 0.189$) aspect.

Conclusion: The model showed good performance and can be used as a guideline and evaluation tool for intervention.

Keywords: Suicide · Artificial intelligence · Social media · Model validation

This study was supported by the grant from the National College Students Innovation and Entrepreneurship Training Program of Wuhan University (202210486105), National Natural Science Foundation of China General Program (72174152), Project of Humanities and Social Sciences of the Ministry of Education in China (20YJCZH204), the Young Top-notch Talent Cultivation Program of Hubei Province.

A. Traina et al. (Eds.): HIS 2022, LNCS 13705, pp. 177–188, 2022.
https://doi.org/10.1007/978-3-031-20627-6_17

1 Background

Suicide is a major public health issue. According to the World Health Organization [1], more than 700,000 people die by suicide every year, indicating that one in every 100 deaths is caused by suicide. Currently, depression is a serious social health challenge in China and worldwide due to its high incidence, disability rates and the following economic and disease burden [2–4]. Now approximately 280 million people worldwide suffer from depression [5]. In China, the lifetime prevalence of depression is 6.9% [2]. Individuals with depression may lose hope in life and eventually choose to end their lives by committing suicide if depression is not treated promptly and effectively.

However, due to the poor public mental health literacy and the social stigma related to psychological problems, most people tend to solve problems by themselves and rarely seek help from relatives, friends or professionals [6, 7], which makes early identification of suicide risk difficult. With the rapid development of the Internet, Chinese people, especially the young ones, tend to express themselves on social media platforms. Therefore, realizing early identification of suicide risk is feasible by analyzing messages on social media platforms.

Suicide is a possible result of the emotional crisis. According to Aguilera's crisis balance theory [8], whether emotional crises can be successfully overcome depends on the individual's cognition of the event, available interpersonal support and coping skills. Individuals with cognitive distortions and without interpersonal support are more likely to experience ineffective coping and thus progress to extreme emotional crises. Therefore, paying attention to the individual's emotional change, cognitive and interpersonal characteristics may provide help for accurate identification of emotional crises and effective interventions in the early stages of the crisis.

Therefore, the objective of this study was to build an automatic crisis balance analysis model based on artificial intelligence which can perform automatic early suicide identification, suicide risk classification and analyze cognitive distortion and interpersonal relationship of users. Then to validate the predictive efficiency of model.

2 Method

2.1 Study Design

This study enriched and quantified Aguilera's crisis balance theory [8] and used deep learning technology to construct an automatic crisis balance analysis model through a multi-task fine-grained deep learning model based on attention mechanism. The model can actively identify and classify emotional crisis in the early stage, analyze psychological characteristics such as cognitive distortion and interpersonal characteristics, provide personalized psychological portrait reports so that it can be used as evaluation tool for the results of changes in psychological characteristics before and after intervention.

2.2 Enriching and Quantifing Aguilera's Crisis Balance Theory

The crisis balance theory was proposed by Aguilera [8], an expert in crisis theory. According to the theory, whether an individual can correctly cope with stressful events is mainly determined by three factors affecting psychological balance: (1) Whether the individual's coping mechanism is sufficient. When a crisis occurs, individuals usually use their previous successful experience to deal with it. When these coping strategies are effective, the crisis will be reversed. If not, the imbalance persists, with increased levels of stress and anxiety, worsening negative emotions and the risk of suicide. (2) Whether individuals can get enough situational support. Situational support refers to interpersonal support that can be obtained in a specific environment. Without adequate support in crisis situations, individuals may feel depressed, helpless and lonely. (3) Whether the individual's perception of events is realistic or distorted. If the individual's perception of the event is realistic, the individual will be more likely to seek enough resources to restore the balance state; if perception is distorted, problem solving tends to be ineffective and balance state cannot be restored. Based on Aguilera's crisis balance theory, this study has enriched and quantified it (Table 1) and built an automatic crisis balance analysis model. The model includes three variables: coping mechanism, cognitive level and interpersonal support.

Table 1. Key variables of the automatic crisis balance analysis model

Crisis balance theory variable	Model indicators	Indicator description
Ineffective individual coping	High risk of suicide (extreme emotional crisis)	Combined with the suicide risk classification in the suicide knowledge graph constructed by Professor Huang [9], high suicide risk refers to suicide plan or suicide attempt
Cognitive level	Cognitive distortions	Ten types of cognitive distortion in Burns' New Mood Therapy [10]
Interpersonal support	Personal characteristics	Interpersonal characteristics in interpersonal Relationship Therapy [11]

2.3 The Construction of Suicide Risk Assessment Model

Data Sources and Processing

This study built a legitimate crawler program to crawl the weibo messages under the "Zoufan Tree Hole". Firstly, we preprocessed the data set, including deleting repetitive data, meaningless emojis and sentences that are too short (less than or equal to five words). Four data sets were constructed: free annotation data set generated by the suicide knowledge graph; easy annotation data set annotated by psychology students; hard annotation data set 1 and 2 annotated by mental psychology experts. These data sets were used to train and test models.

Modeling Process

The task of model is to predict whether a user is at a high suicide risk through the messages posted by the user on a Chinese social media platform, weibo. The classification criteria for suicide risk were proposed by Huang et al. [9] according to the certainty of the suicide methods and the time urgency. We define Level 6 and above as "high suicide risk", which shows users have a suicide plan, and the rest as "low suicide risk".

The modeling process is divided into two main parts: the generation of free annotation data set and classification based on deep learning. Firstly, a set of semantic rules was constructed based on the psychological crisis prevention ontology constructed by Huang [9], and a free annotation data set was generated. The psychological crisis prevention knowledge graph contains four ontologies: suicide, time, space and wish. This free annotation data set can be wrong, which was used to oversee deep learning models. Then, we built a BERT-based model based on the free annotation data set. This new model was used to classify new texts corrected by psychology students to generate an easy annotation data set. The data set had a large number of high suicide risk and low suicide risk messages data, and was used to fine tune the BERT-based model to build a Fine-Tuning Model. At the same time, mental psychology experts provided hard annotation data set. Finally, the model was refined through the hard annotation data set and additional psychological features, combining the prior knowledge gained from the original model and domain expertise to obtain the final Psychology+ model. The detailed process of modeling can be seen in previous article published in 2021 [12].

2.4 The Construction of Cognitive Distortion and Interpersonal Relationship Analysis Model

Preparation of Manual Labeling Guideline

Basis of Cognitive Distortion and Interpersonal Characteristics Labeling

In his book, Feeling good: the new mood therapy [10], the famous American psychologist David Burns summarized ten major types of cognitive distortion, all-or-nothing thinking, overgeneralization, mental filter, disqualifying the positive, jumping to conclusions (mind reading and the fortune teller error), magnification and minimization, emotional reasoning, should statements, labeling and mislabeling and blaming oneself and others.

Interpersonal therapy points out that interpersonal problems are mainly divided into four categories. The first is grief, making it difficult to establish satisfactory interpersonal relationship due to the death of a loved one. The second is role changing, where individuals undergo major life changes, such as illness, child birth, retirement, etc. The third is relationship conflicts, where there is an open or covert conflict in an important personal relationship (such as with spouse or a boss). The fourth is interpersonal deficits, which bring social isolation [11].

Based on the concepts and meaning of the ten major cognitive distortions and four interpersonal characteristics mentioned above, we preliminarily compiled a guideline for manual labeling to guide manual data labeling and improve the accuracy and effectiveness of data labeling.

Expert Discussion

After the preliminary compilation of the labeling guideline, we invited 2 mental psychological experts and 3 nursing experts to discuss the scientificity of the guideline. The discussion covered the framework structure, theoretical support, core concept and related example writing, etc., then we made modifications several times according to the suggestions put forward by the experts, and finally the final version of the cognitive distortion and interpersonal characteristics manual labeling guideline was formed.

Data Labeling and Processing

In order to ensure the consistency and accuracy of data labeling, mental psychological experts were invited to train 10 students with psychosocial backgrounds before the data labeling. Through centralized training, data labelers had a deep understanding of cognitive distortion and interpersonal characteristics, and clearly understood the requirements of data labeling. Ten students were grouped in groups of two to do the labeling synchronously to the same messages under weibo "Zoufan Tree Hole" according to the guideline. After labeling, two students in one group checked if the labeling was consistent. If not, the third person would make judgement. Finally, 91861 pieces of data were labeled. The data labels are showed in Table 2.

Table 2. The data labels of text

Cognitive distortion	Interpersonal characteristics
All-or-nothing thinking	Grief and loss
Overgeneralization	Inter-role conflict
Mental filter	Intra-role conflict
Disqualifying the positive	Role change
Mind reading	Interpersonal deficits
The fortune teller error	
Magnification	
Minimization	
Emotional reasoning	
Should statements	
Labeling and mislabeling	
Blaming oneself	
Blaming others	

The label of every piece of text would include these 18 labels. If the text showed one of the above characteristics, then the corresponding value was set1, and vice versa, was set 0. For example, there was a piece of text, "I always feel that I chose wrong. I should not study science, as if from the moment I changed the label arts to sciences, my life has gone in another way. My reason for change was also extremely naïve. The teacher let me look at the list and I saw a lot of girls. I inexplicable fear, I fear to be bullied again. I hate it when a bunch of girls intrigue against each other. I always live in all kinds of regret, regret step by step, as if wrong can never be changed". It showed this user had the fortune teller error, Should Statements, Blaming himself/herself and Interpersonal Deficits. Therefore, the label of this piece of text is as follows (Table 3).

Table 3. The label of a piece of text

All-or-nothing thinking	Overgeneralization	Mental filter	Disqualifying the positive	Mind reading	The fortune teller error	Magnification	Minimization	Emotional reasoning
0	0	0	0	0	1	0	0	0
Should statements	Labeling and mislabeling	Blaming oneself	Blaming others	Grief and loss	Inter-role conflict	Intra-role conflict	Role change	Interpersonal deficits
1	0	1	0	0	0	0	0	1

2.5 Validation Methods

Evaluation of Suicide Risk Assessment Model

For evaluation of the BERT-based model, Fine-Tuning Model and Psychology+Model, we performed fivefold cross-validation based on every model's corresponding data set respectively, using F1 score, precision, recall and accuracy as evaluation indexes [12].

Evaluation of Cognitive Distortion and Interpersonal Relationship Assessment Model

We used BERT+softmax classifier. Of the 91,861 messages, 3,615 were valid for labels with cognitive distortion or interpersonal characteristics. Some data without label features were randomly selected, and the final data amount is 4500 messages. We performed fivefold cross-validation to the 4500 messages (3600 being used as training set, 900 as verification set). We used F1 score, precision and recall as evaluation indexes, and F1 score was the harmonic average of recall and precision.

Validation of the Automatic Crisis Balance Analysis Model's Predictive Efficacy

Validation of the Suicide Risk Predictive Efficacy Based on Weibo Users in "Zoufan Tree Hole"

We obtained 460,000 messages in "Zoufan Tree Hole" posted by 45,018 users. After the analysis by model, 458 users with a large number of weibo messages and high suicide risk were screened out, and their psychological portraits reports were generated. In order to validate the accuracy of the model's prediction of suicide risk, a psychiatrist was invited to make a judgement of high suicide risk related descriptions in the 458 weibo users' psychological portraits reports, and found that 437 (95.41%) users had a high suicide risk indeed.

Validation of the Cognitive Distortion and Interpersonal Relationship Predictive Efficacy Based on College Students Group

Since this model is constructed based on the messages in "Zoufan Tree Hole", in order to further validate the predictive efficacy of the model on cognitive distortion and interpersonal relationship, semi-structural questions and questionnaires with good reliability and validity were used to investigate in the college student group. We recorded each participant's answer of two semi-structural questions and used the automatic crisis balance analysis model to analyze cognitive distortion and interpersonal characteristics. Then, we compared the results of the model with those of the questionnaires.

We used the following questionnaires as validation tools.

(1) Semi-structural questions: After consulting with psychiatric experts, two semi-structural questions have been formed to collect relevant information as much as possible, "Please record a negative event that has recently made you feel depressed/sad/angry/unhappy. Talk about your feelings and how do you think about it?" "Please list one of the things that makes you feel unpleasant/uncomfortable in your interpersonal interactions with family, friends, teachers, or anyone else. Talk about how you feel".
(2) Cognitive Bias Questionnaire (CBQ): CBQ was compiled by scholars Krantz and Hammen to assess negative cognitive biases associated with depression and was able to measure both depression and cognitive distortion [13, 14]. The questionnaire presents six common situations among college students or psychiatric patients, each with three to four questions that ask participants to answer their personal feelings and experiences when confronted with that situation. These questions cover four different combinations, depression and non-distortion, depression-distortion, non-depression and non-distortion, non-depression and distortion. In this study, depression-distortion scores were used to evaluate cognitive distortion in individuals. Liu et al. [15] used CBQ to measure the cognitive bias of college freshmen and found that the questionnaire had good reliability and validity.
(3) Interpersonal Relationship Assessment Scale (IRAS): The IRAS was developed by Zheng and used to assess participants' interpersonal distress [16]. The scale includes 4 dimensions (interpersonal communication, interpersonal contact, the way how to treat people and heterosexual interaction) and 28 items. For every item, 1 represents yes, 0 represents no. The total score is 0–28 points, and the higher the score, the more serious the degree of interpersonal distress. A score of 0–8 indicates no distress, 9–14 indicates mild distress, and 15–28 indicates severe distress, with a score of ≥ 20 indicating a significant interpersonal disorder. This scale has been shown to have good reliability and validity in several studies [17, 18].

3 Results

3.1 Evaluation of Suicide Risk Assessment Model

The result of final Psychology+ Model was 77.98% F1 score, 80.75% precision, 75.41% recall and 78.68% accuracy. The detailed information of results can also be seen in previous published article [12].

3.2 Evaluation of Cognitive Distortion and Interpersonal Relationship Analysis Model

We obtained a F1 score of 77.26%, a precision of 78.22%, and a recall of 76.33%. All indexes were above 0.75, indicating a good performance of the model.

3.3 Validation of the Automatic Crisis Balance Analysis Model's Predictive Efficacy

Validation of the Suicide Risk Predictive Efficacy Based on Weibo Users in "ZOUfan Tree Hole"
Through judgement of the psychology expert, there was 437 users (95.41%) had high suicide risk indeed in all 458 users automatically identified by the model.

Validation of the Cognitive Distortion and Interpersonal Relationship Predictive Efficacy Based on College Student Group
According to the model analysis, it was found that 55 (78.57%) participants had cognitive distortion and 24 (34.29%) participants had interpersonal relationship problems. Cognitive distortion with higher frequency included magnification, mental filter and labeling and mislabeling Interpersonal relationship problems with higher frequency included grief and loss and interpersonal deficits (Fig. 1).

According to the scale evaluation, it was found that 67 (95.71%) participants had cognitive distortions, and 15 (21.43%) participants had obvious interpersonal relationship problems. The scores for cognitive distortion and interpersonal relationship are presented in Table 4.

Comparing the results of the model analysis with the results of the scale evaluation by chi square test (see Table 5), there were no statistically significant differences in cognitive distortion and interpersonal relationship ($P > 0.05$).

The automatic crisis balance analysis model was highly consistent with expert manual judgment and scale evaluation results in predicting suicide risk, cognitive distortion and interpersonal relationship.

4 Discussion

This study constructed the automatic crisis balance analysis model by enriching and quantifying the Aguilera crisis balance theory and relying on the artificial intelligence

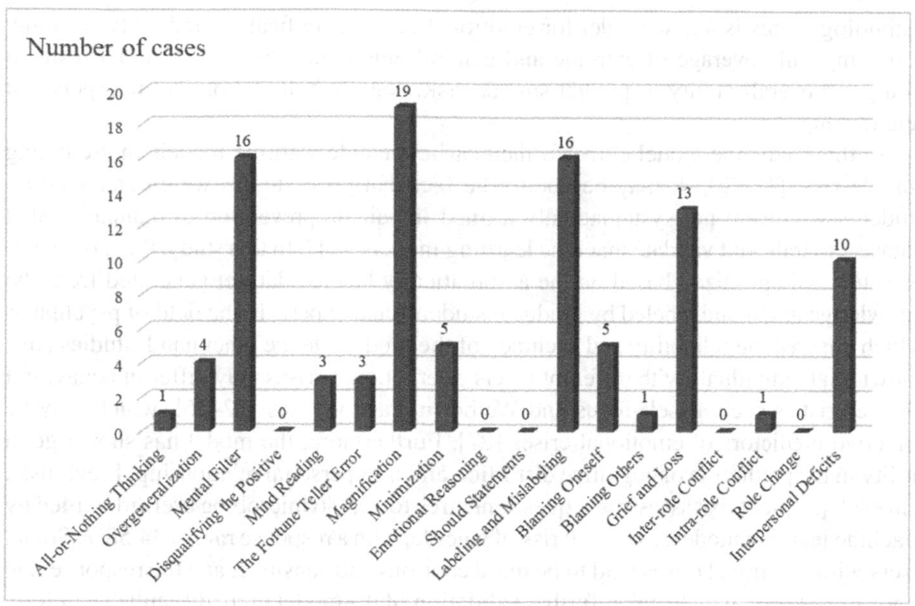

Fig. 1. The frequency distribution of cognitive distortion and interpersonal characteristics

Table 4. Scores of cognitive distortion and interpersonal relationship (N = 70)

Variable	Mean	SD	Frequency	Percentage (%)
CBQ (Depression-Distortion)	3.79	2.34	67	95.71
IRAS (≥20 points)	14.71	5.36	15	21.43

Table 5. Chi square test of model analysis results and scale evaluation results

Item		Cognitive distortion (scale)		Interpersonal relationship (scale)		x^2	P
		No	Yes	No	Yes		
Cognitive distortion (model)	No	1	14	–	–	–	0.521*
	Yes	2	53		–		
Interpersonal relationship (model)	No	–	–	34	12	1.729	0.189
	Yes	–	–	21	3		

* We adopted a Fisher exact test.

technology. This is a new model for emotional crisis identification and early warning, achieving full coverage of extreme and general emotional crises. The model resulted in a good overall ability to predict suicide risk, cognitive distortion and interpersonal relationship.

In this study, the model outperformed earlier suicide warning models in predicting suicide risk. [19, 20]. It may be due to the fact that prior studies were conducted by students who were not systematically trained in suicide prevention to manually label datasets to train and validate machine learning models. [21]. In this study, the model was adjusted and optimized based on the automatically labeled dataset generated from the knowledge graph and labeled by graduate students and experts in the field of psychiatry, which ensured the reliability and accuracy of the model. On the other hand, studies have shown that individuals with different levels of emotional crises may differ in behavioral characteristics such as self-focus and Weibo interaction rates [22–26], which may be effective predictors of emotional crises [27]. Furthermore, the model has shown good utility in the prediction of cognitive distortion and interpersonal relationship. Previously, Liu et al. [27] sent risk assessment questionnaires to 12,486 microblog users identified by machine learning model as being at risk of suicide, with a response rate of 34.58%. Social users with emotional crises tend to be more cautious and sensitive, and the response rate tends to be lower, which makes further validation of the model more difficult. Therefore, this study validated the model by comparing the results of the expert's manual judgment and scale with the prediction results of the model to make it more scientific and reliable.

The model can achieve real-time analysis and rapid response greatly reducing the workload of manual screening, and making up for the shortcomings of traditional screening tools. However, the model needs further improvement. Although the evaluation indexes of this model are above 0.75, the overall performance of the model needs to be further improved. Future studies may consider applying the model to the identification and evaluation of emotional crises, and providing the results to experts or crisis intervention workers for review and follow-up, and further optimizing the model with the feedback from experts [21, 28].

5 Conclusion

In this study, the automatic crisis balance analysis model was constructed using artificial intelligence technology, and the efficacy of the model in predicting suicide risk, cognitive distortion, and interpersonal relationships was validated in the "Zoufan Tree Hole" weibo users group and the college students group.

The automatic crisis balance analysis model showed good performance in predicting suicide risk, cognitive distortion and interpersonal relationship. In addition, the prediction results of the model for suicide risk, cognitive distortion, and interpersonal relationship were in high agreement with the expert manual judgment and scale assessment results. The model can be used as a guideline and an evaluation tool for interventions.

References

1. World Health Organization: Suicide worldwide in 2019. https://www.who.int/publications/i/item/9789240026643. Accessed 16 June 2021

2. Huang, Y.Q., Wang, Y., Wang, H., et al.: Prevalence of mental disorders in China: a cross-sectional epidemiological study. Lancet Psychiatry **6**(3), 211–224 (2019). https://doi.org/10.1016/S2215-0366(18)30511-X
3. World Health Organization: Depression-Fact Sheet. https://www.who.int/news-room/fact-sheets/detail/depression. Accessed 16 Mar 2022
4. Buckman, J.E.J., Underwood, A., Clarke, K., et al.: Risk factors for relapse and recurrence of depression in adults and how they operate: a four-phase systematic review and meta-synthesis. Clin. Psychol. Rev. **64**, 13–38 (2018). https://doi.org/10.1016/j.cpr.2018.07.005
5. World Health Organization: Depression. https://www.who.int/health-topics/depression#tab=tab_1. Accessed 16 Mar 2022
6. Roskar, S., Bracic, M.F., Kolar, U., et al.: Attitudes within the general population towards seeking professional help in cases of mental distress. Int. J. Soc. Psychiatry **63**(7), 614–621 (2017). https://doi.org/10.1177/0020764017724819
7. Bifftu, B.B., Takele, W.W., Guracho, Y.D., et al.: Depression and its help seeking behaviors: a systematic review and meta-analysis of community survey in Ethiopia. Depression research and treatment. 1592596 (2018). https://doi.org/10.1155/2018/1592596
8. Aguilera, D.C.: Crisis intervention: theory and methodology. AORN J. **38**(1), 88 (1971)
9. Huang, Z.S., Hu, Q., Gu, J.G., et al.: Web-based intelligent agents for suicide monitoring and early warning. China Digit. Med. **14**(03), 3–6 (2019). https://doi.org/10.3969/j.issn.1673-7571.2019.03.001
10. Burns, D.: Feeling Good the New Mood Therapy. Scientific and Technical Documentation Press, Beijing (2014)
11. Frank, E., Levenson, J.C.: Interpersonal Psychotherapy. Chongqing University Press, Chongqing (2015)
12. Fu, G., Song, C., Li, J., Ma, Y., Chen, P., Wang, R., et al.: Distant supervision for mental health management in social media: suicide risk classification system development study. J. Med. Internet Res. **23**(8), e26119 (2021). https://doi.org/10.2196/26119
13. Hammen, C.L., Krantz, S.: Effect of success and failure on depressive cognitions. J. Abnorm. Psychol. **85**(6), 577–586 (1976). https://doi.org/10.1037/0021-843X.85.6.577
14. Krantz, S., Hammen, C.: Assessment of cognitive bias in depression. J. Abnorm. Psychol. **88**(6), 611–619 (1979). https://doi.org/10.1037/0021-843X.88.6.611
15. Liu, X.J., Wang, M.P.: The association among childhood psychological abuse and neglect, cognitive bias and self-worth of medical freshmen. Chin. J. Health Psychol. **25**(03), 446–449 (2017). https://doi.org/10.13342/j.cnki.cjhp.2017.03.035
16. Zheng, R.C.: Psychological Diagnosis of College Students. Shandong Education Press, Jinan (1999)
17. Wang, X.L., Xu, N.F., Yang, D.H., et al.: Intercourse vexation among medical students. Chin. Ment. Health J. **04**, 247–250 (2005). https://doi.org/10.3321/j.issn:1000-6729.2005.04.008
18. Chen, Y.J., Huang, S.H., Zhou, Q.A., et al.: Interaction mechanism between boredom proneness, interpersonal disturbance and internet gaming addiction in university freshmen. Med. Soc. **33**(07), 90–93 (2020). https://doi.org/10.13723/j.yxysh.2020.07.021
19. Huang, X.L., Zhang, L., Liu, T.L., et al.: Detecting suicidal ideation in Chinese microblogs with psychological lexicons. In: 2014 IEEE 11th International Conference on Ubiquitous Intelligence and Computing and 2014 IEEE 11th International Conference on Autonomic and Trusted Computing and 2014 IEEE 14th International Conference on Scalable Computing and Communications and Its Associated Workshops, pp. 844–849 (2014). https://doi.org/10.1109/uic-atc-scalcom.2014.48
20. Guan, L., Hao, B., Cheng, Q., et al.: Identifying Chinese microblog users with high suicide probability using internet-based profile and linguistic features: classification model. JMIR Ment. Health **2**(2), e17 (2015). https://doi.org/10.2196/mental.4227

21. Cheng, Q., Li, T.M., Kwok, C.L., et al.: Assessing suicide risk and emotional distress in chinese social media: a text mining and machine learning study. J. Med. Internet Res. **19**(7), e243 (2017). https://doi.org/10.2196/jmir.7276
22. Guan, L., Hao, B.B., Cheng, J., et al.: Behavioral and linguistic characteristics of microblog users with various suicide ideation level: an explanatory study. Chin. J. Public Health **31**(03), 349–352 (2015). https://doi.org/10.11847/zgggws2015-31-03-29
23. Ryan, T., Xenos, S.: Who uses Facebook? An investigation into the relationship between the big five, shyness, narcissism, loneliness, and Facebook usage. Comput. Hum. Behav. **27**(5), 1658–1664 (2011). https://doi.org/10.1016/j.chb.2011.02.004
24. Gosling, S.D., Augustine, A.A., Vazire, S., et al.: Manifestations of personality in online social networks: self-reported Facebook-related behaviors and observable profile information. Cyberpsychol. Behav. Soc. Netw. **14**(9), 483–488 (2011). https://doi.org/10.1089/cyber.2010.0087
25. Cash, S.J., Thelwall, M., Peck, S.N., et al.: Adolescent suicide statements on My Space. Cyberpsychol. Behav. Soc. Netw. **16**(3), 166–174 (2013). https://doi.org/10.1089/cyber.2012.0098
26. Spates, K., Ye, X., Johnson, A.: "I just might kill myself": suicide expressions on Twitter. Death Stud. **44**(3), 189–194 (2020). https://doi.org/10.1080/07481187.2018.1531085
27. Liu, X., Liu, X., Sun, J., et al.: Proactive suicide prevention online (PSPO): machine identification and crisis management for Chinese social media users with suicidal thoughts and behaviors. J. Med. Internet Res. **21**(5), e11705 (2019). https://doi.org/10.2196/11705
28. Agrawal, P.K., Alvi, A.S., Bamnote, G.R.: Natural language-based self-learning feedback analysis system. In: Satapathy, S.C., Raju, K.S., Mandal, J.K., Bhateja, V. (eds.) Proceedings of the Second International Conference on Computer and Communication Technologies. AISC, vol. 380, pp. 99–107. Springer, New Delhi (2016). https://doi.org/10.1007/978-81-322-2523-2_9

Assessing the Utilisation of TELedentistry from Perspectives of Early Career Dental Practitioners - Development of the UTEL Questionnaire

Joshua Lee[1,2(✉)], Joon Soo Park[1,2,3,5], Hua Wang[1], Boxi Feng[2], and Kate N. Wang[4,5,6]

[1] Institute for Sustainable Industries and Liveable Cities, Victoria University, Melbourne, Australia
jleeresearch1@gmail.com
[2] International Research Collaborative - Oral Health and Equity, The University of Western Australia, Crawley, WA, Australia
[3] UWA Dental School, The University of Western Australia, Nedlands, WA, Australia
[4] UWA School of Allied Health, The University of Western Australia, Nedlands, WA, Australia
[5] School of Health and Biomedical Sciences, RMIT University, Melbourne, VIC, Australia
[6] Pharmacy Department, Alfred Health, Melbourne, VIC, Australia

Abstract. Introduction: Teledentistry has allowed for the provision of dental care remotely. It has benefitted people living in regional, rural and remote communities. The use of teledentistry rapidly increased during the COVID-19 pandemic to minimise transmission risk while still allowing for the provision of care, especially during mandated lockdowns. **Aim:** This study aims to pilot and assess the validity of a questionnaire developed to understand early career dental practitioners' opinions regarding teledentistry in Australia. **Method:** Registered early career dental practitioners currently working in Australia were invited to participate. Participants were asked to respond to a series of questions regarding teledentistry on themes containing diagnosis, accessibility, patient care, technology and finances. In addition, participants were asked for feedback upon the conclusion of the questionnaire . **Results:** A total of 23 dental practitioners (60% female, age range 20–34) participated in this study. Work experiences ranged from 0–10 years. A total of 18 participants worked in metropolitan areas, while five worked in regional areas. All participants used teledentistry for approximately 1–9 hours per week. Over 82% of participants believed that telehealth was effective for consultations, and over 90% believed it was more convenient than face-to-face consultations. However, over 78% believed teledentistry was ineffective for diagnosing complex dental cases. Over 95% of participants believed that teledentistry improved patient healthcare access and was beneficial during the coronavirus (COVID-19) pandemic. All participants believed that teledentistry was a useful tool for post-operative care, and over 86% of participants felt that patients accepted teledentistry. **Conclusion:** This questionnaire effectively determines the utilisation of teledentistry during a global pandemic from the perspective of early career dental practitioners.

Keywords: Telehealth · Dentistry · Health science · Digital health · Australia

A. Traina et al. (Eds.): HIS 2022, LNCS 13705, pp. 189–196, 2022.
https://doi.org/10.1007/978-3-031-20627-6_18

1 Introduction

Teledentistry is the usage of information and communication technology to facilitate communication and remote consultations between health professionals and patients [1]. Teledentistry has been beneficial in providing care to patients disadvantaged by distance, frailty, transport and health [2]. Teledentistry saw increased usage during the coronavirus (COVID-19) pandemic as government-mandated lockdowns imposed restrictions on movement and decreased the ability to access healthcare, for example, to remotely consult patients to triage them for eligibility regarding emergency care [3]. Teledentistry allowed the provision of healthcare while reducing social contact and reducing the virus's transmission risk [2]. While teledentistry is beneficial, many dental practitioners have found it challenging to implement due to the technology's complexity and unreliability and the limited diagnostic and interventional capacity of teledentistry [4].

While previous studies have analysed health practitioners' opinions regarding teledentistry, most of this was conducted before the COVID-19 pandemic or in specialised dental services [1, 4]. One study conducted in 2016 by Estai *et al.* demonstrated that 80% of clinicians agreed that teledentistry would improve dental practice through enhanced communication, increasing efficiency of patient management and referrals. The participants also believed that patients had high satisfaction for teledentistry. However, the clinicians were uncertain regarding the reliability of the technology, expenses particularly with setup cost, privacy and diagnostic accuracy [1]. Similarly, Lee *et al.*'s study conducted in 2021 demonstrated that the participants were satisfied with the improved accessibility that telehealth offered however there were concerns regarding diagnostic accuracy and the reliability of the technology. However this study only analysed the opinions of specialist oral and maxillofacial surgeons [4]. Telehealth consultation was provided with a new item number on the Australian Schedule of Dental Services and Glossary to allow clinicians to charge appropriately [5]. Therefore, capturing a more recent understanding of dental practitioners' opinions of teledentistry is important.

2 Aims

This study aims to assess the research protocol to evaluate the efficacy and increase the validity of a questionnaire developed to determine early career dental practitioners' opinions regarding teledentistry.

3 Methods

An anonymous e-questionnaire was created using Qualtrics® XM software (Provo, UT, USA). The e-questionnaire was adapted from Lee *et al.*'s interview questionnaire, which evaluated Australian oral and maxillofacial surgeons' perceptions of telehealth [4]. The first section had questions regarding their demographic and professional background. The second section had 28 questions with a 5-point Likert Scale divided into five sub-sections. The sub-sections were diagnosis, accessibility, patient care, technology and finances.

Convenience sampling was used to identify dental practitioners who would be interested in participating in this pilot study. Participants were recruited from social media, and the survey was distributed via email to those interested. After obtaining consent, the participants completed the questionnaire and were asked to provide feedback.

The collected data from Qualtrics were imported into a comma-separated values (CSV) file. The demographics and answers to the questions were reported as counts and percentages. Descriptive statistics were used to analyse the results.

3.1 Ethics Approval

This study was approved by the Human Research Ethics Committee at the University of Western Australia (Approval Number - ROAP 2022/ET000369).

4 Results

4.1 Demographics

Participants aged 20–34 with 0–10 years of work experience. Nine were males, and 14 were females. Eighteen worked in major cities, and five worked in inner regional cities. Participants spent 1–9 of their working hours using teledentistry.

The results from the study are outlined in Table 1.

Table 1. Results regarding diagnosis, accessibility, patient care, technology and finances. 1 = Strongly agree, 5 = Strongly disagree

	Question	Mean	Standard deviation
Diagnosis	I believe that telehealth is effective for consultations	1.87	0.90
	I believe that patients can reliably self-report symptoms through telehealth	2.43	0.77
	I believe that telehealth is effective for diagnosing simple cases	1.87	0.90
	I believe that telehealth is effective for diagnosing complex cases	3.91	0.93
	I believe that telehealth is effective for diagnosing pathology	3.87	1.03
	I am confident in my diagnosis through telehealth without a tactile exam	3.57	1.01
	Telehealth is convenient e.g., it saves time	1.70	0.86

(*continued*)

Table 1. (*continued*)

	Question	Mean	Standard deviation
Accessibility	Telehealth improves access for remote and rural patients	1.30	0.46
	Telehealth has been beneficial during the pandemic	1.39	0.57
	Telehealth has been convenient for patients	1.65	0.81
	Telehealth has assisted in reducing wait times	1.78	0.78
	Telehealth provides improved flexibility compared to in-person	1.78	0.66
	Telehealth is easily accessible for older patients	2.52	1.25
Patient care	Telehealth is useful for triaging patients	1.48	0.58
	Telehealth has effective interventional capacity	2.74	0.99
	Telehealth is comparable to face-to-face	3.74	1.07
	Telehealth is useful for post-op care	1.52	0.50
	I am able to build patient rapport over telehealth	2.17	0.76
	Patients are accepting of telehealth	1.91	0.58
Technology	I prefer telehealth over face-to-face	3.30	1.33
	The quality of the technology used in telehealth is adequate	2.61	0.87
	I believe that data is secure over telehealth	2.65	0.96
	I am happy that medicolegal issues are not a problem over telehealth (Consent)	2.65	0.87
	Patients are able to use the technology	2.65	0.81
	Telehealth technology is reliable	2.26	0.61
Finances	There are no issues regarding billing with telehealth	2.91	0.65
	The cost for delivering telehealth is similar to face-to-face	3.26	0.74

4.2 Diagnosis

Over 82% of participants believed teledentistry was effective for consultations and diagnosing simple cases. Only 60% of participants somewhat agreed that patients were reliable at self-reporting their symptoms through teledentistry, with 21% neither agreeing nor disagreeing and 13% disagreeing. Over 78% of participants believed that teledentistry was unable to diagnose complex cases, and over 69% believed that they were unable to diagnose pathology. Approximately 60% were not confident in their diagnosis due to the inability to conduct a tactile exam. However, 91% believed that teledentistry was convenient (Fig. 1).

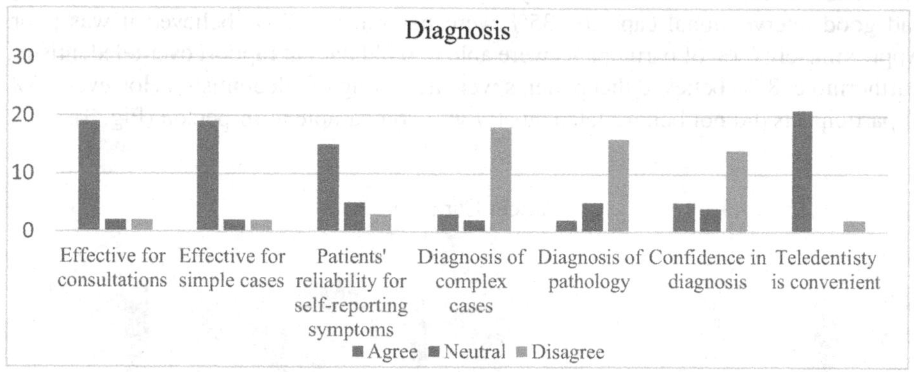

Fig. 1. Practitioners' opinions regarding diagnosis through teledentistry

4.3 Accessibility

All participants agreed that teledentistry improved access for patients living in rural and remote regions. Over 95% believed that teledentistry was beneficial during the coronavirus pandemic, 86% believed that teledentistry was convenient for patients, and 77% stated that teledentistry assisted in the reduction of waiting times for patients accessing treatment. In addition, approximately 86% of the participants believed that teledentistry was more flexible compared to in-person consultations, and around 60% believed that teledentistry was easily accessible for older patients (Fig. 2).

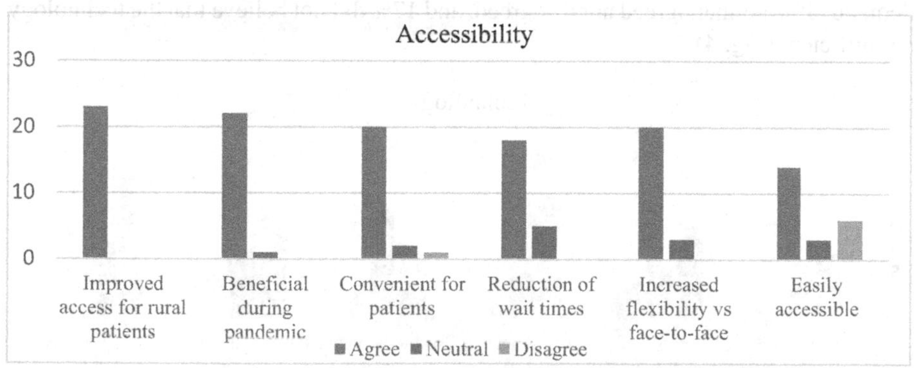

Fig. 2. Practitioners' opinions regarding accessibility

4.4 Patient Care

Teledentistry was useful for 95% of the participants, and all participants believed it was good to deliver post-operative care. However, there were mixed opinions regarding the interventional capacity of teledentistry. Approximately 39% believed that teledentistry had good interventional capacity, 35% were neutral, and 26% believed it was poor. Approximately 69% of participants were able to build patient rapport over teledentistry. Furthermore, 87% believed that patients were accepting of teledentistry. However, 65% of participants did not believe teledentistry was comparable to in-person (Fig. 3).

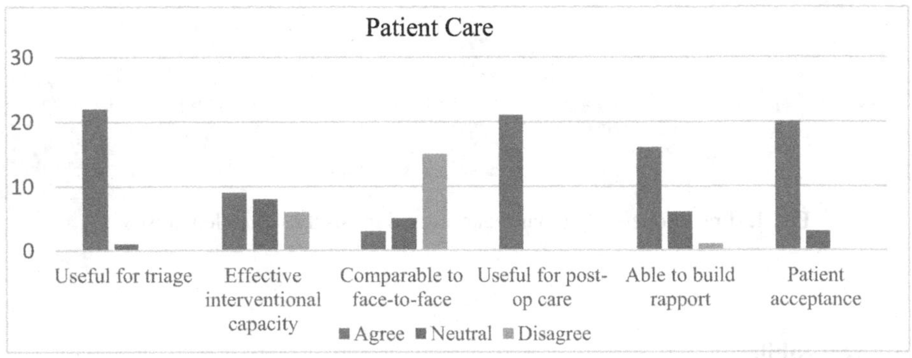

Fig. 3. Practitioners' opinions regarding patient care

4.5 Technology

Approximately 65% of participants strongly or somewhat agreed that the technology behind teledentistry was reliable. However, most participants somewhat or strongly disagreed that they preferred teledentistry over in-person consultations. Approximately 52% of participants felt neutral that medicolegal issues were not an issue over teledentistry. Regarding the quality of the technology, 48% believed that the current technology was adequate, 35% neither agreed nor disagreed, and 17% did not believe that the technology was sufficient (Fig. 4).

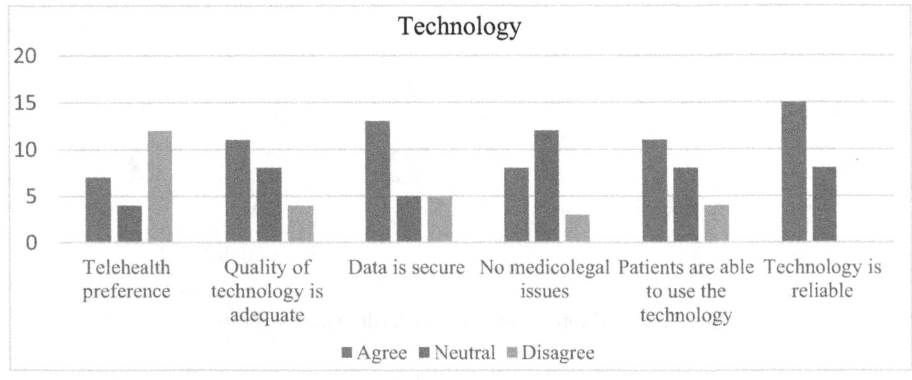

Fig. 4. Practitioners' opinions regarding technology of teledentistry

4.6 Finances

Regarding billing, 57% of the participants neither agreed nor disagreed that there were no issues over teledentistry. Approximately 26% agreed that there were no issues, and 17% felt there were some issues. Around 17% of participants agreed that the cost of delivering teledentistry was similar to in-person consultations, while 39% neither disagreed nor agreed, and 43% disagreed (Fig. 5).

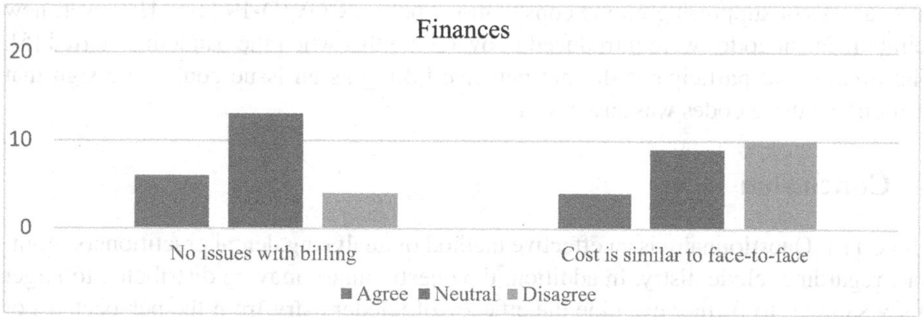

Fig. 5. Practitioners' opinions regarding finances

5 Discussion

This study was developed to assess the efficacy of the developed UTEL (Utilisation of Telehealth) e-questionnaire. All participants were satisfied with the questionnaire and stated that they could effectively outline their opinions regarding teledentistry. The UTEL questionnaire appears to be effective.

The preliminary findings showed that early career dental practitioners viewed teledentistry favourably. The participants liked teledentistry for non-complex consultations and believed that patients could reliably self-report symptoms. However, teledentistry was reported to have limitations in managing more complex cases such as pathology, which is consistent with telehealth across various health disciplines [4, 6].

Most participants agreed that teledentistry increased accessibility for patients, especially those living in rural and regional communities. This is most likely due to patients not having to travel a long distance to access health services. This has been a documented benefit of telehealth, particularly for specialist services, as there is a shortage of specialist health care workers in regional, rural and remote communities [7]. Previous studies also indicated that clinicians believed that telehealth would be beneficial for rural and regional communities, hence our results further support this [4, 8].

Teledentistry was also useful in providing post-operative care and building patient rapport, especially since patient acceptance was high. However, most participants did not believe teledentistry was comparable to in-person services. This is likely due to the inability to conduct a tactile exam which is a crucial part of diagnosing complex cases such as pathology [4]. Another common issue reported in the literature was the quality of technology available such as internet connections and cameras, which have been perceived to be inadequate [8]. In our study, the participants found that the technology was reliable, and this may be due to the improvements in infrastructure and technology allowing for smoother delivery of teledentistry. However, most participants still preferred in-person consultations. Participants were neutral regarding medicolegal issues, which could be due to the new technology leading to a lack of a clear legal and regulatory framework [9].

Billing was not noted to be an issue by the participants of this study. Finances were seen as an issue in previous studies, which stated that reimbursement was a large barrier to telehealth implementation. This is likely due to many private health insurance companies not supporting online consultations before COVID-19 [10]. However, new reimbursement codes were introduced to overcome this when the pandemic started [5]. The finding that participants did not perceive billing as an issue could be a sign that introducing these codes was successful.

6 Conclusion

The UTEL Questionnaire is an effective method of analysing dental practitioners' opinions regarding teledentistry. In addition, the questionnaire may be distributed to larger study samples to further examine the efficacy of teledentistry from the perspectives of dental practitioners.

References

1. Estai, M., et al.: The efficacy of remote screening for dental caries by mid-level dental providers using a mobile teledentistry model. Commun. Dent. Oral Epidemiol. **44**, 435–441 (2016)
2. Kayyali, R., Hesso, I., Mahdi, A., Hamzat, O., Adu, A., Nabhani Gebara, S.: Telehealth: misconceptions and experiences of healthcare professionals in England. Int J. Pharm. Pract. **25**, 203–209 (2017)
3. Zimmermann, M., Nkenke, E.: Approaches to the management of patients in oral and maxillofacial surgery during COVID-19 pandemic. J Craniomaxillofac Surg. **48**, 521–526 (2020)
4. Lee, J., Park, J.S., Wang, K.N., Feng, B., Tennant, M., Kruger, E.: The use of telehealth during the coronavirus (COVID-19) pandemic in oral and maxillofacial surgery–a qualitative analysis. EAI SIS e10-e10 (2022)
5. Australian Dental Association. Dentists now have new item number for telehealth consultations (2020). https://www.ada.org.au/News-Media/News-and-Release/Latest-News/New-item-number-for-telehealth-consultations. Accessed 19 Apr 2022
6. Kichloo, A., et al.: Telemedicine, the current COVID-19 pandemic and the future: a narrative review and perspectives moving forward in the USA. Fam. Med. Commun. Health **8** (2020)
7. Northridge, M.E., et al.: Feasibility and acceptability of an oral pathology asynchronous tele-mentoring intervention: a protocol. J. Public Health Res. **9**, 1777 (2020)
8. Estai, M., Kruger, E., Tennant, M., Bunt, S., Kanagasingam, Y.: Challenges in the uptake of telemedicine in dentistry. Rural Remote Health **16**, 3915 (2016)
9. Becker, C.D., Dandy, K., Gaujean, M., Fusaro, M., Scurlock, C.: Legal perspectives on telemedicine part 1: legal and regulatory issues. Perm J. **23** (2019)
10. Almathami, H.K.Y., Win, K.T., Vlahu-Gjorgievska, E.: Barriers and facilitators that influence telemedicine-based, real-time, online consultation at patients' homes: systematic literature review. J. Med. Internet Res. **22**, e16407 (2020)

Genetic Algorithm for Patient Assignment Optimization in Cloud Healthcare System

Xinyu Pang[1], Yong-Feng Ge[2(✉)], and Kate Wang[3]

[1] Guangdong Technion Israel Institute of Technology, Shantou, China
[2] Institute for Sustainable Industries and Liveable Cities, Victoria University, Melbourne, Australia
yongfeng.ge@vu.edu.au
[3] School of Health and Biomedical Sciences, RMIT University, Melbourne, Australia

Abstract. The cloud healthcare system is achieved based on the integration between Internet technologies and the traditional healthcare system. By combining online diagnosis and offline treatment, such a system can effectively reduce patients' waiting time and also improve idle medical resources' utilization ratio. In this paper, to optimize the balance of patient assignment (PA) in the cloud healthcare system, a genetic algorithm (GA) is proposed. Each individual in the proposed GA represents a solution for the PA optimization problem. Better solutions are generated by executing crossover, mutation, and selection operators in GA. Experiments verify that the proposed GA is effective in optimizing the PA problem.

Keywords: Patient assignment optimization · Genetic algorithm · Cloud healthcare system

1 Introduction

With the development of the Internet and information technologies [5,14,16,29,33], there is increasing demand for a cloud healthcare system [17,19,27,28] that satisfies all medical services [23,26,31]. Based on the combination of online diagnosis and offline treatment, a cloud healthcare system will likely save patients' time and improve the utilization of idle medical resources. However, the patient assignment (PA) problem is crucial in developing such a cloud healthcare system.

To solve this PA problem, various strategies have been proposed. In [15], a queuing model was developed using discrete event simulation, which could reduce the patient waiting time and increase the system's overall throughput. In [19], a Petri net was presented to describe the relationship between the medical process and resources in this integrated healthcare system. In [22], the hybrid ant agent algorithm was developed to identify the optimal path, thus reducing the patient's waiting time and cycle time. In the previous work, patients' waiting time is a crucial objective. The cloud healthcare system have continuously

A. Traina et al. (Eds.): HIS 2022, LNCS 13705, pp. 197–208, 2022.
https://doi.org/10.1007/978-3-031-20627-6_19

ongoing patients admissions. Thus, the balance of assignments among different doctors will improve the efficiency of the cloud healthcare system and should be considered.

To optimize the PA problem, genetic algorithm (GA) [6,30] can be utilized. GA is one kind of evolutionary algorithms (EAs) [3,9,12,34]. They are mostly utilized in computer mathematics to solve optimization issues. Several evolutionary biology phenomena, including heredity, mutation, natural selection, and hybridization, are used to build EAs [10,11,21]. GAs can find reasonable solutions quickly, even in complex spatial solutions. Chromosome sets are based on parallel studies, selection operations, alteration operations, and guessing mutation functions. In the previous work, EAs, including GAs, have been utilized in various scenarios [7,8,18], and have shown their advantages in reliability and performance.

In this paper, GA is utilized to optimize the PA problem. Each individual in the proposed GA represents a solution to the PA optimization problem. Several individuals in the proposed GA form a population. During the evolution of such a population, information included in different solutions is exchanged by the crossover operator. Solutions are randomly adjusted in the mutation operator. After that, the competitiveness of different solutions is evaluated in the selection operator, and the most competitive solutions are kept in the population. Finally, the optimal solution is outputted.

The organization of this paper is as follows. In Sect. 2, we review the related work about the PA problem. Then, a formal problem definition is given in Sect. 3. Afterward, the proposed GA is introduced in detail. In Sect. 5 and Sect. 6, the experimental study is executed. Finally, we conclude this paper.

2 Related Work

In [1], a positive model of the public hospital waiting lists was established. According to the studies, doctors did not necessarily treat the mildest cases on the waiting list in order to have the shortest overall hospital stay. In [4], Conforti *et al.* defined that the scheduling objective of radiotherapy patients in the oncology department was to ensure the best treatment in the shortest possible time. As a result, the waiting time should be minimized, and device utilization should be maximized. Various criteria were added to the optimization model. In [24], the dynamic patient scheduling with different priorities in a public healthcare setting was tackled. The proposed method dynamically assigns available capacity to incoming demand to achieve cost-effective wait-time targets. In [32], Takakuwa and Wijewickrama created a discrete-time simulation model and integrated the simulation model into the optimization algorithm to reduce patient waiting and physician idle time without adding any additional resources. This study collected real-time data from Nagoya University Hospital's outpatient clinic to create a simulation. In [13], the Lean Six Sigma (LSS) method was used to solve the problem of the long waiting time of patients. The entire procedure was covered, from patient registration to prescription distribution. A causal map was created for patients with longer waiting times, and data collected during the process were used to verify the reasons. In [20], a system was designed to reduce the doctors' idle time instead of the patients' waiting time. This study aimed to improve resource efficiency and modify how doctors schedule visits. The results showed that patients' waiting time might could be lowered without affecting doctors' work efficiency. In [15], a queuing model was developed using discrete event simulation, which could reduce the patient waiting time and improve the system's overall throughput. To resolve ambiguities in the present system, required data was collected, and alternative scenarios were generated and examined. Furthermore, the best solution with concerning patient satisfaction was proposed. In [19], a Petri net was presented to describe the relationship between the medical process and resources in this integrated healthcare system. A PA scheduling problem was investigated and studied to efficiently allocate this system's bottleneck medical resource. A mathematical model was established, and a greedy-based heuristic algorithm was designed. In [2], Chawasemerwa *et al.* developed a constraint satisfaction and penalty minimization scheduling model that satisfied "hard constraints" and minimized the cost of "soft constraints" violations. Furthermore, since multiple schedules may be obtained using the same parameters defined by users, an optimization protocol can be added to the system to reduce the search space and obtain the optimal schedule while satisfying the constraints. In [22], the real-time walk-in patient scheduling optimization problem was addressed. An overall patient scheduling model was integrated. The status and information of all outpatient departments were combined. The hybrid and agent algorithm was developed to identify the best path for the patient while also lowering cycle time (from registration to exit).

3 Problem Definition

In the PA problem, the optimization objective is to minimize the diagnosis time difference among different doctors.

Specifically, in PA, the i-th patient is represented by P_i; D_j represents the j-th doctor. The estimated diagnosis time of i-th patient is indicated by $\widetilde{T}_i$.

The total diagnosis time of j-th doctor (represented by T_j) is calculated as follows:

$$T_j = \sum_{i=1}^{nP} \widetilde{T}_i \times S_i^j \tag{1}$$

where nP is the number of patients; S indicates a status matrix. S_i^j equals to one when the i-th patient is allocated to the j-th doctor; S_i^j equals to zero when the i-th patient is not allocated to the j-th doctor.

Thus, the mean value of diagnosis time is calculated as:

$$\overline{T} = \sum_{j=1}^{nD} T_j \tag{2}$$

where nD is the number of doctors.

The time factor (TF) is then obtained by calculating the standard deviation of diagnosis time of all the doctors. Formally,

$$\mathrm{TF} = \sqrt{\frac{\sum_{j=1}^{nD}(T_j - \overline{T})^2}{nD}} \tag{3}$$

As mentioned above, the optimization objective is to balance the doctors' diagnosis time. Therefore, the optimization objective is to minimize the value of TF.

4 GA for PA

This section illustrates the proposed GA for optimizing the PA problem. Firstly, we introduce the representation manner of GA. Secondly, the crossover and mutation operators of GA are described. Afterward, the entire procedure of GA is described.

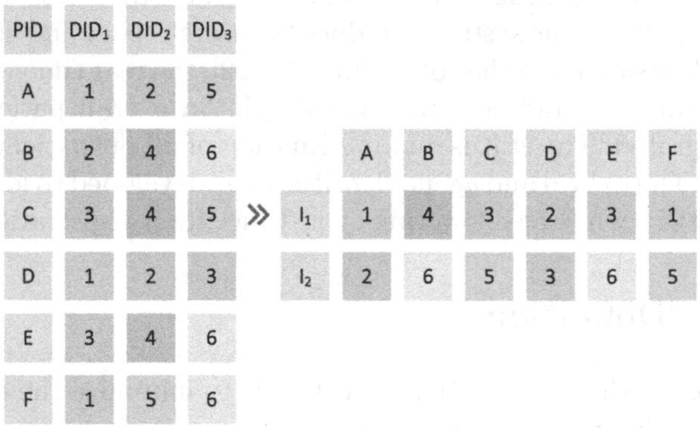

PID	DID_1	DID_2	DID_3
A	1	2	5
B	2	4	6
C	3	4	5
D	1	2	3
E	3	4	6
F	1	5	6

»

	A	B	C	D	E	F
I_1	1	4	3	2	3	1
I_2	2	6	5	3	6	5

Fig. 1. Illustration of the representation manner in GA.

4.1 Representation

In GA, each individual represents a solution for PA. In each individual, each gene indicates the assignment of each patient. An example of this representation manner is given in Fig. 1. In this example, three doctors allocated to for each patient (represented by A, B, ..., F). Different digits with different colors represent different doctors. In total, six doctors are included in this example. Therefore, one doctor is chosen from the candidature lists for each patient. In this example, two individuals are given (represented by I_1 and I_2). For the first patient (patient A), doctor 1 is allocated to in individual I_1, while doctor 2 is allocated to individual I_2. For each complete individual, it can be directly evaluated according to the definition of the PA problem.

4.2 Crossover Operator

In genetics, the crossover operator is an algorithmic procedure that encapsulates the phenomena of chromosomal crossover exchange and biological hybridization. For example, the act of recombining and assigning genes on the chromosomes of two parents to form the next generation of humans may combine the dominant genomes of the two parents to produce new individuals more adaptable and closer to the ideal solution via crossing over.

Similarly, the core of GAs is the internal operation of genetic manipulation. By crossover, we mean the function of replacement and recombination of parts of the structure of biparental individuals, resulting in new individuals. The searchability of GAs is greatly improved by crossover. First, general GAs have a mating probability (crossover probability). This mating probability reflects the probability of two selected individuals mating. Each pairing produces two new individuals that replace the original individuals, while the unmated individuals remain unchanged. Second, the parents' chromosomes pair to produce two new chromosomes. The first half is the father's chromosome, the second half is the mother's chromosome, and the second is the opposite. However, the halves here are not halves but a random part of the chromosome, a place called the mating point.

An example of the crossover operator in GA is given in Fig. 2. In the example, two individuals (represented by I_1 and I_2). The information included these two individuals is then exchanged. In this example, each individual includes six genes representing six patients. The values on six genes indicate the assignment of these six patients. For each gene, with the same possibility, one value is randomly chosen from two individuals during the crossover operator. For instance, on the first gene (gene A), the value in individual I_1 is chosen. Thus, in the child individual (represented by C), the value on the first bit is 1. Similarly, on the second gene (gene B), the value in C comes from individual I_2.

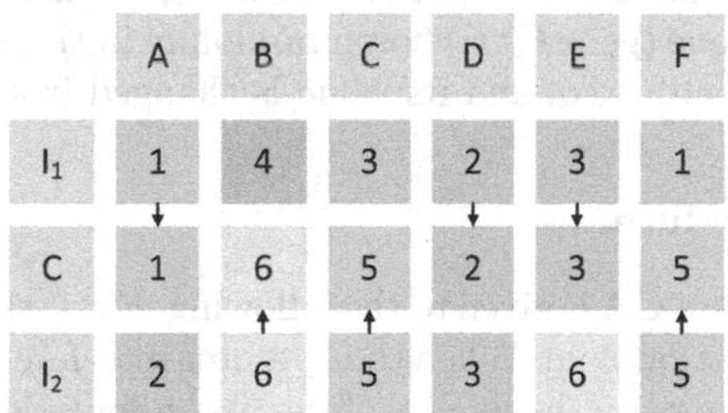

Fig. 2. Illustration of crossover operator in GA.

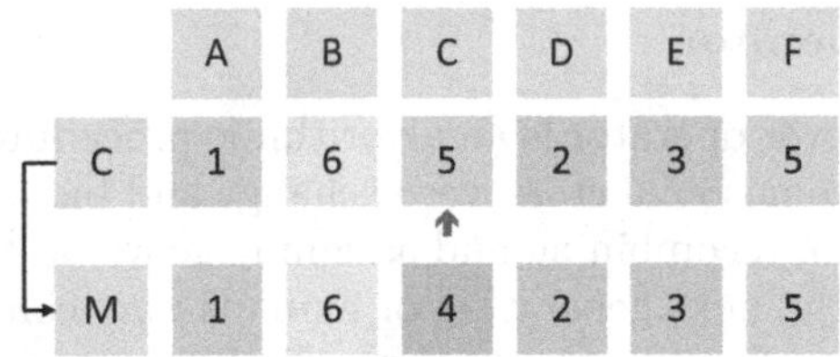

Fig. 3. Illustration of mutation operator in GA.

4.3 Mutation Operator

There are always individual differences between the parents and offspring of an organism, i.e., differences in the genetic material of different individuals in the same gene pool are called mutations.

The mutation operator's primary goal is to change the gene values at specific location in individual strings in the population. The probability of the mutation operator is represented by a constant in the general GA for fixed mutations (the probability of mutation). Based on this probability, a random mutation on the chromosome of a new individual is usually a change of one byte of the chromosome. There are two reasons for introducing mutations into GAs: First, give the GA a local random search function. The variation operator's local random search capability can speed up the convergence in the optimal solution when the GA approximates the optimal solution neighborhood by the crossover operator. In this case, the variance probability should take a small value. Otherwise, the variation will destroy the building blocks close to the optimal solution. The second is to enable the GA to maintain population diversity and prevent premature convergence. In this case, the convergence probability should take a more meaningful value.

In Fig. 3, an example of the mutation operator is given. With the mutation rate MR, each gene of the child individual (represented by C) is randomly adjusted. The third gene (gene C) is chosen randomly in this example. Therefore, its value is randomly adjusted, and its value is changed from 5 to 4.

4.4 Overall Procedure

The overall procedure of GA is given to the following. First, the program creates a set number of people at random. When the operator interferes with this randomly produced process to increase the quality of the first population, the quality of the initial population improves. After that, each generation's individuals are given a value, and the fitness value is calculated using the fitness function. Compared to the population's poor fitness, individuals with superior fitness are rated first.

The next step is to generate the next generation of individuals to form the population. This process is done by selection and replication, where replication involves crossover and mutation in algorithmic studies. Selecting the winners from the population and eliminating the inferior ones is called selection. The goal of selection is to pass on their directly optimized genes to the next generation or generate new people through crossover pairing and generation, which are then passed on to the next generation. Selectivity is based on assessing the physical condition of the people in the population. Selection is based on the fitness of new individuals. However, it does not mean at the same time that it is entirely oriented toward fitness because simply selecting individuals with high fitness will lead to a rapid local conversion of the algorithm to the optimal solution rather than to the optimal global solution, which we call the initial stage. As a compromise, GAs follow the principle that the higher the fitness, the higher the chance of being selected, and the lower the fitness, the lower the chance of being selected. The initial data can be selected to form a relatively optimal group. After that, the selected individuals enter the mating process. The core of biological evolution in nature is the recombination of biogenetics (coupled with mutation).

After this series of processes (selection, crossover, mutation), a new generation of individuals differs from the first generation. Each generation moves toward improved overall fitness since selecting the best individuals to produce the next generation is always more common. Conversely, poorly adapted individuals are gradually eliminated.

Table 1. Properties of 16 test instances

Test instances	nP	nD	T
T_1	100	10	[5, 20]
T_2	100	20	[5, 20]
T_3	100	30	[5, 20]
T_4	100	40	[5, 20]
T_5	200	10	[5, 20]
T_6	200	20	[5, 20]
T_7	200	30	[5, 20]
T_8	200	40	[5, 20]
T_9	300	10	[5, 20]
T_{10}	300	20	[5, 20]
T_{11}	300	30	[5, 20]
T_{12}	300	40	[5, 20]
T_{13}	400	10	[5, 20]
T_{14}	400	20	[5, 20]
T_{15}	400	30	[5, 20]
T_{16}	400	40	[5, 20]

5 Experimental Setup

This section illustrates the test instances, parameter settings, and algorithm implementation in the following experiments.

In the subsequent experimental studies, 16 test instances are utilized to investigate the performance of the proposed GA. Table 1 outlines the properties of these test instances, including the number of patients nP, the number of doctors nD, and the range of estimated diagnosis time T.

In the proposed GA, the population size N is set as 20; mutation rate MR is set as 0.1. The maximum fitness evaluation number is set as $nP \times nD$.

GA and all the compared algorithms in this paper are implemented in C++.

6 Experimental Result

Table 2. Comparison with existing approaches

Test instances	Random		Greedy	DE		GA	
	Avg	Std	Result	Avg	Std	Avg	Std
T_1	1.28E+01	1.81E+00	2.40E+01	1.11E+01	1.90E+00	**6.90E+00** †	9.27E−01
T_2	1.49E+01	1.01E+00	1.22E+01	1.24E+01	8.55E−01	**7.45E+00** †	6.43E−01
T_3	1.40E+01	8.01E−01	9.66E+00	1.13E+01	8.18E−01	**7.30E+00** †	4.94E−01
T_4	1.37E+01	5.67E−01	8.98E+00	1.14E+01	6.25E−01	**8.05E+00** †	2.76E−01
T_5	1.91E+01	1.72E+00	4.83E+01	1.60E+01	1.80E+00	**9.42E+00** †	1.26E+00
T_6	2.03E+01	1.47E+00	2.54E+01	1.64E+01	1.16E+00	**1.00E+01** †	1.05E+00
T_7	1.91E+01	1.01E+00	1.73E+01	1.50E+01	7.02E−01	**9.50E+00** †	6.93E−01
T_8	1.86E+01	7.84E−01	1.22E+01	1.51E+01	6.48E−01	**9.69E+00** †	4.59E−01
T_9	2.08E+01	3.02E+00	8.06E+01	1.63E+01	2.31E+00	**1.05E+01** †	1.23E+00
T_{10}	2.61E+01	1.91E+00	3.58E+01	1.96E+01	1.50E+00	**1.22E+01** †	8.68E−01
T_{11}	2.43E+01	1.04E+00	2.54E+01	1.94E+01	1.30E+00	**1.22E+01** †	8.33E−01
T_{12}	2.07E+01	9.75E−01	1.33E+01	1.72E+01	8.47E−01	**1.11E+01** †	5.24E−01
T_{13}	2.24E+01	3.51E+00	9.62E+01	1.91E+01	3.23E+00	**1.12E+01** †	1.64E+00
T_{14}	2.93E+01	2.25E+00	3.89E+01	2.24E+01	2.05E+00	**1.37E+01** †	9.76E−01
T_{15}	2.78E+01	1.28E+00	2.61E+01	2.15E+01	1.44E+00	**1.34E+01** †	9.04E−01
T_{16}	2.57E+01	1.18E+00	1.91E+01	2.03E+01	1.03E+00	**1.32E+01** †	9.04E−01

6.1 Comparison with Existing Approaches

To verify the performance of the proposed GA algorithm, it is compared with three existing algorithms, i.e., Random, Greedy, and differential evolution (DE) [25]. These algorithms are described as follows:

1. Random: This algorithm uses a random manner to solve the PA problem. Random solutions are continuously generated and compared with the best solution. The best solution is replaced once a more competitive solution is generated.

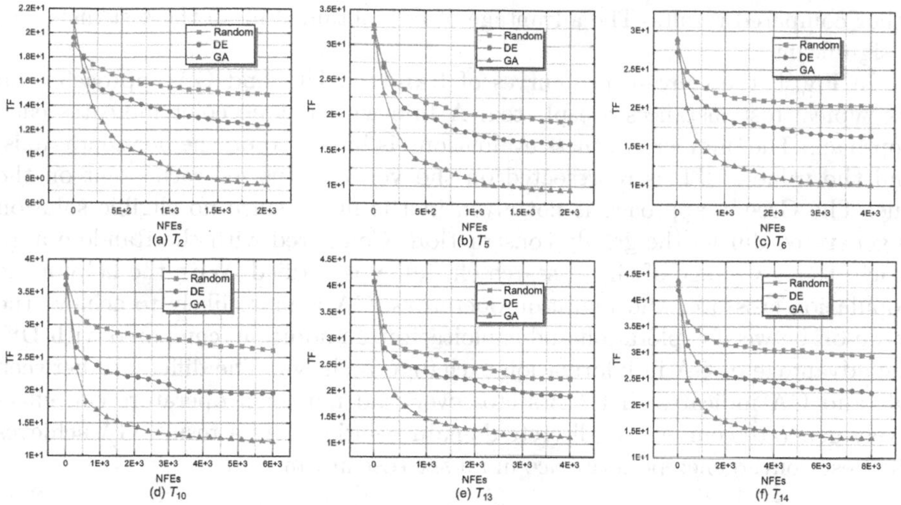

Fig. 4. Convergence curves of GA and compared algorithms on six typical test instances.

2. Greedy: This algorithm uses a greedy manner to solve the PA problem. Each patient is greedily allocated to a doctor about the value of TF.
3. DE [25]: This DE algorithm utilizes the "DE/best/1" mutation schema to generate the mutant individuals, which can help accelerate the exploitation search ability during the optimization of the PA problem.

Table 2 lists the mean and standard deviation of TF values over 25 independent runs. The Greedy approach only lists its results since it can generate deterministic results. In Table 2, the best results are highlighted in **boldface**. Our proposed GA can outperform the competitors on all 16 test instances. The benefit of GA in population recombination and mutation operators is confirmed compared to Random. With the help of these two operators, the allocation of information among different individuals is effectively exchanged, and more competitive solutions are generated and inserted into the population. Compared with Greedy, the advantage of GA in population diversity is verified. The greedy technique is more likely to get trapped by the local optima during the PA problem optimization. Unlike the Greedy approach, the population diversity of GA can effectively guarantee the exploration search ability of GA. The benefit of GA in discrete-domain optimization is demonstrated when compared to DE. The mutation strategy of DE, such as "DE/best/1", is efficient in the continuous-domain calculation. However, for this discrete PA problem, its mutation strategies are difficult to transfer the information among individuals.

Besides, the Wilcoxon rank-sum test with a 0.05 level is utilized to investigate the performance of these algorithms in a statistical sense. In Table 2, the symbol † shows that the corresponding result is significantly better than the other compared results. The advantage of GA obtained in all the test instances is significant.

In Fig. 4, the convergence curves of Random, DE, and GA approaches on six typical test instances are plotted. A line with unique color indicates each approach. The number of fitness evaluations is indicated on the horizontal axis, and the value of TF is represented on the vertical axis for each point on the line. The Greedy approach is not given in the figure since no eligible solution is generated during the greedy construction. Compared with the Random approach, the advantage of GA in search efficiency is verified. With the help of the population crossover and mutation operators, GA is more likely to achieve the trade-off between exploration and exploitation. In addition, compared with DE, the advantage of GA in information exchange is shown. The difference between DE and GA indicates that GA's crossover and mutation operators can effectively generate competitive discrete-domain solutions. As a result, GA achieves the best convergence performance in all six test instances.

7 Conclusion

In this paper, a GA has been proposed to optimize the balance of PA schedules. Each individual in the proposed GA represents a solution for the PA optimization problem. Furthermore, three operators in the proposed GA, i.e., crossover, mutation, and selection, have been utilized to improve the competitiveness of these solutions. Through the analysis of the experimental results, we have verified that the proposed GA effectively optimizes the PA problem.

In the future, it would be crucial to include more objectives in PA problem. Thus, some practical multi-objective optimization algorithms should be designed accordingly.

References

1. Barros, P.P., Olivella, P.: Waiting lists and patient selection. J. Econ. Manage. Strategy **14**(3), 623–646 (2005). https://doi.org/10.1111/j.1530-9134.2005.00076.x
2. Chawasemerwa, T., Taifa, I., Hartmann, D.: Development of a doctor scheduling system: a constraint satisfaction and penalty minimisation scheduling model. Int. J. Res. Ind. Eng. 7(4), 396–422 (2018). https://doi.org/10.22105/riej.2018.160257.1068
3. Chen, Z.G., Zhan, Z.H., Wang, H., Zhang, J.: Distributed individuals for multiple peaks: a novel differential evolution for multimodal optimization problems. IEEE Trans. Evol. Comput. **24**(4), 708–719 (2020). https://doi.org/10.1109/tevc.2019.2944180
4. Conforti, D., Guerriero, F., Guido, R.: Optimization models for radiotherapy patient scheduling. 4Or, **6**(3), 263–278 (2007). https://doi.org/10.1007/s10288-007-0050-8
5. Du, J., Michalska, S., Subramani, S., Wang, H., Zhang, Y.: Neural attention with character embeddings for hay fever detection from Twitter. Health Inf. Sci. Syst. **7**(1), 1–7 (2019). https://doi.org/10.1007/s13755-019-0084-2

6. Ge, Y.F., et al.: A benefit-driven genetic algorithm for balancing privacy and utility in database fragmentation. In: Proceedings of the Genetic and Evolutionary Computation Conference, pp. 771–776. ACM (2019). https://doi.org/10.1145/3321707.3321778
7. Ge, Y.-F., Cao, J., Wang, H., Zhang, Y., Chen, Z.: Distributed differential evolution for anonymity-driven vertical fragmentation in outsourced data storage. In: Huang, Z., Beek, W., Wang, H., Zhou, R., Zhang, Y. (eds.) WISE 2020. LNCS, vol. 12343, pp. 213–226. Springer, Cham (2020). https://doi.org/10.1007/978-3-030-62008-0_15
8. Ge, Y.F., Orlowska, M., Cao, J., Wang, H., Zhang, Y.: Knowledge transfer-based distributed differential evolution for dynamic database fragmentation. Knowl.-Based Syst. **229**, 107325 (2021). https://doi.org/10.1016/j.knosys.2021.107325
9. Ge, Y.F., Orlowska, M., Cao, J., Wang, H., Zhang, Y.: MDDE: multitasking distributed differential evolution for privacy-preserving database fragmentation. VLDB J. **31**, 1–19 (2021). https://doi.org/10.1007/s00778-021-00718-w
10. Ge, Y.F., et al.: Distributed memetic algorithm for outsourced database fragmentation. IEEE Trans. Cybern. **51**(10), 4808–4821 (2021). https://doi.org/10.1109/tcyb.2020.3027962
11. Ge, Y.F., Yu, W.J., Zhan, Z.H., Zhang, J.: Competition-based distributed differential evolution. In: 2018 IEEE Congress on Evolutionary Computation (CEC). IEEE (2018). https://doi.org/10.1109/cec.2018.8477758
12. Ge, Y.F., Yu, W.J., Zhang, J.: Diversity-based multi-population differential evolution for large-scale optimization. In: Proceedings of the 2016 on Genetic and Evolutionary Computation Conference Companion. ACM (2016). https://doi.org/10.1145/2908961.2908995
13. Gijo, E.V., Antony, J.: Reducing patient waiting time in outpatient department using lean six sigma methodology. Qual. Reliab. Eng. Int. **30**(8), 1481–1491 (2013). https://doi.org/10.1002/qre.1552
14. He, J., Rong, J., Sun, L., Wang, H., Zhang, Y., Ma, J.: A framework for cardiac arrhythmia detection from IoT-based ECGs. World Wide Web **23**(5), 2835–2850 (2020). https://doi.org/10.1007/s11280-019-00776-9
15. Hossain, N.U.I., Debusk, H., Hasan, M.M.: Reducing patient waiting time in an outpatient clinic: a discrete event simulation (DES) based approach. In: Proceedings of IIE Annual Conference, pp. 241–246. Institute of Industrial and Systems Engineers (IISE) (2017)
16. Jiang, H., Zhou, R., Zhang, L., Wang, H., Zhang, Y.: Sentence level topic models for associated topics extraction. World Wide Web **22**(6), 2545–2560 (2018). https://doi.org/10.1007/s11280-018-0639-1
17. Lee, J., Park, J., Wang, K., Feng, B., Tennant, M., Kruger, E.: The use of telehealth during the coronavirus (COVID-19) pandemic in oral and maxillofacial surgery - a qualitative analysis. ICST Trans. Scalable Inf. Syst. **9**, 172361 (2021). https://doi.org/10.4108/eai.2-12-2021.172361
18. Li, J.Y., Du, K.J., Zhan, Z.H., Wang, H., Zhang, J.: Distributed differential evolution with adaptive resource allocation. IEEE Trans. Cybern. (2022). https://doi.org/10.1109/tcyb.2022.3153964
19. Li, Y., Wang, H., Li, Y., Li, L.: Patient assignment scheduling in a cloud healthcare system based on petri net and greedy-based heuristic. Enterp. Inf. Syst. **13**(4), 515–533 (2018). https://doi.org/10.1080/17517575.2018.1526323
20. Mardiah, F.P., Basri, M.H.: The analysis of appointment system to reduce outpatient waiting time at Indonesia's public hospital. Hum. Resour. Manage. Res. **3**(1), 27–33 (2013)

21. Mirjalili, S.: Evolutionary Algorithms and Neural Networks. SCI, vol. 780. Springer, Cham (2019). https://doi.org/10.1007/978-3-319-93025-1
22. Munavalli, J.R., Rao, S.V., Srinivasan, A., van Merode, G.: Integral patient scheduling in outpatient clinics under demand uncertainty to minimize patient waiting times. Health Inform. J. **26**(1), 435–448 (2019). https://doi.org/10.1177/1460458219832044
23. Pandey, D., Wang, H., Yin, X., Wang, K., Zhang, Y., Shen, J.: Automatic breast lesion segmentation in phase preserved DCE-MRIs. Health Inf. Sci. Syst. **10**(1), 1–19 (2022). https://doi.org/10.1007/s13755-022-00176-w
24. Patrick, J., Puterman, M.L., Queyranne, M.: Dynamic multipriority patient scheduling for a diagnostic resource. Oper. Res. **56**(6), 1507–1525 (2008). https://doi.org/10.1287/opre.1080.0590
25. Price, K.V.: Differential evolution. In: Zelinka, I., Snášel, V., Abraham, A. (eds.) Handbook of Optimization, pp. 187–214. Springer, Heidelberg (2013). https://doi.org/10.1007/978-3-642-30504-7_8
26. Sarki, R., Ahmed, K., Wang, H., Zhang, Y.: Automated detection of mild and multi-class diabetic eye diseases using deep learning. Health Inf. Sci. Syst. **8**(1), 1–9 (2020). https://doi.org/10.1007/s13755-020-00125-5
27. Sarki, R., Ahmed, K., Wang, H., Zhang, Y., Wang, K.: Convolutional neural network for multi-class classification of diabetic eye disease. ICST Trans. Scalable Inf. Syst. **9**, 172436 (2021). https://doi.org/10.4108/eai.16-12-2021.172436
28. Singh, R., Zhang, Y., Wang, H., Miao, Y., Ahmed, K.: Investigation of social behaviour patterns using location-based data - a Melbourne case study. ICST Trans. Scalable Inf. Syst. **8**, 166767 (2020). https://doi.org/10.4108/eai.26-10-2020.166767
29. Siuly, S., et al.: A new framework for automatic detection of patients with mild cognitive impairment using resting-state EEG signals. IEEE Trans. Neural Syst. Rehabil. Eng. **28**(9), 1966–1976 (2020). https://doi.org/10.1109/tnsre.2020.3013429
30. Srinivas, M., Patnaik, L.: Genetic algorithms: a survey. Computer **27**(6), 17–26 (1994). https://doi.org/10.1109/2.294849
31. Supriya, S., Siuly, S., Wang, H., Zhang, Y.: Automated epilepsy detection techniques from electroencephalogram signals: a review study. Health Inf. Sci. Syst. **8**(1), 1–15 (2020). https://doi.org/10.1007/s13755-020-00129-1
32. Takakuwa, S., Wijewickrama, A.: Optimizing staffing schedule in light of patient satisfaction for the whole outpatient hospital ward. In: 2008 Winter Simulation Conference. IEEE (2008). https://doi.org/10.1109/wsc.2008.4736230
33. Vimalachandran, P., Liu, H., Lin, Y., Ji, K., Wang, H., Zhang, Y.: Improving accessibility of the Australian my health records while preserving privacy and security of the system. Health Inf. Sci. Syst. **8**(1), 1–9 (2020). https://doi.org/10.1007/s13755-020-00126-4
34. Wang, Z.J., et al.: Automatic niching differential evolution with contour prediction approach for multimodal optimization problems. IEEE Trans. Evol. Comput. **24**(1), 114–128 (2020). https://doi.org/10.1109/tevc.2019.2910721

Research on the Construction of Psychological Crisis Intervention Strategy Service System

Yahong Yao[1], Shaofu Lin[1](✉), Zhisheng Huang[2], Shushi Li[1], Chaohui Guo[1], and Ying Wu[1]

[1] Faculty of Information Technology, Beijing University of Technology, Beijing, China
{yaoyh,guochaohui}@emails.bjut.edu.cn, linshaofu@bjut.edu.cn
[2] Department of Computer Science, Vrije University Amsterdam, Amsterdam, The Netherlands

Abstract. Purpose: Traditional psychological crisis intervention requires one-to-one and long-term consultation by psychotherapists, which has high time cost and expense. The public has a strong realistic demand for more convenient psychological crisis intervention services. In order to solve the above problem, this paper presents an approach which transforms the actual professional psychological consultation data into knowledge graph, establishes a terminology/ontology of psychological crisis intervention, and constructs an automatic service prototype system of psychological crisis intervention. Method: This paper takes actual professional psychological crisis intervention cases as prior knowledge, expresses and stores them in the form of triples. The natural language generation model based on GPT-2 model is constructed by using the data in PsyQA as the training set for several rounds of training. The terminology of psychological crisis intervention is constructed. Then the psychological crisis intervention system is constructed, including modules as keyword extraction, deep semantic matching, knowledge graph retrieval crisis intervention strategy providing module and natural language generation. Result: The test results show that for the users which can correctly input the psychological problem description text, the system can Identify crisis types, provide the corresponding intervention strategies and return the targeted crisis intervention text. Conclusion: This system avoids the constraints of traditional crisis intervention such as high price, poor timeliness and few professionals, and provides a feasible method for people who need to get simple crisis intervention services in time.

Keywords: Mental health · Psychological crisis intervention · Knowledge graph · Natural language processing

1 Introduction

At present, while the pace of life in society is getting faster and faster, people are facing more pressure from work and study, and thus they are prone to mental diseases. The psychological pressure, panic and anxiety brought by COVID-19 epidemic have exacerbated the prevalence of mental diseases, which has become a major global public health problem [1]. People with psychological diseases need to be treated in time, otherwise the

A. Traina et al. (Eds.): HIS 2022, LNCS 13705, pp. 209–216, 2022.
https://doi.org/10.1007/978-3-031-20627-6_20

negative emotions it brings will cause immeasurable consequences if they accumulate for a long time [2]. For example, suicides of students in colleges and middle schools are common [3]. The reason for this is complicated. On the one hand, it is due to people's lack of basic knowledge of mental diseases, a clear understanding of the harm of mental diseases. On the other hand, the lack of psychological counselors leads to the fact that counselors can't get effective help in time [4]. And the lack of a scientific theoretical system to solve psychological problems intelligently also counts.

Knowledge graph is a better method for storing information intelligently at present [5]. This method was proposed by Google in 2012 and quickly used in intelligent semantic search. At present, artificial intelligence technology is gradually mature, and has penetrated into all aspects of society [6]. Especially with the development of natural language processing technology, knowledge graph has more application prospects.

The purpose of psychological crisis intervention is to reduce the psychological trauma of psychological crisis events and reduce the possibility of causing long-term psychological crisis. It plays a decisive and key role in helping the victims get out of the dilemma [7]. Some researchers have applied computer technology in the field of crisis intervention. However, most of the existing studies only apply computer technology to the judgment of psychological crisis or the identification of intervention opportunities [8]. There have been no Chinese studies that apply computer technology to the implementation stage of psychological crisis intervention. The specific implementation still mainly depends on offline manual intervention.

In order to solve the above problems, this paper constructs a prototype system that can simulate the crisis intervention process. The users input text describing their psychological state, life experiences and encounters, and the system can identify whether there are crisis and the type of crise, give strategies for crisis intervention and the text of crisis intervention. This paper combines knowledge graph with natural language generation technology, to store actual crisis intervention texts by using the characteristics that knowledge graph can describe complex graph relational data. When the system encounters the situation that the existing knowledge can't cover, it calls the neural network model to generate personalized crisis intervention text.

2 Construction of Knowledge Graph

2.1 Data Sources

The data source for the knowledge graph is PsyQA [9], a data set composed of real records of psychological Q & A in Yixinli community. The data set contains questions, keywords, answers and other information, including about 22,000 pieces of psychological counseling data. Topics included in the PsyQA data set include: growth, emotion, love, interpersonal relationship, behavior, family, treatment, marriage and career. The questions in PsyQA data set cover a variety of user groups. The answers in PsyQA data set are highly professional. About 8% of the answers come from national second-class psychological counselors; 35% of the responses come from volunteers recruited by Yixinli community.

2.2 Structure Design of Knowledge Graph

After analyzing the structure of PsyQA, it is found that all the questions in the data set are marked with 2–4 keywords by the questioner, which are closely related to the content of questions and answers. There are many questions with the same keywords and their corresponding answers, which have significant overlap in terms of semantic similarity and the help strategies used. Therefore, we can use keywords to improve the speed of retrieving information in the knowledge graph, and store keywords and the description and solutions of psychological problems into the knowledge graph.

Then the knowledge graph structure represented by the triples of Eqs. 1, 2 and 3 is designed.

$$(\text{Question},\ \text{Keyword},\ \text{topic}) \tag{1}$$

$$(\text{Answer},\ \text{Question},\ \text{reply}) \tag{2}$$

$$(\text{Vector},\ \text{Question},\ \text{embedding}) \tag{3}$$

2.3 Calculation of Sentence Vector

When users input the description of their psychological problems, they need to calculate the semantic similarity between the description and the existing knowledge stored in the knowledge graph, so as to select the available knowledge [10]. Semantic similarity calculation is based on sentence vector calculation of questions.

In this paper, BERT pre-training model is used to calculate sentence vectors. In the specific operation, we directly install the BERT-as-service tool and start the service, load the downloaded BERT pre-training model, and input text information to get the corresponding sentence vector result, which has 728 dimensions.

2.4 Storage of Knowledge Graph

The Py2Neo, a python driven tool of the Neo4j is used to store our knowledge graph.

PsyQA data sets are provided in the string format of JSON format, so Python programs are written and run to identify the corresponding entity data from JSON files. RDFLib library is used to create graph instance, establish corresponding triples of entity and relationship data extracted from data set and add them to knowledge graph instance. Then the BERT as service pre training model is called to, calculate the sentence vector of the psychological problem description in each data set, and save it to the knowledge graph instance. Finally, the knowledge graph instance is exported to RDF file in JSON-LD format.

The Neo4j graph database is used as the storage carrier of knowledge graph. The Py2Neo library is used to connect to Neo4j database, and a new instance of Neo4j database is created. Then the neosemantics (n10s) component is called with cypher [18] statement as shown in Table1, and the knowledge graph saved in JSON-LD format is imported into Neo4j.

Table 1. Key functions of cypher statement

Cypher statement	Functions
CREATE CONSTRAINT n10s_unique_uri ON (r:Resource); ASSERT r.uri IS UNIQUE;	Create uniqueness constraints to ensure the uniqueness of resources through URIs
CALL n10s. rdf. import. fetch(file:///D:\\Desktop\\BS\\Bertutilsmaster\\knowledgegraph_vec.rdf, "JSON-LD");	Import RDF data and persist it to Neo4j
MATCH (k:kwords) where k.name = '' create (:question{name:"Q", text:""})-[:keyword]- > (k);	Correct triples by predicate

3 Construction of Psychological Crisis Intervention System

3.1 Keyword Extraction Module

The keyBERT is selected for keyword extraction of psychological problems raised by users. It uses BERT to extract the document vectors (embedding) to obtain document level representation. Then, the word vectors are extracted for N-ary grammatical words or phrases. Finally, the cosine similarity algorithm is used to find the most similar words or phrases with the document.

3.2 Knowledge Graph Retrieval Module

After the psychological problem description text input by the user passes through the keyword extraction module, the topic domain to which it belongs has been acquired. Then we need to retrieve the information in the knowledge graph according to the acquired keywords.

1. First, we need to use the extracted keywords to retrieve information in the graph, and then calculate the semantic similarity between the retrieved questions and the questions entered by the user. The system uses Py2Neo package to connect to Neo4j database and retrieve it through cypher statement.
2. For the matched question text Q_{k1}, …, Q_{kn}, the semantic similarities with Qu are calculated in turn. For many different texts or short text dialog messages, we need to calculate the similarity between them. This paper maps the words in these texts to the vector space to form the mapping relationship between the text and the vector data in the text, and calculates the similarity of the text by calculating the difference of several or more different vectors. The cosine similarity of vector space uses the cosine value of the angle between two vectors in vector space as a measure of the difference between two individuals. The closer the cosine value is to 1, the closer the included angle is to 0°, that is, the more similar the two vectors are.

The calculation formula of cosine similarity is shown in formula (4).

$$\cos\theta = \frac{\sum_{i=1}^{n}(A_i \times B_i)}{\sqrt{\sum_{i=1}^{n}(A_i)^2} \times \sqrt{\sum_{i=1}^{n}(B_i)^2}} = \frac{A \cdot B}{|A| \times |B|} \tag{4}$$

3.3 Generation of Intervention Text Module

GPT-2 model is used in this paper to generate intervention texts. The core idea of GPT-2 is to use unsupervised pre-training model to do supervised tasks. It also has a strong one-way language ability to automatically generate classes from text models. All languages used in the structure of its one-way language model are decoder models based on the transformer language model.

In this paper, the GPT-2 model is improved as follows.

1. The GPT-2-Chinese project open source by Zeyao Du is used as the basis [20], in which the GPT-2-Chinese model with 117m parameters is used as the basis, and the general GPT-2-Chinese small model after pre-training is used.
2. At the same time, the data in PsyQA data set is used as the training set to fine tune the parameters of the general GPT-2-Chinese small model. However, considering the reason of computing power, the system did not carry out enough rounds of full training. Therefore, in the later experiments, the generated texts still tend to the style of the original pre-training model, but does not affect the smoothness of the generated texts.

Because the word vector of the input text is calculated and the keywords are extracted by using the BERT model in advance, the effect of omitting the word vector embedding module of the original word2vec part is achieved by using a linear layer instead. At the same time, this change makes it possible to map the 256 dimensional word vector into a word vector suitable for the given dimension 768 in the position encoder. In the part of the position encoder, each dimension is encoded separately, and finally the stacking operation is adopted.

Because the tokenizer of the Chinese version of GPT-2 language model is not open sourcing by OpenAI, and the original word2vec has poor semantic expression effect, we have to adopt the word representation method adopted by BERT model, considering the feasibility and the advantages of BERT bidirectional generation. After the modification of the model combination, we use PsyQA data set to train it. In the training process, the loss function is given as MSE (Mean Square Error), and the optimization algorithm adopts Adam algorithm.

3.4 Crisis Intervention Strategy Providing Module

In this paper, a lexicon of psychological crisis intervention is constructed. The crisis type of the text input by the user is judged through the crisis intervention lexicon, including psychological crises such as interpersonal relationship, academic pressure, loss of relatives and friends, financial theft, internet addiction disorder, accidents and sexual assault. The corresponding intervention strategies are collected the from a book named Adolescent Crisis Intervention and were converted them into electronic data. Part of the Lexicon of Psychological Crisis Intervention is shown in the Table 2.

Table 2. Part of lexicon of psychological crisis intervention

Type of psychological crisis	Words
Interpersonal relationship	Contradiction, quarrel, repression, alienation, indifference, conflict, competition
Academic pressure	Impatience, emotional ups and downs, low learning efficiency, anxiety, irritability
Loss of relatives and friends	Pain, fear, guilt, helplessness, grief, mourning, funeral, commemoration, crying, wailing, die, death
Financial theft	Guilt, anxiety, anger, money, blow, imbalance, shock, fidgeting
Internet addiction disorder	Introverted, solitary, nervous, lonely, rebellious
Accident	Fear, loss of control, grief, stress reaction, deformity
Sexual assault	Pregnancy, rape, indecency, suicide, sex, injury, infection

3.5 System Performance Analysis

This system is an application software for the people who are in psychological crisis. Because they need to obtain crisis intervention services as soon as possible, the front-end interactive interface should be simple and easy to use so that users can obtain the services quickly and directly. This system uses the FLASK front-end framework and is written in HTML and JavaScript languages. Figure 1 shows the interface style of the front-end interface before the user submits the description.

The test results show that the system can return the type of the psychological crisis, the strategies and targeted crisis intervention text correctly after the user input the psychological problem description (Fig. 2).

Psychological Crisis Intervention Strategy Service System
Feelings and confusion
Four years ago, my parents died of cancer. The family situation is getting worse and worse. I started working three years ago, but my work didn't go well, and I felt more and more inferior. Without any relatives, the only biological brother has become indifferent to himself. Because the family economy became difficult four years ago, the family house was gone. No one in the world loves me anymore, and no one needs me. More and more, I feel that there is no point in living. I feel that I have been alone, struggling in the dark but no one can give me a hand, desperate and confused about the future.
Access intervention
The type of Psychological crisis
Strategies should be adopted
Text of intervention

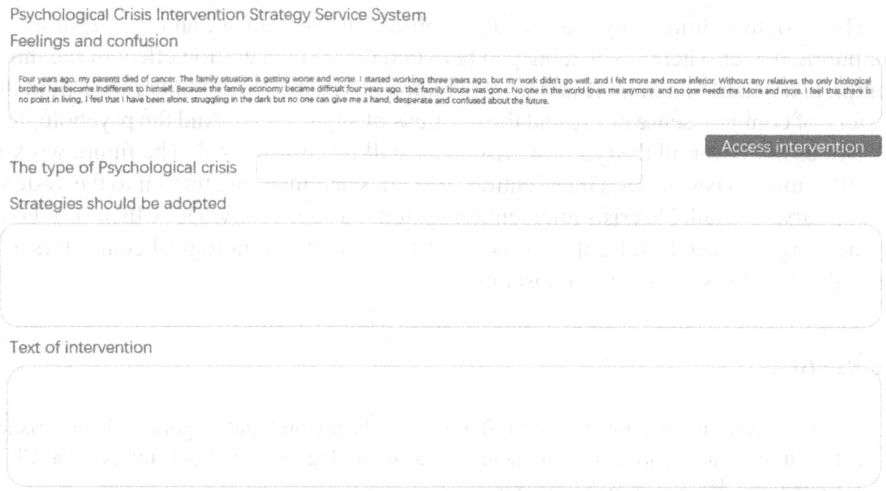

Fig. 1. Display of system

Psychological Crisis Intervention Strategy Service System
Feelings and confusion
Four years ago, my parents died of cancer. The family situation is getting worse and worse. I started working three years ago, but my work didn't go well, and I felt more and more inferior. Without any relatives, the only biological brother has become indifferent to himself. Because the family economy became difficult four years ago, the family house was gone. No one in the world loves me anymore, and no one needs me. More and more, I feel that there is no point in living. I feel that I have been alone, struggling in the dark but no one can give me a hand, desperate and confused about the future.
Access intervention
The type of Psychological crisis
Loss of relatives and friends
Strategies should be adopted
1. Encourage him to express his feelings. Talking about the feeling of losing his family, we can let him express his inner grief, sadness and even regret through words and paintings. Don't criticize or even satirize some negative emotions expressed by him, such as "You shouldn't think that way", "You shouldn't hurt yourself" and "How can you do that?" But listen
2.Help him get rid of his guilt. Some people will think that the death of their families is self-inflicted. We must let him know that everyone can make mistakes, and he has tried his best to behave well. He is not responsible for anyone's death. At the same time, help him remember the happy days with his deceased relatives, and remind him that he made his family feel very happy.
Text of intervention
I am very distressed by your experience and give you a warm hug ~ You mentioned in the message: 1. Because of the death of your parents and your brother's indifference to you, you feel very helpless; 2. Unfavorable work coupled with financial difficulties, has added a lot of pressure to you.
Share some of my own views: 1. Family support is really very important to us. Without the love of parents, you and your brother depend on each other. You might as well talk to your brother and listen to the reason why he snubbed you. In addition, it should be clear that family members depend on each other and help each other. Parents love you very much. On the one hand, because you are their child, they also have enough resources and financial ability to give you what you want at that time. However, unlike your brother, he grew up with the care of his parents just like you, and it is hard for him to lose his parents. For him, his situation is similar to yours, and he has to face the test of life, so he can't give you all the dependence and support. Mutual support is the better way for you to get along with each other. 2. After leaving your parents, you have to learn to grow up by yourself. Not many family members can give you support. You have to gradually establish and run your own circle of friends. When you are in trouble, your friends can give you a hand; in addition, when life is difficult, the society still provides us with a lot of resources and help, just as low-income groups have set up relief funds, venture funds for those who start businesses, etc. We don't live in an isolated society. As long as you are in need, there are always people in the society who lend you a helping hand. If you don't know how to find these resources, you might as well ask social workers in community service centers for help. We are not alone, but you have to take the initiative to find the allies who will go with you. Good luck! The world and I love you.

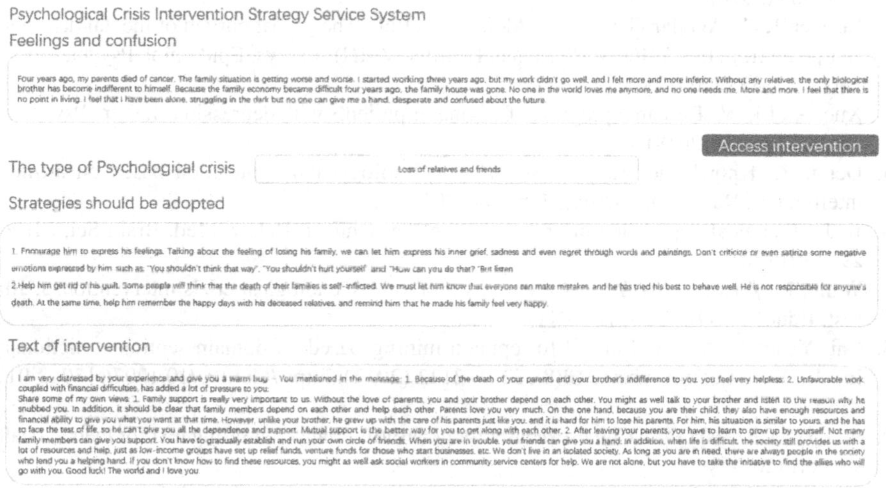

Fig. 2. Display of test case

4 Conclusion

This paper constructs a knowledge graph based on professional actual psychological crisis intervention knowledge. On the basis of GPT-2-Chinese model, we train it by using the data in PsyQA data set as the training set. A terminology of psychological crisis intervention is established to identify crisis types. Then we establish a service system that can automatically carry out basic psychological crisis intervention at any time.

The system is limited by the low data volume of the data set and the pre training computing power. There is still a big gap between the text generation effect of the intervention text generation module and words spoken by real people, mainly reflected in the mastery of common sense of life and the richness of suggestions. And the psychological crisis does not cover all the types of crises that will be encountered. The future work is to collect more types of crisis intervention strategies and integrate them into the system. In summary, an available crisis intervention system has been provided, which is of great practical significance to solve the problems of the lack of psychological counselors and the high cost of psychological counseling.

References

1. Guan, L., Hao, B.: A pilot study of differences in behavioral and linguistic characteristics between Sina suicide microblog users and Sina microblog users without suicide idea. Chin. J. Epidemiol. **36**(5), 421–425 (2015)
2. Li, J., Tong, H., Zhang, Y., et al.: Study on the relationship between the pathological time of Heyi and the onset time of depression in Mongolian medicine. Global Chin. Med. **9**(6), 678–683 (2016)
3. Kessler, R.C., Aguilar-Gaxiola, S., Alonso, J., et al.: The global burden of mental disorders: an update from the WHO World Mental Health (WMH) surveys. Epidemiol. Psychiatric Sci. **18**(1), 23–33 (2009)
4. Xue, X., Li, W.: Research progress of stigma in patients with depression. J. Clin. Psychiatry **28**(3), 212–214 (2018)
5. Deng, Z.: Knowledge graph construction technology and application based on artificial intelligence. Radio Eng. **52**(05), 766–774 (2022)
6. Ji, J.: Technical application of crisis intervention. Chin. J. Behav. Med. Brain Sci. **21**(04), 299–301 (2016)
7. Wang, L., Zhao, J., Xu, Y.: Review of research on psychological crisis intervention. J. Jilin Inst. Educ. **27**(09), 139–141 (2011)
8. Cai, Y., et al.: A hybrid model for opinion mining based on domain sentiment dictionary. Int. J. Mach. Learn. Cybern. **10**(8), 2131–2142 (2017). https://doi.org/10.1007/s13042-017-0757-6
9. Sun, H, et al.: PsyQA: a Chinese dataset for generating long counseling text for mental health support (2021)
10. Huang, Z., Min, Y., Lin, F., et al.: Temporal characteristics of suicide information in social media. Chin. Digit. Med. **14**(3), 7–10 (2019)

Towards a Perspective to Analyze Emergent Systems in Health Domain

Sandro Luís Freire de Castro Silva[1](✉), Bruno Elias Penteado[3], Rodrigo Pereira dos Santos[2], and Marcelo Fornazin[3]

[1] Brazilian National Cancer Institute, Rio de Janeiro, Brazil
sandro.freire@inca.gov.br
[2] Federal University of the State of Rio de Janeiro, Rio de Janeiro, Brazil
rps@uniriotec.br
[3] Oswaldo Cruz Foundation, Rio de Janeiro, Brazil
bruno.penteado@fiocruz.br, marcelo.fornazin@ensp.fiocruz.br

Abstract. The digital transformation has enabled substantial technological innovations in the health care practice. As a result, a myriad of technological devices and applications emerged in the hands of health care practitioners, patients, and laypeople. However, once the emergent systems and technologies do not follow a planned and managed process, it is difficult to understand how they can be applied. This article aims to review the literature of emergent systems in healthcare to investigate the plurality of terms and approaches and synthesize definitions and properties for these systems and technologies. Based on the results, this study also proposes a research agenda and discusses directions for researchers and practitioners dealing with emergent systems in the health domain. The main findings support that emergence has a direct relationship with collaboration and action performed by different actors. In addition, emergent systems cannot be isolated and observed without considering issues regarding the context in which a technological artifact is inserted.

Keywords: Emergent systems · Health informatics · Information systems

1 Introduction

The technologies based on the Internet of Things (IoT), big-data analytics, Artificial Intelligence (AI), robotics, blockchain, additive manufacturing, and cyber-security have been transforming health practice and medicine [1]. Topics such as efficiency [2], productivity [3], and optimization [4], give rise to other relevant questions, e.g., the nature of digital transformations, the development within the organizations, and the impacts caused in health practice.

On the other hand, the focus only on business health limits the analysis of these technologies in other areas of study, such as organizational sciences, sociology, public health, and information systems (IS) [5]. Specific phenomena, in most cases, are ignored. One of these little-discussed themes in digital transformations is emergent systems in

A. Traina et al. (Eds.): HIS 2022, LNCS 13705, pp. 217–228, 2022.
https://doi.org/10.1007/978-3-031-20627-6_21

the health domain. The emergent systems phenomenon occurs when an artifact, which is not explicitly designed for a given task, is appropriate by the actors and used to achieve socially defined goals. These systems become a significant part of a given context and consequently live without controls or regulation. An example is instant messaging [6].

Nowadays, it is impossible to think about health practice without using an IS for shared decision-making [7]. When we observe this phenomenon, there are countless reasons to explain the use of an instant messaging application: timeliness, the need for timely collaboration, and the cost; nevertheless, emergent systems in the health domain are not limited to messaging applications. Office suites, pen drives, wikis, social networks, and the most unexpected technologies can become an emergent system and enable an infinity of discussions on this theme [6].

The complexity and emergence of technologies have been discussed for the last 30 years [8, 9]. However, to the best of our knowledge, there is consensus to a definition of emergent systems in healthcare in the literature related to medical informatics, computer science, and IS. The lack of studies to analyze aspects of emergent systems in health motivates further investigations. There are open questions regarding how these systems arise? Why do the actors involved choose to use them? What are the risks when adopting informal artifacts in healthcare organizations?

Furthermore, the plurality of terms and approaches to emergent systems makes it difficult to understand how they can be applied to analyze specific technological domains, including health [10, 11]. Several opinions behind emergent systems have been investigated, and it was called the "great eclipse", which represents a distortion of vision when the term is used to analyze specific domains [12].

Another problem is the fact that some studies present cases that address emergent systems but do not use this category, which makes the task of studying emergent systems even more complex [13]. It is also necessary to understand the properties of emergent systems, specifically, because that comprehension could be considered critical to know their particularities. The concept of emergent properties is consolidated when the perspective comes from software engineering studies, but few and widespread forms of observation are considered when we treat properties as a characteristic of something.

This article aims to define consensus between the different approaches of emergent systems to clarify the conceptualization of emergent systems and reduce these theoretical gaps. From that point on, our study focuses on formulating a perspective to analyze specific domains. This study chose the health domain based on the argument that it is a global subject and has attracted attention in computing and engineering [14]. Despite the constant evolution of technologies developed exclusively for health practice, the health domain has been increasingly dependent on these emergent systems. In addition, there are no known studies in the literature that developed works with this focus.

To achieve the goal of our study, a review was planned and executed based on guidelines for conducting systematic mapping studies [15, 16]. Based on the results, this study also proposes a research agenda and discusses the directions for researches in emergent systems in the health domain. The article is organized as follows: Sect. 2 presents the article background; Sect. 3 explains the review procedure; Sect. 4 shows results; Sect. 5 brings some discussion and presents the literature common factors; Sect. 5.1 presents the chosen perspective to analyze emergent systems in the health domain and presents a research agenda; Sect. 5.2 present study limitations; and Sect. 6 concludes the article.

2 Background

Studies analyzing emergence in complex systems can be found in the exact and social sciences, with applications in physics, chemistry, biology, medicine, economics, and sociology [17]. One of the emergence perspectives is that they are associated with dynamic systems whose behavior arises from the interaction among its parts and cannot be predicted from knowledge about the parts in isolation [18]. In Economic Sciences, that concept is presented as the emergence of new and coherent structures, patterns, and properties during self-organization processes in complex systems [19].

The IS studies address emergent systems through a systemic view, treating those systems as a product of the interaction between the parties [18]. This view seems coherent when complex systems are analyzed as something static and linear. However, the perspective may seem incomplete when considering the interactions between systems, actors, and the context in which they belong. Therefore, it is necessary to define what can be treated as emergent systems in IS since the term is used deliberately and confused as a synonym for "appearance" or "growth," different from something similar to its essence built upon philosophical concepts of complex systems.

In emergent systems approaches, emergent properties are mostly cited, and several studies present emergent properties as a result of the interaction between components. Nevertheless, little is discussed on the interactions between actors and the context in which the systems are established. An emergent property can be defined as a collection or complex system property but not its decoupled parts. They belong to a group of items, whether insects, atoms, or buildings, that someone would not find in any of the items if analyzed in isolation [8]. Otherwise, in the literal definition of the Oxford English Dictionary, a property can be defined as a quality or characteristic that something has. An emergent property can also be interpreted as a particularity of these systems.

In the Economic Sciences definition [19], the emergent properties were summarized in: (1) radical novelty (features not previously observed in the system); (2) coherence or correlation (meaning integrated wholes that maintain themselves over a while); (3) a global or macro "level" (i.e., there is some property of "wholeness"); (4) being the product of a dynamical process (it evolves); and (5) being "ostensive" (it can be perceived). However, these definitions possibly make more sense when we consider that in analyzing specific domains in IS, including health.

Based on the conceptualization originated in the Economic Sciences, in our study, emergent systems in the health domain should not be considered static artifacts: they must be part of a context, with multiple interactions between their actors and other systems. From this current of thought, it was noticed that the literature on health information systems addresses several emergent systems. However, it does not use this taxonomy. Several reasons for using these systems could also be identified and implications that can make this choice a negative thing.

The highest frequency and the best example to start understanding emergent systems are smartphones. They were incorporated in the context to meet the particular need of different actors. According to some studies, the use of this emergent system was mainly motivated to allow communication among individuals, promote agility of healthcare, and suppress the geographical problem to provide healthcare [11, 12].

It is worth reflecting that the presence of smartphones may be related to the easy access to this device and its popularization and reduction of production cost. Other studies argue that the evolution of technologies and easy access to this device have contributed to this reality [20]. Even with the experiences reported in the literature, there are essential reflections to be carried out in this scenario, such as patient privacy, timeliness of responses, and work relations. The following section presents details on a systematic mapping study that aims to identify studies in the literature that address emergent systems and emergent properties.

3 Research Method

Our research was conducted based on Kitchenham and Charters' guidelines for performing literature reviews in a systematic way [21]. We initially ran specific queries of health and emergent systems against online databases to gain an initial understanding of the coverage offered by literature in different disciplines. After that, we define that our question was formulated following the PICOC criteria (Population, Intervention, Comparison, Outcomes, Context). In the context of our study, only PO was used since this review consists of a systematic mapping study. The population was: **emergent systems and emergent properties**; and the outcomes were: **studies reporting cases, models, methods, or theories about emergent systems**.

The objective was formalized based on GQM (Goal-Question-Metric) [29]: to **analyze** reports from research groups **in order to** characterize with respect to concepts and approaches for emergent systems concepts as well as emergent properties **from the point of view** of researchers and practitioners **in the context** of the studies.

Based on [16], our work defined two research questions (RQ1) and (RQ2) and six sub-research questions (Sub-Q) (Table 1). These Sub-Qs were formulated to aid the analysis of the information collected and consequently the discussions of the results.

Table 1. Research questions.

Research question	Sub-question
(RQ1) What do we know about emergent systems?	• (Sub-Q1) Which definitions exist? • (Sub-Q2) Which properties are reported? • (Sub-Q3) Which areas are explored?
(RQ2) What are the implications to the health domain?	• (Sub-Q4) How does the literature contribute to emergent systems in healthcare? • (Sub-Q5) What kind of analysis does the literature present? • (Sub-Q6) What are the research challenges in the health domain?

3.1 Define Research Terms

The search terms were pooled into a search string. After some iterations, we refined a term that better represented the purpose of our research. Thus, the search string and the logical operators used were: ("emergent system") OR ("emergent properties"). In the search bases, two search filters were applied, delimiting the area for technological studies (in general). Next, we executed the search string in the selected digital libraries.

3.2 Inclusion, Exclusion, and Selection Criteria

According to Kitchenham and Charters [16], inclusion criteria (IC) and exclusion criteria (EC) should be defined and applied to the retrieved studies. For the selection of a study, it should address at least one IC. In turn, the exclusion would be for any study attending at least one EC. The criteria were described in Table 2.

Table 2. Inclusion and exclusion criteria.

Inclusion criteria	IC 1	• The study refers to an emergent system
	IC 2	• The study describes emergent properties
Exclusion criteria	EC 1	• The solution has no technology area relationship

Three researchers conducted this review. These researchers have had practical experience in the industry and health information systems research for at least five years. In addition, researchers #2 and #3 supported the data analysis and discussion of results, given their experience of 15 years in literature studies. The selection process was operationalized based on five steps: (1) search execution; (2) first filter: reading titles, abstracts, and keywords; (3) second filter: reading introduction and conclusion; (4) third filter: complete reading; and (5) data extraction.

After step 5, data were extracted and organized into a table that recorded the items from the reading and analysis of each study. This table has recorded data required to respond Sub-Qs. The fields were: (1) study ID, (2) title, (3) year, (4) authors, (5) object of the case study, (6) emergent system concept, (7) emergent properties presented, and (8) analysis if emergent system concept could be applied to the context of the study.

4 Results

Initially, this research found 1,298 studies that approach emergent systems between 1994 and 2021. Then, they were analyzed if it was valid for the study following the criteria presented in Sect. 3. Each study received a category that defined the study area in which the study belonged during this step. After that, duplicate studies were removed to pass through new reading filters (steps 2–4) until the relevant studies were defined. After that, 46 studies [21] were considered for discussion, and obtaining the definitions of emergent systems (Sub-Q1) and 15 emergent systems areas (Sub-Q3) were listed in this study (Table 3).

The highest frequency of emergent systems concepts appeared in System of Systems. Therefore, this result has an origin from the concept of emergent behavior in System of Systems and, according to the definitions found [S33] [S36] [S44], it can be defined as a new behavior from the interactions among constituent systems but cannot be deduced from the behaviors of the constituent systems themselves.

Table 3. Table captions should be placed above the tables.

Area	Id	Frequency
System of systems	S8, S10, S11, S13, S15, S18, S21, S22, S27, S33, S35, S36, S41, S42, S43, S44	16
System engineering	S5, S6, S7, S12, S20, S23, S24, S29, S30, S45	10
Complex systems	S1, S14, S16, S32	4
Algorithms	S19, S26, S40	3
Internet of Things	S34, S37	2
Intelligent robotic system	S2, S3	2
Computer security	S31	1
Organizational perspective	S17	1
E-government	S38	1
Communication protocols	S39	1
CSCW	S9	1
Ubiquitous computing systems	S28	1
Human-centered computing	S46	1
Non-functional requirements	S25	1
Mobile media	S4	1

The perspective of System Engineering presents emergent properties [S7] [S30] [S40] associated with a set of components at one level in a hierarchy that are related to constraints upon the degree of freedom of those components. In Systems Engineering, another study points the same in System of Systems [S10]: if the architectural style of an emergent system could be predicted in advance, the system architect could make necessary changes to ensure that the quality attributes dictated by the system requirements were satisfied before the actual system was deployed. This topic is important because it points to the possible investigation of predictability characteristics for this type of system. However, it seems contradictory to predict an emergent system, given that one of the factors that characterize these systems in some views is unpredictability.

In Computer Supported Cooperative Work (CSCW) [S9], emergent systems, also referred to as Complex Adaptive Systems (CAS), comprise a significant number of actors which can interact with one another and with an environment in such a way that system functions may be accomplished despite some degree of individual agent failures and unexpected environmental changes. The Computer Security area [S31] presents a relevant perspective to emergent properties. The literature of emergent systems in Information Security has mostly been restricted to isolated cases, rarely with a perspective on reacting to the broader picture of the possibilities of emergent vulnerabilities, attacks, defenses, and diagnostics. The most common example in this area is that human consciousness is hard to understand or predict by studying individual neurons.

Socio-technical Design of Ubiquitous Computing Systems area [S28] presents emergent properties such as something not limited to computer systems but are also known in other disciplines such as biology, physics, and chemistry. In Applied Computing to e-government, the notion of emergent properties [S38] could also be attributed to the non-deterministic behavior of e-government. A property is called emergent if it comes from the properties and relations characterizing its simpler constituents. It is neither predictable nor reducible to lower-level characteristics. The definition is usually interpreted using the famous quote "the whole is greater than the sum of the parts", suggesting that such properties or structures arose from the interactions among smaller parts. However, these parts do not exhibit such properties or structures alone [S38].

The interaction among smaller parts of pattern and process at a smaller, faster scale produces a fundamentally new organization at a more extensive, slower scale. Understand the emergent properties in e-government is essential. E-government, as an enterprise, is a complex system. It is composed of multiple components (sub-systems) with multiple interactions between them [S38]. Interaction between people, processes, technology, and the environment may produce new emergent properties that only could be monitored and controlled at the level of the whole system [S38]. The e-government perspective is important to understand emergent systems in the health domain, given that most health technologies initiatives have government investments.

Regarding the domain applications, the Mobile Media area [S4] brings subsidies for emergent properties comprehension. The study relates to the use of emergent properties for music sharing. In addition, the studied artifact is a mobile platform, which shows the possibility of linking the perspectives when observing a complex system.

Once the results are found, the next section synthesizes concepts to define emergent systems to healthcare. Emergent properties (Sub-Q2) are also addressed to show the most relevant findings to this study.

5 Consensus on Emergent Systems from the Literature

This work proposes to present a theoretical approach to emergent systems. Even though several concepts and approaches were found, the results show common factors between the areas. Regardless of the area, it is possible to recognize that the phenomenon of emergent systems starts specifically from structures of complex systems, with the hierarchy between the actors and at levels that, if observed superficially, do not even allow the recognition of the existence of an emergent system. Therefore, it is the fundamental premise for a deep investigation on the theme: observing a technological artifact in isolation does not allow analyzing an emergent system.

The second basic premise is the evidence that analyzing a technological artifact without observing the context to which it belongs is a useless task for emergent systems. The context is fundamental to understand behaviors, actions, and characteristics, setting the definition of an emergent property. Based on this perspective, a common factor from the literature is organized below so that an approach to specific domains is identified. Considering the systematic mapping study results and the basic premises presented previously, some common factors could be reported for the emergent systems. Initially, it is possible to confirm that an emergent system is a system or behavior that originated from something unexpected [S14].

An emergent system is consensually part of a whole, which makes sense when observing an emergent system in a systemic view [19]. An emergent system may emerge for the most varied possible reasons. Fundamentally, they may originate from systemic failures or behaviors resulting from the actions of the operators of these systems (in this case, humans). Emergent systems are a phenomenon in which a system behavior is a novel in comparison to the behavior of its parts. An emergent system comes essentially from some behavior or action and, as a result, an action result.

Another property of emergent systems is that this phenomenon cannot be predicted from a superficial system analysis. Therefore, to observe an emergent system, it is necessary to analyze from the deepest to the highest levels. After the analysis, five main emergent systems factors towards a consensus found in our study were identified to answer RQ1: **[F1]** Emergent systems occurs at lower levels; **[F2]** Emergent systems changes system behavior; **[F3]** Emergent systems are something unexpected; **[F4]** Once an emergent system appears, it becomes a natural part of the functioning of the system; **[F5]** An emergent system is always a part of a whole. The factors are explained next. The goal is to build a theoretical link with the gap between emergent systems and the health domain.

5.1 Perspective Do Analyze the Health Domain

After analyzing the systematic mapping study results and identifying the factors as a consensus from the literature on emergent systems, our study seeks to present its state-of-the-art use of the concept formed to analyze the emergent system phenomenon in the health domain. Initially, it is important to consider that it is impossible to imagine the healthcare domain without technological support, such as electronic medical record systems, teleradiology, and medical knowledge portals. The technological innovations in the health domain are as diversified as possible, and the relevance of analyzing it and promoting complementary ways of observing the phenomena cannot be ignored.

The first factor is the fact that emergent systems occur at lower levels **[F1]**. It seems evident that a complex phenomenon can only be analyzed when observed at its lowest hierarchical levels. However, when the health domain is approached, this perspective makes more sense. Medical practice in a nursery scenario can be an example. If the medical practice is observed from a superficial point of view, the interactions between actors are limited to recording data in hospital medical records. However, if this process is analyzed in the lowest levels, considering the system is not something static, it can unexpectedly change the dynamics as a whole, making it possible to consider that this can be mediated through an emergent system.

From this fact, it is possible to think about the second factor found in the literature **[F2]**. If the structured practice is modified by the emergent system, the complete changes, and that system becomes a crossing point for the process to happen. For example, if medical conduct is subject to an endorsement by a more experienced professional, an exchange of messages via smartphones can be the way to support this task, instead of an electronic signature in an electronic medical record system. In this case, the innovation behind the signature tool does not matter, and the option will be the emergent system.

The third factor **[F3]** suggests that emergent systems, in general, are somewhat unexpected. When we point to the health domain, some hypotheses can be considered. If an emergent system appears unexpectedly in a process defined in the health practice, this dystopia may represent a need for improvement or an innovation opportunity. In other cases, the emergent system use may prove to be a way of circumventing norms, rules, or regulations that govern the health practice.

Therefore, the vast number of actors and their frequent collaboration take the emergent system to a natural part of the system's functioning **[F4]**. For example, from the idea of a smartphone as an emergent system in medical practice, it is possible to see that this behavior is repeated in several studies and probably in several organizations worldwide. Nowadays, it is impossible to think of communication between individuals without the mediation of a smartphone. In this case, the incorporation of the emergent system in medical practice may result from an appropriation of the social communication implemented for organizations.

The last presented factor is that an emergent system can effectively change the behavior of the whole **[F5]**. For example, suppose the actors involved in the health practice decide to use an emergent system instead of a non-emergent system (formal). In that case, the standard IS flow receives a deviation that can improve the performance of that medical practice (e.g., quick service or rapid diagnosis), or a worsening such as increased bureaucracy. One of the main reflections is that the domain processes are not static. Therefore, the interaction between the actors enables the most varied behaviors, with technologies mediating these relationships, including systems that emerge. Table 4 proposes theoretical perspectives based on the consensual factors to analyze each emergent system's common point (Sub-Q4).

The study also relates that emergent system concepts can be connected to IS studies in the health domain, as it has been established in research those emergent systems are a reality in technological innovations studies (Sub-Q5). Thus, it provides not only theoretical perspectives for analysis but also offers relevant reflections for future investigations. Emergent systems and emergent properties should be complementary to observe the complexity of the innovations in the health domain and to look at the complexity of systems in other contexts. By characteristic, these systems, in some cases, become a vital part of the functioning of the whole (Sub-Q5).

Some insights were obtained to propose a research agenda on the topic (Sub-Q6). These ideas indicated the need for dedicated studies that provide perspectives for analyzing technologies in the health domain, as shown in Table 5.

Table 4. Common factors and perspectives to emergent systems in the health domain.

Common factor	Perspective to analyze health domain
[F1] Emergent systems occur at lower levels	Researches involving health technologies need to be multidisciplinary; this perspective should consider the health practice and the organizational context with the artifact
[F2] Emergent systems changes system behavior	This common factor in the health domain points to the need to observe emergent systems as mandatory crossing points for health practice processes
[F3] Emergent systems are something unexpected	Sometimes the emergent systems can be treated as a risk, but they must be treated to something positive, looking for innovations and opportunities for improvement
[F4] Emergent systems become a natural part of the functioning of the system	An emergent system can become regular in a given context. Once used by the health professionals, the system becomes part of the natural functioning of the system
[F5] An emergent system is always part of a whole	Observing an emergent system is essential to consider the whole; in the health domain, it is crucial to observe multidisciplinary

Table 5. Research agenda.

Motivation	Research directions
Organizational context	1. Investigate theories in organizational studies to understand digital transformation in health and emergent systems 2. Investigate theories in the organizational studies that deal with health practice as part of the context of organizations in this field and the role of emergent systems 3. Discuss health data privacy issues based on emergent systems
Emergent properties	4. Investigate ways to represent emergent systems through diagrams 5. Investigate ways to catalogue emergent properties in health
Specific domains	6. Develop methods to investigate emergent systems in the health domain through exploratory studies 7. Develop an exploratory study on the role of emergent systems amid pandemic situations

5.2 Limitations

The first limitation refers to the identification of published studies. In our study, we opted for some digital libraries that only include studies in Computer Science and can be insufficient to collect studies from other areas that can provide multidisciplinary insights for this study. The second limitation is that some factors can lead to errors in the disclosed data, such as the possibility of error in the extraction and compilation of the system data. Several data were selected for manual checking to avoid this threat, such as a complete reading of some works in the screening step. Finally, the inclusion criteria may have occasionally excluded some relevant studies. However, due to the low number of studies in the first search step and the extensive manual checking, we believe that such inconsistencies have been minimized at the end of the study.

6 Conclusion and Future Research

Our study aimed to define the factors for consensus on the emergent systems approaches in the literature (RQ1) and seek a perspective to analyze the phenomenon in the health domain (RQ2). To answer (RQ1), the discussions from the results of the systematic mapping study helped us to point five critical factors for a common sense on emergent systems and emergent properties found in the literature: **[F1] Emergent systems occurs at lower levels; [F2] Emergent systems changes system behavior; [F3] Emergent systems are something unexpected; [F4] Once they appear, an emergent system become a natural part of the functioning of the system, and [F5] Emergent system is always a part of a whole**.

To answer (RQ2), our study presented common factors and perspectives to emergent systems in the health domain connecting with the factors for a common sense on the emergent systems approaches in the literature presented in (RQ1). To [F1], we suggested that research involving health technologies must be multidisciplinary; this perspective should consider the artifact's health practice and organizational context. To [F2], we recommend that the health domain point to the need to observe emergent systems as mandatory crossing points for health practice processes. Finally, to [F3], we recommend treating emergent systems as something unexpected, but we point out that sometimes, the emergent systems can be treating as a risk, but they must be treated to something positive, looking for innovations and opportunities for improvement.

To [F4], we suggest that an emergent system can become regular in a given context. Once used by the health professionals, the system becomes part of the system's natural functioning, and, to [F5], we recommend observing that an emergent system is essential to consider the whole; in the health domain, it is crucial to observe multidisciplinary.

As future work, we intend to conduct a complementary systematic mapping study to consider the organizational perspective. Another future work refers to conduct case study research in health organizations from different contexts. This work will be grounded on the theoretical findings from our previous studies. Health professionals should conduct interviews to identify and analyze emergent systems and their role as mediators of political, social, labor, and economic issues.

References

1. Iizuka, M., Ikeda, Y.: Regulation and innovation under the 4th industrial revolution: the case of a healthcare robot, HAL by Cyberdyne. Technovation **108**, 102335 (2021)
2. Beaulieu, M., Bentahar, O.: Digitalization of the healthcare supply chain: a roadmap to generate benefits and effectively support healthcare delivery. Technol. Forecast. Soc. Change **167**, 120717 (2021)
3. Balta, M., Valsecchi, R., Papadopoulos, T., Bourne, D.J.: Digitalization and co-creation of healthcare value: a case study in occupational health. Technol. Forecast. Soc. Change **168**, 120785 (2021)
4. Miyake, N., Lu, H., Kamiya, T., Aoki, T., Kido, S.: Optimizing early cancer diagnosis and detection using a temporal subtraction technique. Technol. Forecast. Soc. Change **167**, 120745 (2021)
5. Marques, I.C.P., Ferreira, J.J.M.: Digital transformation in the area of health: systematic review of 45 years of evolution. Health Technol. **10**(3), 575–586 (2020)
6. Silva, S.L.F.C., Antônio, N.P., Fornazin, M., Santos, R.P.: Looking for emergent systems in computer-based medical systems: a review from the last decade. In: IEEE 32nd International Symposium on Computer-Based Medical Systems (CBMS), pp. 229–232 (2019)
7. Sousa, M.J., Pesqueira, A.M., Lemos, C., Sousa, M., Rocha, Á.: Decision-making based on big data analytics for people management in healthcare organizations. J. Med. Syst. **43**(9), 1 (2019). https://doi.org/10.1007/s10916-019-1419-x
8. Morin, E.: La méthode 2: La vie de la Vie, Le Seuil (2001)
9. Johnson, S.: Emergence: The Connected Lives of Ants, Brains, Cities, and Software. Scribner, New York (2001)
10. Filho, R.V.R.: Emergent software systems (2018)
11. Corning, P.A.: The re-emergence of emergence?: A venerable concept in search of a theory. Complexity **7**(6), 18–30 (2002)
12. Iwaya, L.H., Fischer-Hübner, S., Åhlfeldt, R.M., Martucci, L.A.: mHealth: a privacy threat analysis for public health surveillance systems. In: 2018 IEEE 31st International Symposium on Computer- Based Medical Systems (CBMS), pp. 42–47 (2018)
13. Difrancesco, S., et al.: Out-of-home activity recognition from GPS data in schizophrenic patients. In: 2016 IEEE 29th International Symposium on Computer-Based Medical Systems (CBMS), pp. 324–328 (2016)
14. Nambisan, S.: Digital entrepreneurship: toward a digital technology perspective of entrepreneurship. Entrep. Theory Pract. **41**(6), 1029–1055 (2017)
15. Petersen, K., Vakkalanka, S., Kuzniarz, L.: Guidelines for conducting systematic mapping studies in software engineering: an update. Inf. Softw. Technol. **64**, 1–18 (2015)
16. Kitchenham, B.A., Charters, S.: Guidelines for performing systematic literature reviews in software engineering (2007)
17. Coleman, T.: Would-Be Worlds. How Simulation is Changing the Frontiers of Science, vol. 71, no. 5, p. 336 (1998)
18. Meadows, D., Wright, D.: Thinking in Systems. Chelsea Green Publishing (2008)
19. Goldstein, J.: Emergence as a construct: history and issues. Emergence **1**, 49–72 (1999)
20. Ranjan, P., Soman, S., Ateria, A.K., Srivastava, P.K.: Streamlining payment workflows using a patient wallet for hospital information systems. In: 2018 IEEE 31st International Symposium on Computer- Based Medical Systems (CBMS), pp. 339–344 (2018)
21. Basili, V.: Software modeling and measurement: the goal/question/metric paradigm. University of Maryland, CS-TR-2956, UMIACS-TR-92-96, September 1992

Health and Medical Data Mining via Graph-based Approaches

Food Recommendation for Mental Health by Using Knowledge Graph Approach

Chengcheng Fu[1,2,3], Zhisheng Huang[3(✉)], Frank van Harmelen[3], Tingting He[2], and Xingpeng Jiang[2(✉)]

[1] National Engineering Research Center for E-Learning, Central China Normal University, Wuhan, China
[2] School of Computer, Central China Normal University, Wuhan, China
xpjiang@mail.ccnu.edu.cn
[3] Department of Computer Science, Vrije Universiteit Amsterdam, Amsterdam, The Netherlands
z.huang@vu.nl

Abstract. There are many social factors have led to the crises of human mental health. Series of mental disorders, such as the depression, anxiety, and autistic disorder, have seriously affect human life. However, healthy diet can be a recommended way for improving mental health. The gut-brain axis, which is a bi-directional pathway that promotes diets work and regulates mental health in the body. As recent nutritional researches, food can be transformed into nutrients for feeding the gut microbiota. Furthermore, the nutrients can be metabolized as activators for mental health through the gut-brain axis. In this case, integrating these complex associations is necessary for exploring the function of food on mental health. Although there is a large scale of researches about food, gut microbiota and mental disorders that have been published but seldom been further reorganized. In this paper, we curate heterogeneous data sets from multiple sources and propose a framework about food recommendation for mental health by using knowledge graph approach. There are two available case studies, which are designed for demonstrating the application about food recommendations based on SPARQL query. The results have shown that our system have integrated useful knowledge and can be used to design proper diet patterns for patients with mental disorders. It's worth mentioning that our knowledge graph can also be extended to general human health and provide more convincing results for food researches and disease interventions.

Keywords: Knowledge graph · Diet · Gut microbiota · Mental health

1 Introduction

With the increasing of mental disorders in the world, that brings serious burden on the human health and social life [1]. Taking the depression disorder as an example, as the World Health Organization[1] (WHO) recorded, there are around

[1] https://www.who.int/health-topics/depression.

A. Traina et al. (Eds.): HIS 2022, LNCS 13705, pp. 231–242, 2022.
https://doi.org/10.1007/978-3-031-20627-6_22

5% of adults worldwide suffered from depression. The traditional intervention of mental disorder is hardly implemented widely due to its high cost in most countries [2]. As a result, healthy dietary patterns are being encouraged more often on the intervention of various mental disorders [3]. Many mental diseases, such as depression disorder [4], anxiety [5] and Parkinson syndrome have been verified to be associated with diet pattern [6]. For example, the Mediterranean diet, has been confirmed as a recommendation diet pattern for depressive patients [7]. Thus, the researches about biological function of food could have significant promotion for the prevention and therapy of mental disorders [8].

The effect of food on mental health are bi-directional, which be explained by the its biological characteristics. Although human mood can temporarily affect the choices of food, the diet and nutrition are long-term contributors to mental health [9]. There are different types of components about food, which can be divided into vitamins, minerals, lipid, proteins, sugars, etc. Due to its diversity of components, food can have multiple biological functions [10]. The digestion of food in human gut transform the nutrition compounds into the functional activators in gut microbiota. Furthermore the gut brain axis also promotes an effective transportation of metabolic nutrients between gut and brain community [11]. For example, the food with polyunsaturated fatty acids (e.g. omega-3 fatty acids), such as fish oil [12], have increased the proportion of beneficial bacteria (e.g. Bifidobacteria [13]) in gut community. Through the gut-brain axis, the bacterial metabolisms have been confirmed to promote the consumption of the pro-inflammatory factors in the brain and relief the depressive symptom [14]. In this case, our work is dedicated to integrating existing knowledge and designing applications around the food recommendation on mental health.

There are strong relations between mental diseases, gut microbes, and dietary nutrients according to biomedical experiments. There also have deep learning methods applied on mental health researches [15]. As huge numbers of related literatures have been published, it is necessary to integrate existing knowledge for further research [16]. There already have related works, such as a database named VMH [17], which is a metabolic database developed based on human metabolism associations with Mendelian diseases. Another database called MENDA [18], which also focus on the associations between metabolism and depression. These database are constructed based on text mining in biomedical literature manually, which is hard for further updating. In recent researches, knowledge graph has been introduced for representation learning on the intricate associations. For example, Ting Liu et al. [19] proposed a knowledge graph based on gut microbes and neurotransmitters about depression. Fu et al. [20] also used knowledge graph approach for mining relationships between depression and its complications. And Haussmann et al. [21] constructed a knowledge graph based on food recipes and properties, which can provide recipe proposals through on semantic queries. However, there is still a lack of research about using knowledge graph for food recommendation on mental health.

Thus, we propose a more generic knowledge graph around food, gut microbes, and mental health. The work in this paper are mainly focus on two aspects. (i)

The integration and transformation of heterogeneous data sets into structured knowledge, which is about food, gut microbiota and mental disorders. (ii) There are case studies designed based on knowledge graph provide the applications for food recommendations on human disorders. Finally, we also draw conclusions about our work and discuss future possibilities in food and human health.

2 Knowledge Enrichment

This paper works on the knowledge about the effect of food on human mental health, which is based on the hypothesis proposed in recent researches. That is the food consists of nutrients can promote gut microbial metabolism, which also have further effect on mental health through the gut brain axis.

2.1 Data Source

The data sets consist of the interactions and ontology, which has been shown in Table 1 as the detailed sources and descriptions. It will demonstrate the multi-sources data about knowledge graph from three areas: food, gut microbiota and mental disorders. We will also introduce the detailed statistics of the integration.

Table 1. Statistics of integrated data sets in knowledge graph.

Source	Relation	Entity	Triples	Description
FoodData Center	9	1,220,480	2,332,603	Food and components
FoodOn	56	56,079	79,769	Food ontology
Chinese products	7	160,802	215,863	Food ontology
KEGG	5	23,212	74,286	Microbial metabolites
NCBI taxonomy	5	984,031	1,306,152	Microbial ontology
MENDA	5	2,367	2,633	Depression and metabolic
MiKG	3	1,138	1,234	Mental diseases and microbes
SNOMED CT	63	2,064,178	4,291,226	Disease ontology
MESH	3	483,663	261,556	Disease ontology
Total	140	1,637,915	13,346,991	Total statements (4,741,023 inferred)

- ***FoodData Central (FDC).***[2] The FDC dataset provides a large amount of description on general and experimental food. We have integrated a total of 34,250 specific food, in which each item has its unique identifier and a standard weight of 100g. More specifically, the food comes from various brands and has particular components, which can be used to classified into various food categories.
- ***FoodOn.***[3] FoodOn is a food-centered ontology, which is contributed by the curators within academia and the OBO Foundry consortium. And we take use of the FoodOn for entity linking.

[2] https://fdc.nal.usda.gov/download-datasets.html.
[3] https://github.com/FoodOntology/foodon.

- ***Chinese Product.***[4] Chinese Product is a general list around food that is released by the China National Bureau of Statistics. We also use this for mapping our food samples to food ontology manually.
- ***KEGG.***[5] KEGG is a database consists of the whole metabolic pathway maps both in human and microorganisms. We have mapped around 230 nutrients components into gut metabolites and got related bacterial metabolism pathways.
- ***NCBI taxonomy.***[6] NCBI taxonomy focus on classification of microorganisms. We have integrated the phylogenetic trees of 322,917 bacteria from the NCBI taxonomy as gut microbial ontology.
- ***MENDA.*** There are 5,675 metabolite associations with depression from MENDA that have been compiled in our knowledge graph. We also integrate 157 gut microbes that have association with mental disorders from the database.
- ***MiKG.*** MiKG is also a knowledge graph around mental health, in which we integrate 1,234 gut microbes associated with mental diseases.
- ***MeSH.***[7] MeSH provides comprehensive disease terminology, which can be used for disease entity linking in our knowledge graph.
- ***SNOMED CT.***[8] It is a global common language standards for clinical terms contributed by the domain experts, and we also use their unique identifiers for disease items.

In conclusion, there are ontology and associations around foods, gut microbes, and diseases in our knowledge graph, which can be well represented through the knowledge graph structure.

2.2 Data Preprocessing

There are a huge number of heterogeneous knowledge in our knowledge graph after data integration. During data processing, entities from different knowledge bases may have various descriptions, which need to be linked to standard unique identifiers. In our knowledge graph, we use the Uniform Resource Identifier (URI) to represent each entity, and retain their description and attributes from the different knowledge bases.

We use the unique identifier from the FDC as the representation of each item of food, which can be mapped to other data sources through the label. The label of food from FDC may be a food name or a paragraph of food description. Firstly, we take use of the exact matching to map some simple names of food. And for the complex food descriptions, they will be split by the comma into strings, and we will use the first word in the string as the food label. The others are mostly unnecessary and will be retained as description labels or removed

[4] http://www.stats.gov.cn/tjsj/tjbz/tjypflml/.
[5] https://www.genome.jp/kegg/compound/.
[6] https://www.ncbi.nlm.nih.gov/taxonomy.
[7] https://www.nlm.nih.gov/mesh/meshhome.html.
[8] https://www.snomed.org/snomed-ct/.

directly. For example, the food description in FDC is "Chocolate milk, ready to drink, low fat", in which only "Chocolate milk" is what we need, and can be used to map in the FoodOn and Chinese Product knowledge bases with the unique representation. We also define some rules for mapping the food categories. For example, we sort the description of class with "drinks" (i.e. Soft drinks, Diet soft drinks) into a sub-class of "Beverages". However, due to the complexity and variety of category descriptions, we also make some manual efforts. For example, "Cakes and pies" and "Rolls and buns" are both the sub-classes of "Baked products". In general, we take use of a semi-automatic method and integrate food knowledge of 128 food categories and 34,250 food labels.

Similarly, the nutrient of food can be linked to the metabolites with the unique identifier in KEGG, in which their semantic relationships can be represented as "owl: sameAs" through the rules in OWL. Finally, we have mapped 123 nutrients to gut metabolites. We also link diseases to the ontology from MeSH or SNOMED CT through their labels. In this case, the description with "'s" that will be removed to ensure the exact matching. Such as the "Alzheimer's Disease" will be mapped to the Alzheimer Disease. Similar way with mapping compounds, the matching process also ignores the effects of case, singular and plural, and the sequence of the words. In a word, we have integrated the 277 diseases with their ontology.

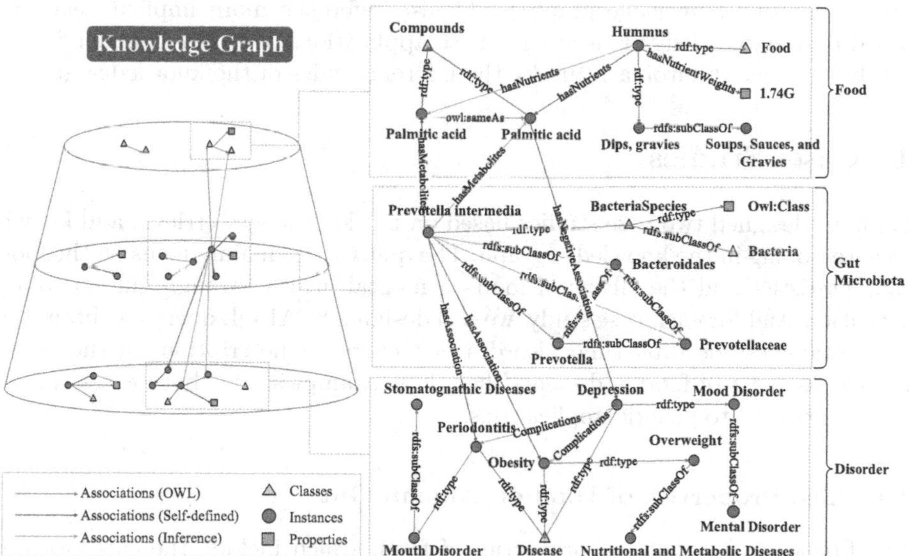

Fig. 1. An example of the graph structure in knowledge graph. The ontologies are mainly food, gut microbiota, and disorder. Associations are mainly from OWL (well-defined general relations), self-defined relations, and inference (relations that inferred from knowledge reasoning). And Knowledge graph also includes multiple entities as classes, instances, and properties. This figure has shown an example of the food could affects complicated disorders through the gut microbial metabolisms, which has been represented as a graph structure comprehensively.

3 Knowledge Graph Construction

Based on the hypothesis that food could affect mental disorders through gut microbial metabolisms, we design the general architecture of our knowledge graph. An example of network in our knowledge graph is shown in Fig. 1.

After the integration of heterogeneous data, there is a large number of binary associations originally, which need to be further transformed into triples. The triples are represented by the format of Resource Description Framework (RDF), which consists of subject, predicate, and object. Specifically, both subject and object are the factual concepts or property descriptions, the predicates are associations. And our knowledge graph could be well understood through the structured representations as triples.

There are also some ontological associations can be acquired from the original data sets. For example, apple products are the subclass of the general fruits, which can be represented in knowledge graph as (apple products, rdfs: subclassOf, fruits). That relation represents an inclusion relationship between classes, such as fruit is a general class that includes apple, banana products, etc. Besides, the apple juice is an instance of the apple products, and their association can be represented as the "rdf: type". After the binary relations are transformed into the format of RDF, the heterogeneous data are given more semantic representations based on the graph structure. Except for well representing our original knowledge, our knowledge graph could also inference more implicit relations based on the knowledge reasoning. Those applications of food recommendation can be completed automatically by the inference rules of the knowledge graph.

4 Cases Studies

We have designed two case studies based on the knowledge retrieval and knowledge reasoning in the knowledge graph. The query cases mainly focus on the food characteristics and the effects of food on mental health through gut microbial activities. And for each case study, we will design a SPARQL query to obtain the associations as the table, and also drawn picture for description. In the cases, we just use part of food and mental health as examples, that both cases can be easily extended to generic applications.

4.1 The Properties of Food on Human Gut

The first case is about the properties of food, which include the categories of food, the weight of nutrient and the associations between nutrients and gut metabolites. Taking the question for example: how much Vitamin B can be absorbed from the mixed meal as the milk with the egg products. Based on the natural language question, we have designed the SPARQL query:

SPARQL case 1: How much Vitamin B can be absorbed from the mixed meal as the milk with the egg products.

```
select distinct ?Eggname?Milkname?Nutrientname((?eggweight + ?milkweight) AS ?Weight) where
{ {?egg pq:hasNutrients ?nutrient;
pq:hasNutrientWeights ?eggunit;
rdf:type ?eggclass;
rdfs:label ?eggname.}
{?milk pq:hasNutrients ?nutrient;
rdfs:label ?milkname.}
?eggclass rdfs:label ?eggclassname.
{?nutrient rdfs:label ?nutrientname;
pq:hasNutrientWeights ?eggunit;
pq:hasNutrientWeights ?milkunit.}
?eggunit rdf:value ?eggweight.
?milkunit rdf:value ?milkweight.
filter regex(?nutrientname,"Vitamin B","i")
filter regex(?eggname,"Egg","i")
filter regex(?milkname,"Milk","i") }
```

Table 2. The properties of food on human gut.

No	Egg products	Milk products	Gut metabolites	Weight (mg/200 g)
0	Potato salad with egg	MILK, 1%	Vitamin B-12	0.082
1	Egg omelet or scrambled egg	Milk, skim	Vitamin B-12	0.071
2	Roll, egg bread	Soy milk, light	Vitamin B-12	0.082
3	Egg, whole, fried with butter	Milk, whole	Vitamin B-6	6.591
4	Shrimp-egg patty	Chocolate milk	Vitamin B-6	6.766
5	Egg, whole, boiled or poached	Yogurt, coconut milk	Vitamin B-6	6.602

Through the SPARQL query, we have obtained 254 egg products and 402 milk products. As part of results have been shown in Fig. 2, the milk and egg products are various in different brands or characteristics, which is random paired in the results. Totally, we have acquired around 80,000 results in this case. We assume that the weight of each food instance is 100 g. And the results is the sum of the vitamin B (taking Vitamin B6 and Vitamin B12 as examples) in mixed diet. The unit of vitamin B is milligram in 200 g diet (100 g milk and 100 g egg products). The detailed results shown in Table 2, the sum of the Vitamin B12 in the mixed meal is about 0.08 mg (in the mixed diet of egg salad and 1% milk), varying slightly from food pairs. It is worth mentioning that according to the WHO [22] reported, the recommended intake of Vitamin B12 for adults is 2.4 g per day. And it can demonstrate this mixed diet is suitable for the intake of Vitamin

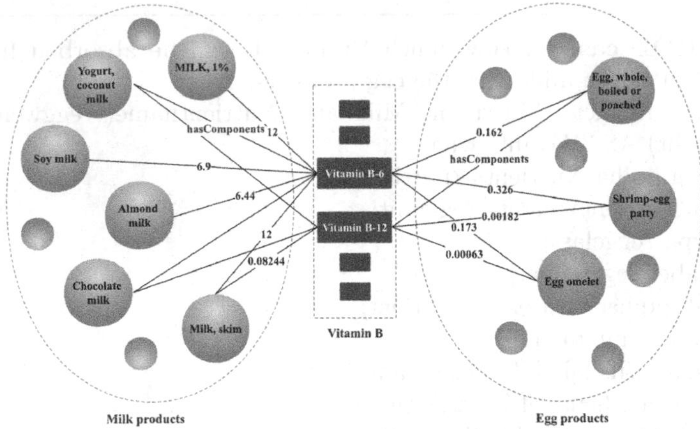

Fig. 2. The properties of food on human gut. In both circles are food with same category, as milk products and egg products. And in the square box are components of the food, as vitamin B. Their links are the weight of compounds in food.

B12 to an adult per day. We can use this conclusion as a reference for further nutritional experiments.

4.2 The Effects of Food on Mental Disorder

This case is about the effects of food on mental disorder through gut microbiota. Based on the hypothesis, there are nutrients from food that have positive effects on mental health, which could also participate in the gut microbial metabolism in human body. Taking the depression disorder as an example, this case is about which gut metabolism pathway could have effect on food and depression. Based on the natural language description, the SPARQL query is as follows.

SPARQL case 2: Which gut metabolism pathway could have effect on food and depression.

```
select distinct ?foodname?fcategory?comname?weight?bacname where
{ ?depression npq:hasNegativeAssociation ?compound;
rdfs:label ?depressionname.
?compound rdfs:label ?comname.
?nutrition owl:sameAs ?compound;
pq:hasNutrientWeights ?unit.
{?food pq:hasNutrients ?nutrient;
pq:hasNutrientWeights ?unit;
rdfs:label ?foodname.}
?unit rdf:value ?weight.
?food rdf:type ?foodclass.
```

```
?foodclass rdfs:label ?fcategory.
?depression npq:hasPositiveAssociation ?bacteria.
?bacteria npq:hasMetabolites ?compound.
?bacteria rdfs:label ?bacname.
filter regex(?depressionname,"depression | depressive | depressed","i") }
```

Table 3. The effects of food on depression based on the gut microbiota.

No	Food name	Food category	Compound	Weight (mg/100 g)	Bacteria	Mental disorder
0	FLOUR, SOY	Legumes and legume products	Glutamic acid (+)	8,870	Enterococcus faecalis	Depression
1	Broccoli, raw	Vegetables and vegetable products	Glycine (+)	89	Enterococcus faecalis	Depression
2	Grape juice	Fruits and fruit juices	Citric acid (+)	216.7	Adlercreutzia equolifaciens	Depression
3	Kiwi	Fruits and fruit juices	Ascorbic acid (+)	84	Bifidobacterium longum	Depression
4	Lettuce, Romaine	Vegetables and vegetable products	Ascorbic acid (+)	7.5	Bifidobacterium longum	Depression
5	BEEF SAUSAGE	Sausages and luncheon meats	L-Threonine (−)	500	Bacteroides ovatus	Depression
6	BEEF SAUSAGE	Sausages and luncheon meats	L-Threonine (−)	500	Bacteroides vulgatus	Depression
7	Whole wheat bread	Baked products	Choline (−)	27.2	Bifidobacterium longum	Depression

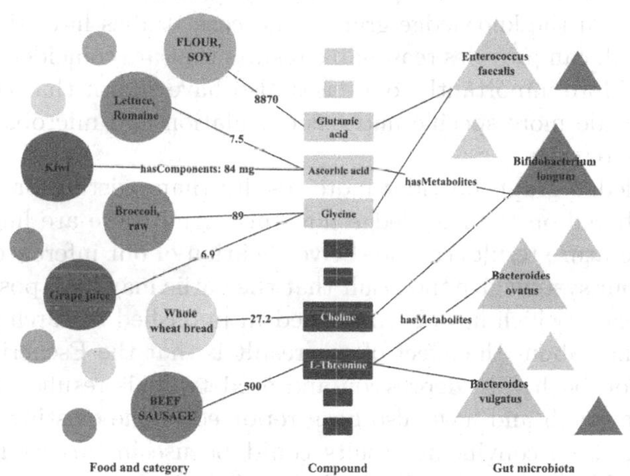

Fig. 3. The effects of food on mental disorder. The triangles are the gut microbiota that could have effects on depression through their metabolites. The various color of the food represent the categories, of gut microbiota represent different genus.

Specifically, we have acquired 9,512 food, which can be divided into 182 food categories, 14 compounds, and 4 microbes that have association with depression. Totally, we obtained around 10,000 results, part of which have been shown in Table 3, Such as the soy flour, which belongs to the legume products, contains around 8.87 g Glutamic acid per 100 g. We have obtained the food instances and categories containing these nutrients, which is based on the premise of the food effect on mental health. And the component in those food may have various effects on depression, which have shown in Fig. 3. Such as the Glutamic acid has been confirmed that has positive effect on depression as reactants in metabolisms of Enterococcus faecalis. The community of gut microbiota is also altered through the metabolites and may affect depression. In this case, we could have more verification results through the multi-pathway effects of food on the mental disorder. These results conducted by our knowledge graph can be further verified through the experimental researches.

5 Conclusion and Discussion

In this paper, we construct the knowledge graph around the effects of food on mental disorders via gut microbes, which provides applications on knowledge retrieval and knowledge reasoning. We make more efforts on the integration and construction of knowledge graph, which can lay foundations on the following applications. According to the effects of food on mental disorders, the factors around gut brain axis are necessary for designing the framework of our knowledge graph. For the validation of the quality of our system, we also design two cases as applications on the knowledge graph. The case studies have shown that our knowledge graph can provides reasonable results that are coincident for our daily food pattern. More importantly, our cases also have shown that the knowledge graph can provide more specific nutrient calculation and microbial evidence in food recommendations.

Our knowledge graph provides more results than existing data sets, which is conducted based on the knowledge inference. And there are huge number of biomedical literature results can be the verification of our inference conclusions. For example, our system give the result that the garlic may have positive effect on Alzheimer disease, which have been verified in published research [23]. And the another evidence about the effect of our result is that the Escherichia coli may have association both with depression and anxiety. This result is inferred from our knowledge graph and have also been reported in the existing research [24]. In conclusion, these convincing results could be use in further researches, as well as being able to provide reliable design directions for future experimental validation.

6 Future Work

We have made some efforts on extracting the effects of food on multiple mental health and construct a framework to build the knowledge graph for obtaining significant query results. In future work, our knowledge graph could have more extensions. It worth mentioning that knowledge graph mainly provides applications, such as the food recommendation and diet designing, which just focus on the mental disorders in this work. Because there are limited structured associations between human diseases (more than mental disorders) and gut microbiota. Furthermore we plan to add more relations between human disease and metabolites, which can promote the designing of food recommendations on general human diseases based on the knowledge inferences. For further experimental validation, more biologists who are still expected to use the results obtained through our knowledge graph as references in their experiments in the future. Knowledge graph will continue being used to work on the effects of food on human health around gut microbiota. We also encourage that our work can provide general knowledge services for human health.

Acknowledgements. This research is supported by the National Natural Science Foundation of China (61872157 and 61932008), the Key Research and Development Program of Hubei Province (2020BAB017), and the China Scholarship Council.

References

1. Cosgrove, L., Morrill, Z., Karter, J.M., Valdes, E., Cheng, C.P.: The cultural politics of mental illness: toward a rights-based approach to global mental health. Community Mental Health J. **57**(1), 3–9 (2021)
2. Merlo, G., Vela, A.: Mental health in lifestyle medicine: a call to action. Am. J. Lifestyle Med. **16**, 7–20 (2022)
3. Marx, W., et al.: Diet and depression: exploring the biological mechanisms of action. Mol. Psychiatry **26**(1), 134–150 (2021)
4. Campisi, S.C., Cost, K.T., Korczak, D.J.: Food intake reporting bias among adolescents with depression. Eur. J. Clin. Nutr. **76**(6), 904–906 (2022)
5. Coffino, J.A., Spoor, S.P., Drach, R.D., Hormes, J.M.: Food insecurity among graduate students: prevalence and association with depression, anxiety and stress. Public Health Nutr. **24**(7), 1889–1894 (2021)
6. Dinan, T.G., et al.: Feeding melancholic microbes: MyNewGut recommendations on diet and mood. Clin. Nutr. **38**(5), 1995–2001 (2019)
7. Petersson, S.D., Philippou, E.: Mediterranean diet, cognitive function, and dementia: a systematic review of the evidence. Adv. Nutr. **7**(5), 889–904 (2016)
8. Mafra, D., Borges, N.A., Lindholm, B., Shiels, P.G., Evenepoel, P., Stenvinkel, P.: Food as medicine: targeting the uraemic phenotype in chronic kidney disease. Nat. Rev. Nephrol. **17**(3), 153–171 (2021)
9. Ezra-Nevo, G., Henriques, S.F., Ribeiro, C.C.: How nutrients lead the gut brain axis: the diet-microbiome tango. Curr. Opin. Neurobiol. **62**, 122–132 (2020)
10. Parker, G., Brotchie, H.: Mood effects of the amino acids tryptophan and tyrosine: 'food for thought' III. Acta Psychiatr. Scand. **124**(6), 417–426 (2011)
11. Stower, H.: Gut-brain communication. Nat. Med. **25**(12), 1799 (2019)
12. Appleton, K.M., et al.: Omega-3 fatty acids for depression in adults. Cochrane Database Syst. Rev. (11) (2021)
13. Desbonnet, L., Garrett, L., Clarke, G., Bienenstock, J., Dinan, T.G.: The probiotic bifidobacteria infantis: an assessment of potential antidepressant properties in the rat. J. Psychiatr. Res. **43**(2), 164–174 (2008)
14. Pei-Yu, W., Chen, K.-M., Belcastro, F.: Dietary patterns and depression risk in older adults: systematic review and meta-analysis. Nutr. Rev. **79**(9), 976–987 (2021)

15. Alvi, A.M., Siuly, S., Wang, H.: Developing a deep learning based approach for anomalies detection from EEG data. In: Zhang, W., Zou, L., Maamar, Z., Chen, L. (eds.) WISE 2021. LNCS, vol. 13080, pp. 591–602. Springer, Cham (2021). https://doi.org/10.1007/978-3-030-90888-1_45
16. Haro, C., et al.: Consumption of two healthy dietary patterns restored microbiota dysbiosis in obese patients with metabolic dysfunction. Mol. Nutr. Food Res. **61**(12), 1700300 (2017)
17. Noronha, A., et al.: The virtual metabolic human database: integrating human and gut microbiome metabolism with nutrition and disease. Nucleic Acids Res. **47**(D1), D614–D624 (2019)
18. Juncai, P., et al.: MENDA: a comprehensive curated resource of metabolic characterization in depression. Brief. Bioinform. **21**(4), 1455–1464 (2020)
19. Liu, T., Pan, X., Wang, X., Feenstra, K.A., Heringa, J., Huang, Z.: Predicting the relationships between gut microbiota and mental disorders with knowledge graphs. Health Inf. Sci. Syst. **9**(1), 1–9 (2021)
20. Fu, C., Jiang, X., He, T., Jiang, X.: MDepressionKG: a knowledge graph for metabolism-depression associations. In: Proceedings of the 2nd International Symposium on Artificial Intelligence for Medicine Sciences, pp. 63–68 (2021)
21. Haussmann, S., et al.: FoodKG: a semantics-driven knowledge graph for food recommendation. In: Ghidini, C., et al. (eds.) ISWC 2019. LNCS, vol. 11779, pp. 146–162. Springer, Cham (2019). https://doi.org/10.1007/978-3-030-30796-7_10
22. Pawlak, R., James, P.S., Raj, S., Cullum-Dugan, D., Lucus, D.: Understanding vitamin B12. Am. J. Lifestyle Med. **7**(1), 60–65 (2013)
23. Chauhan, N.B.: Multiplicity of garlic health effects and Alzheimer's disease. J. Nutr. Health Aging **9**(6), 421–432 (2005)
24. Tiller, J.W.G.: Depression and anxiety. Med. J. Aust. **199**(6), S28–S31 (2013)

Medical Knowledge Graph Construction Based on Traceable Conversion

Wei Hou[1], Wenkui Zheng[1(✉)], Ming Sheng[2], Peng Ren[2], Baifu Zuo[1], Zhentao Hu[3], Xianxing Liu[1], and Yang Duan[2,4]

[1] Henan University, Kaifeng 475004, China
{houwei,liuxianxing}@henu.edu.cn, zwk@vip.henu.edu.cn
[2] BNRist, DCST, RIIT, Tsinghua University, Beijing 100084, China
{shengming,renpeng}@tsinghua.edu.cn
[3] Henan University, Zhengzhou 450046, China
hzt@henu.edu.cn
[4] University of Illinois Urbana-Champaign, Champaign, IL, USA
yangd4@illinois.edu

Abstract. Medical knowledge graph (MKG) can provide ideal technical support for integrating multi-structure data and enhancing graph-based services. The construction of MKG usually requires information extracted from a large number of data sources, including structured data from medical databases (MDBs) and unstructured data from medical texts. However, the previous works used single data sources and simple format conversion when constructing MKG, and the MKG information constructed in this way is incomplete and untraceable. This paper proposes a method to build MKG based on traceable conversion to solve the above problems. For the structured data from MDB, the DB data is automatically converted into MKG nodes in the form of the RDF, which not only reduces the DB information loss in the conversion process but also enriches the types of graph nodes. When the data is efficiently converted, the converted nodes can also be traced back to the source. For the unstructured data from medical text, a strong deep learning model is used for entity and relation extraction. On the basis of avoiding the exposure bias and ensuring consistency of model training and prediction, the medical texts information is maximally extracted, and traceability is added, which reduces medical texts information loss and further complements the MKG. Based on the traceable conversion method for MKG construction, medical multi-structure data can be used more effectively to construct MKG.

Keywords: Traceable conversion · Structured data · Unstructured data · Medical knowledge graph

1 Introduction

The advent of the information technology makes the data storage service in the medical field more convenient [1], and many data processing methods for the medical field have appeared [2–6]. Meanwhile, the stored medical data has also laid a foundation for the

A. Traina et al. (Eds.): HIS 2022, LNCS 13705, pp. 243–257, 2022.
https://doi.org/10.1007/978-3-031-20627-6_23

construction of MKG. Some of the data used to construct MKG is stored in the database (DB) in the structured form, and some are stored in medical text in the unstructured form. How to fully mine the semantic information and construct a more complete MKG is an urgent problem to be solved in MKG research [7].

As an important data storage method for MKG construction, relational databases (RDBs) still have certain advantages in the storage efficiency but lack semantics. Resource Description Framework (RDF) is a framework proposed by the World Wide Web Consortium (W3C) for normalizing the content of the Semantic Web [8]. However, the data in the medical domain is different from other data, its characteristic of scale and complexity makes the process of RDB to RDF more difficult. Moreover, due to the limitation of RDF representation, in the process of mapping RDB to RDF, the traditional mapping methods do not have an ideal effect when mapping the semantic information embedded in RDB to RDF, and many of them cannot be traceable, resulting in more information loss of data. Therefore, it is necessary to design a mapping rule that reduces the data information loss to a minimum extent and constructs MKG with more sufficient information.

For medical text data, information extraction is generally performed first. In order to extract information from medical text data, researchers have done some work by neural network-based approaches [9, 10]. These works have achieved some good results, but when extracting relations between entities, entity pair overlap and individual entity overlap can lead to incomplete information extraction. Thus, the final MKG has a situation with information loss.

Contributions. The main contributions are summarized as follows.

1. For structured medical database (MDB) data, we propose a method to map RDB data to traceable medical fine-grained knowledge graph nodes. We have designed a custom approach to automatically and traceably convert the RDB to RDF.
2. For unstructured medical text data, we have combined the idea of information traceability with a joint entity and relation extraction model. We add traceability markers to the model, and then the model is used to extract information from medical text.
3. By integrating information extracted from structured and unstructured data separately, we propose a traceable method for constructing large-scale MKG, and demonstrate that our method can construct traceable and more complete MKG.

This paper is organized as follows. In Sect. 2, we introduce the related work. In Sect. 3, we present the method in detail. In Sect. 4, we show the application. In the end, we summarize the paper and propose future work in Sect. 5.

2 Related Work

The research in this paper involves data traceability, MKG construction, medical RDB to RDF conversion, and medical text information extraction, so we provide some overviews from these directions.

Data Traceability. Medical data information is an important medical basic resource. Therefore, remaining data source information is crucial for data reuse and preventing data loss when processing medical data.

Metadata information embedding and traceable model design are two existing methods of knowledge graph data traceability. The metadata information embedding approach is relatively simple, and it is only necessary to embed metadata information into the generated graph nodes. For the traceable model, ISO has developed a model called ISO 19115 [11], which directly applies elements in the nodes to describe resource types, processing steps and data sources. The PROV model developed by W3C is simplified by packaging simple and detailed descriptions separately [12]. The core terms of PROV are used for simple traceable descriptions, and more detailed traceable descriptions are explained by using extended and modified terms.

However, the traceable model-based approach interprets the traceability by adding nodes to the original nodes, which is inefficient. Therefore, the method of embedding meta-information has been adopted in RDF node generation to achieve traceability. It can ensure less data loss and achieve a concise MKG representation at the same time.

MKG. MKG construction is the purpose of this study, which is also crucial in the medical field. As shown in Table 1, there are some knowledge graph construction methods for the non-medical domain and the medical domain. In these methods, different from our construction methods that consider structured and unstructured data together, they all construct knowledge graph by one data type. In addition, the rules and node types classification methods they use in structured data have no more fine-grained consideration. However, our method focuses on the integration of the problems of the above methods while having the 6 functional points involved shown in Table 1.

Although the knowledge graphs mentioned above have specific roles for different data sources, they rarely consider integrating DB data and medical text data. Unlike them, the method proposed in this paper can extract the semantic information contained in DB data and medical text data traceably, constituting a more complete MKG.

RDB to RDF. Converting RDB data to RDF data can make it easy for medical applications to access and manipulate these data. Sequeda et al. [19] considered information preservation and query preservation in the mapping process. With DB models, Spanos et al. [20] reviewed the RDB-RDF approach and classified it into disjoint categories. However, the method does not describe the explicit characteristic and expressiveness of characteristic mapping language.

Different from the above methods, the method proposed in this paper is a custom mapping for a specific DB, which also has clear semantic expressiveness under the premise of the integrity of the information in the conversion process.

Medical Text Information Extraction. Extracting information from unstructured medical texts is another key point in constructing large-scale MKG. At present, machine learning technology is widely used in medical text information extraction, which can be classified into supervised [21], semi-supervised [22], and unsupervised approaches [23]. Moreover, their results are difficult to interpret and map to existing relations.

Table 1. Comparison of different methods.

Method	Domain	Data source	Traceability	Entity recognition	Relation extraction	ER/RDF mapping	Rules-based	Node type classification
PGMKG [13]	Power Grid	RDB	✗	✗	✗	✗	✗	✗
AliMeKG [14]	Business	Item articles	✗	✓	✓	✗	✗	✗
EEAKG [15]	Business	General	✗	✓	✓	✗	✗	✗
REMK [16]	Medical	Medical text	✗	✓	✓	✗	✗	✗
COVID19 [17]	Medical	Medical text	✗	✓	✓	✗	✗	✗
TCMKG [18]	Medical	Medical text	✗	✓	✓	✓	✓	✗
Ours	Medical	RDB + Medical text	✓	✓	✓	✓	✓	✓

In addition to the shortcomings mentioned above, entity nesting and relation overlap are rarely considered when the text information is extracted, which results in information extraction loss. We introduce a joint entity and relation extraction model into medical text information extraction, which can well solve the above problems.

3 Methodology

To address the challenging problems of current MKG construction methods, we design a MKG construction method based on traceable conversion. The framework of our construction method is shown in Fig. 1.

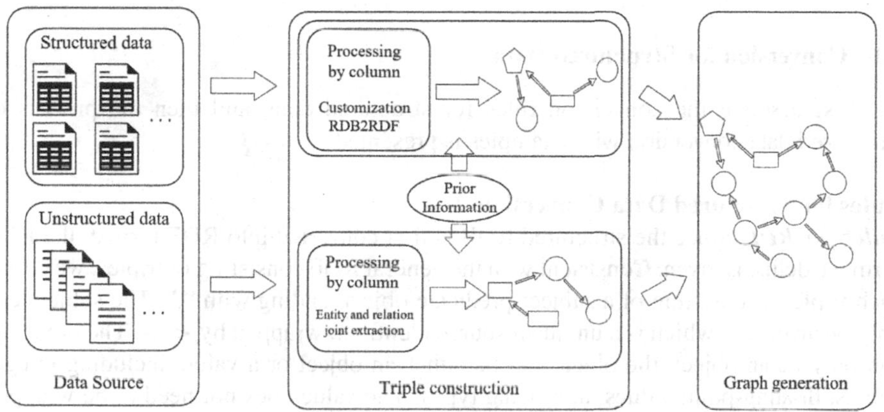

Fig. 1. The overall framework.

For structured data, we use a custom approach to convert the data to RDF by column, and then expand the tables, columns, and values into finer-grained graph triple nodes. Meanwhile, the formal definition of the traceability graph for structured data is as follows:

$$provenance = graph(E, C, I)$$

where $E \in Table1 \cup Table2 \cup Table3 \cup \cdots \cup TableN$
$C \in TableColumn1 \cup TableColumn2 \cup TableColumn3 \cdots \cup TableColumnM$
$I \in Value1 \cup Value2 \cup Value3 \cdots \cup ValueK$

For unstructured data, we perform the joint extraction of entities and relations according to the text sequences, and the text IDs are used as the traceable markers. Thus, the formal definition of traceable graph for unstructured data is as follows:

$$provenance = graph(ID, S, P, O)$$

where $S_1, O_1 \in Text1$

$S_2, O_2 \in Text2$

$S_3, O_3 \in Text3$

$\ldots$

$S_n, O_n \in TextN$

In particular, the data is transformed and processed under the addition of prior information, which also ensures the reliability of the generated graph triples.

3.1 Conversion for Structured Data

We first describe the conversion rules for structured data, and then the process of structured data conversion with examples is presented.

Rules for Structured Data Conversion

Rules for RDF. Since the structured RDB is first converted into RDF format, the RDF form we define is given. Consistent with the general RDF consisting of triples, we define each triple as consisting of a subject-predicate object, ending with ".". The subject can only be an object, which is a unique resource identifier, wrapped by $< >$. The predicate can only be an object, the object can be either an object or a value, including integer values, floating-point values, and string types. The value does not need to be wrapped by $< >$. Example is as follows:

@prefix rdf: <http://www.tsinghua-west.com/mimic03>

"<rdf:/Patient/31567> <rdf:/PatientMaster> <rdf:/instance/ETHNICITY-WHITE>."

The above triple represents patients with ID 31576 corresponding to Caucasians.

Conversion Rules. Based on the definition of RDF, we define the rules from the perspective of data conversion. Among them, coarse subdivision rules give the overall conversion, and subdivision is further defined on the basis of coarse subdivision.

(1) The rules in rough: The DB is first converted to RDF type, and the RDF type then corresponds with the nodes of the graph. When converting to RDF, the elements of the DB tables are used as subjects and objects in the RDF triples, and the pre-defined relations are used as predicates in the RDF triples.
(2) The rules in detail: Divide the table names in DB to graph event nodes. Divide the column names in DB to concept nodes. Divide the concrete values in DB to instance nodes.

In the current RDF formats of the HIS system, the main prefixes include Patient, times, pte, ptel, ptela. The Patient indicates the patient, times indicates the visit ID, pte(Patient|times|event) indicates a visit corresponding to the subject of an event (the table in which the visit ID is located), ptel indicates the subject of each record in a pte (a column in the table), and ptela indicates the subject of the information subdivided under a ptel (for example, the number of the same visit ID in the same table).

For each RDF triple actually converted, the event node is represented concretely when the last character of each RDF tuple string is the table name. The following table shows the triples containing event (table name) nodes. But it does not mean that whenever a table name appears, it is an event node (Table 2).

Table 2. Triples with event (table name) nodes.

No	Subject	Predicate	Object
1	rdf:/pte/Visit ID-event	rdf:/PTE#TLINK	rdf:/times/Visit ID
2	rdf:/pte/Visit ID-event	rdf:/PTE#ELINK	rdf:/event/event name
3	rdf:/pte/Visit ID-event	rdf:/PTE#LLINK	rdf:/ptel/ Visit ID-event –column name for processing (CNP)

For each RDF actually converted, a concept node is represented concretely when the last character of each RDF tuple string is a column name. The following table shows the triples containing concept (column name) nodes, but it does not mean that whenever a column name appears, it is a concept node (Table 3).

Table 3. Triples with concept (column name) nodes.

No	Subject	Predicate	Object
1	rdf:/instance/CNP - field value of the column name for processing (FVCNP)	rdf:/valueOf	rdf:/concept/ FVCNP

For each RDF that is actually converted, the instance node is specified when the last character of each RDF tuple is a field value. The following table shows the triples containing instance (field value) nodes, but it does not mean that whenever a field value appears, it is an instance node (Table 4).

Table 4. Triples with instance (field value) nodes.

No	Subject	Predicate	Object
1	rdf:/ptela/Visit ID -event- FVCNP -number of same visit IDs	rdf:/PTELA#ILINK	rdf:/instance/CNP- FVCNP
2	rdf:/instance/ CNP- FVCNP	rdf:/valueOf	rdf:/concept/ CNP
3	rdf:/instance/ CNP- FVCNP	rdf:/valueIs	FVCNP
4	rdf:/ptel/Visit ID-Parent table- FVCNP	rdf:/PTEL#RLINK	rdf:/ptela/ Visit ID - event - FVCNP
5	rdf:/ptel/Visit ID - event - FVCNP	rdf:/PTEL#INCLUDE	rdf:/ptela/ Visit ID - event - FVCNP - number of same visit IDs
6	rdf:/ptela/Visit ID - event - FVCNP - number of same visit IDs	rdf:/PTELA#Num	number of same visit IDs
7	rdf:/ptela/Visit ID - event - FVCNP - number of same visit IDs	rdf:/PTELA#ILINK	rdf:/instance/ CNP - FVCNP

The Process of Structured Data Conversion. According to the conversion rules for structured data, an example is presented to elaborate on the process of conversion. As shown in Fig. 2, for a patient with ID 2, the events include icustays and admissions of the icustays's parent table, and the column name to be processed is hospital_expire_flag. In Fig. 2, the pentagon stands for the event node, the rectangle indicates the concept node and ellipse is the instance node.

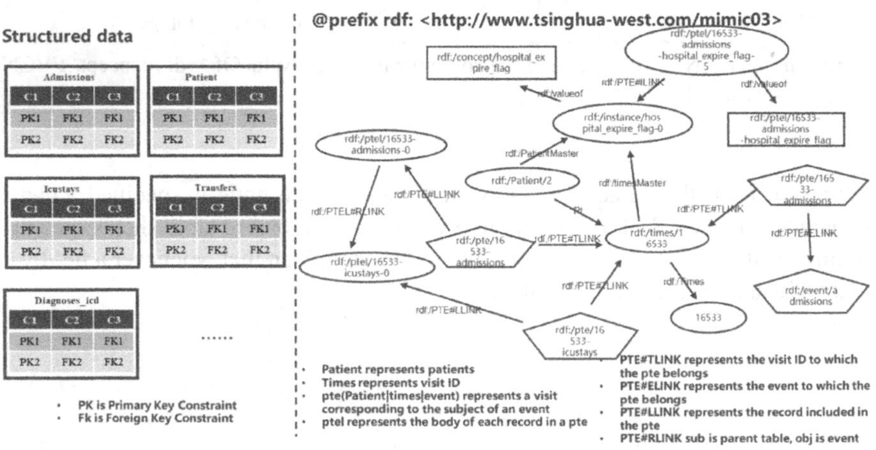

Fig. 2. Example of structured data conversion process.

3.2 Conversion for Unstructured Data

Unstructured data in the medical field is mainly based on medical text data, and TPLinker [24], a cutting-edge deep learning model, is used to extract entity and relation information from medical text, laying the foundation for completing MKG nodes.

Rules for Unstructured Data Conversion. We define conversion rules for unstructured data in a way that is a combination predefined by us and complemented by doctors. For this purpose, we have developed an active annotation method for unstructured data [25].

The Process of Unstructured Data Conversion. According to our defined unstructured data rules, as shown in Fig. 3, we take two records, Discharge Instructions and Hospital Course, which the hospital produced to a patient with ID 2 during his hospitalization. Then an example is given to illustrate the conversion process.

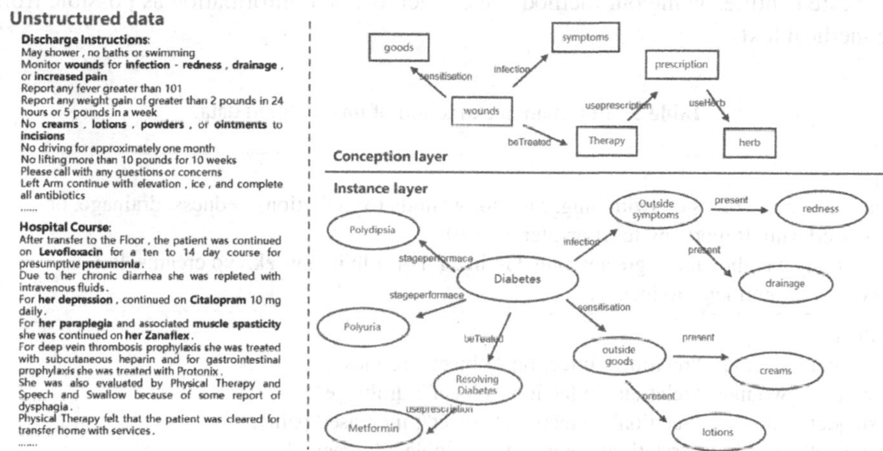

Fig. 3. Example of conversion process for unstructured data.

3.3 Conversion for Both Types of Data

According to the conversion process of structured and unstructured data in the previous two sections, we first describe the conversion process mechanism of the two kinds of data separately, and finally the converted example is given.

Structured Data. The conversion of structured data starts by connecting to the DB and executing DB statements to obtain table metadata. Next, the different data types in the DB are mapped into Jena's data types to better come to query and modify the information. Finally, the rules we defined for converting RDBs to graph nodes are used as the basis for first converting to RDF data types, and then each RDF triple is corresponding to a graph node. The specific conversion algorithm is as follows:

Algorithm 1: Structured data conversion algorithm.

```
Input: DB table T to be processed, column C to be processed
Output: RDF triple sets
sqlcon ← getConnection(DataBaseName)
statement ← creatStatement
sqlx ← select * from T
metadata ← sqlcon.prepareStatement(sqlx)
jenatype(metadata)
for each c in C do
RDF ← jenatype(metadata) with the rules in section 3.1.1
end for
```

Unstructured Data. As shown in Table 5, for a medical text, traditional information extraction methods often only output one result when there are overlapping relations and nested entities while our method can extract as much information as possible from the medical text.

Table 5. Information extraction of unstructured data.

Input: May shower, no baths or swimming. Monitor wounds for infection - redness, drainage, or increased pain. Report any fever greater than 101 Report any weight gain of greater than 2 lb in 24 h or 5 lb in a week. No creams, lotions, powders, or ointments to incisions
Output: {"subject": wounds, "relation": infection, "object": redness}, {"subject": wounds, "relation": infection, "object": drainage}, {"subject": wounds, "relation": infection, "object": increased pain}, {"subject": incisions, "relation": sensitisation, "object": creams}, {"subject": incisions, "relation": sensitisation, "object": lotions}, {"subject": incisions, "relation": sensitisation, "object": powders}, {"subject": incisions, "relation": sensitisation, "object": ointments}

As shown in Fig. 4, after getting the structured and unstructured data converted with formatted manner, we use the visit ID as the connection point to link the structured data converted mapping nodes and the unstructured data converted mapping nodes to finally form our MKG.

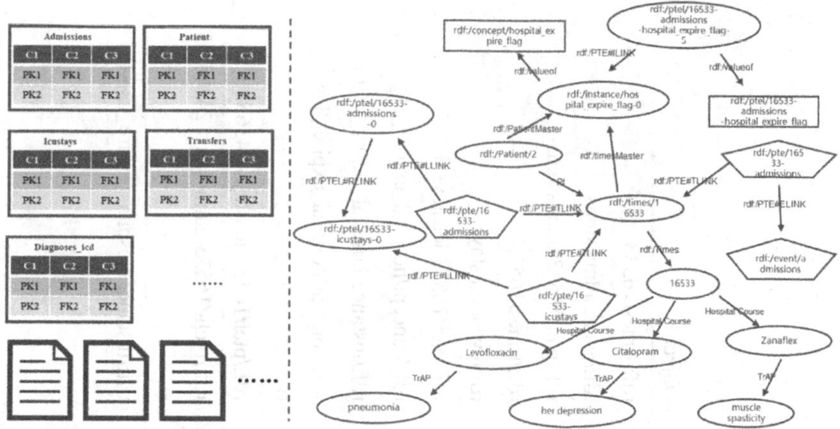

Fig. 4. Example of conversion process for structured and unstructured data.

4 Application

To verify the utility of our approach, we conducted experiments on the MIMIC-III DB and the text data associated with it. This DB contains 26 tables, which are connected by patient ID (subject_id), record ID (hadm_id) and ICU ID (icustays_id). According to the data format, the data can be divided into structured data (laboratory measurements, vital signs, etc.) and unstructured data (medical advice information, etc.).

4.1 Applications for Structured Data

We first give the metadata of the MIMIC-III DB to show the information of the DB itself, and then for one of the processes, we show the process of RDF triples generated from the DB data. Besides, these generated RDF triples are used as the components of the final knowledge graph nodes.

In the experiments, we take two tables, admissions and icustays, as an example. As shown in Table 6, RDF triples involving event (table), concept (column) and instance (field values) are obtained according to the rules defined in 3.1.1.

Table 6. RDF triple example.

Type	Subject	Predicate	Object
Event nodes involved	rdf:/pte/16533-admissions	rdf:/PTE#TLINK	rdf:/times/16533
	rdf:/pte/16533-admissions	rdf:/PTE#ELINK	rdf:/event/admissions
	rdf:/pte/16533-admissions	rdf:/PTE#LLINK	rdf:/ptel/16533-admissions-1
	rdf:/pte/16533-icustays	rdf:/PTE#TLINK	rdf:/times/16533
	rdf:/pte/16533-icustays	rdf:/PTE#ELINK	rdf:/event/icustays
	rdf:/pte/16533-icustays	rdf:/PTE#LLINK	rdf:/ptel/16533-icustays-1
Concept nodes involved	rdf:/instance/hospital_expire_flag-0	rdf:/valueOf	rdf:/concept/hospital_expire_flag
Instance nodes involved	rdf:/ptela/16533-icustays-hospital_expire_flag-5	rdf:/PTELA#ILINK	rdf:/instance/hospital_expire_flag-0
	rdf:/instance/hospital_expire_flag-0	rdf:/valueOf	rdf:/concept/hospital_expire_flag
	rdf:/instance/hospital_expire_flag-0	rdf:/valueIs	0
	rdf:/ptel/16533-admissions-243653	rdf:/PTE#RLINK	rdf:/ptel/16533-icustays-243653
	rdf:/ptel/16533-admissions-243653	rdf:/PTEL#INCLUDE	rdf:/ptela/16533-admissions-243653-5
	rdf:/ptela/16533-admissions-243653-5	rdf:/PTELA#Num	5
	rdf:/ptela/16533-admissions-243653-5	rdf:/PTELA#ILINK	rdf:/instance/hospital_expire_flag-0

4.2 Applications for Unstructured Data

For unstructured data, we use predefined and doctor-supplemented ways as rule. The predefined entity and relation types are shown in Table 7, and the doctor-supplemented entity and relation types through the annotation system are shown in Table 8.

Table 7. Predefined entity and relation types.

Type	Concepts to be extracted
Entity	goods; nausea; wounds; symptoms; Therapy; prescription; herb. (7 items)
Relation	sensitization; beTreated; useprescription; useHerb; stageperformace; present; TrAP (7 items)

Table 8. Supplementary entity and relation types based on annotation system.

Type	Concepts to be extracted
Entity	disease incentive; accompany symptoms; wounds location. (3 items)
Relation	lead to; suggest; co-occur with. (3 items)

According to our defined rules, for the Discharge Instructions medical text of a patient with ID 2 during hospitalization, we give the information extraction process and the mapping process of the graph triad as shown in Fig. 5.

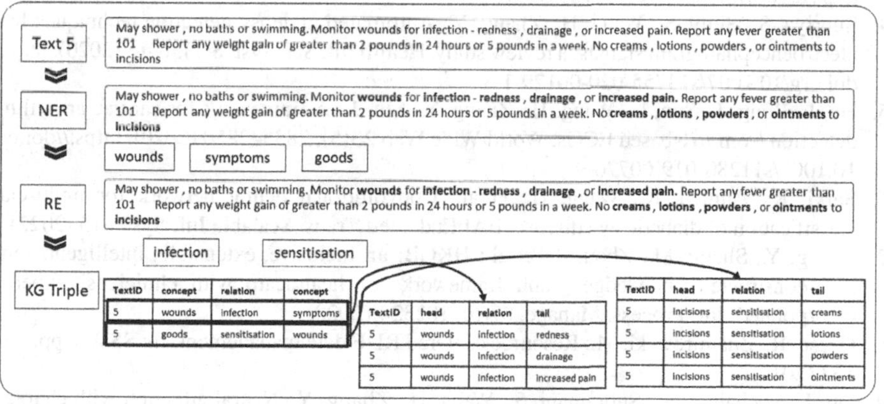

Fig. 5. Example of the mapping process of information extraction to the graph triple

5 Conclusion

In this paper, we propose a MKG construction method based on traceable conversion. This method not only considers the semantics of the data but also the constraints in DB when coping with structured data conversion. The contained semantic information can be fully extracted in DB. The mapping process implemented based on this method can complete the automated mapping of the DB without a lot of user interaction. It can also perform information traceability based on the converted mapping nodes to ensure no information loss. For dealing with unstructured medical text for extracting information, the problem of nested entity and relation can be better solved. On the basis of ensuring information traceability, more information is extracted, and the quality and scale of constructing MKG is improved.

MKG, as a technical tool to assist physicians in decision support in the medical field, requires content in multiple modalities, including but not limited to text, images and videos. Therefore, combining the MKG with other technologies [26, 27] is our next step.

Acknowledgements. This work was supported by National Key R&D Program of China (2020AAA0109603).

References s

1. Vimalachandran, P., Liu, H., Lin, Y., Ji, K., Wang, H., Zhang, Y.: Improving accessibility of the Australian my health records while preserving privacy and security of the system. Health Inf. Sci. Syst. **8**(1), 1–9 (2020). https://doi.org/10.1007/s13755-020-00126-4
2. Pandey, D., Wang, H., Yin, X., et al.: Automatic breast lesion segmentation in phase preserved DCE-MRIs. Health Inf. Sci. Syst. **10**(1), 1–19 (2022)
3. Sarki, R., Ahmed, K., Wang, H., Zhang, Y.: Automated detection of mild and multi-class diabetic eye diseases using deep learning. Health Inf. Sci. Syst. **8**(1), 1–9 (2020). https://doi.org/10.1007/s13755-020-00125-5
4. Supriya, S., Siuly, S., Wang, H., Zhang, Y.: Automated epilepsy detection techniques from electroencephalogram signals: a review study. Health Inf. Sci. Syst. **8**(1), 1–15 (2020). https://doi.org/10.1007/s13755-020-00129-1
5. He, J., Rong, J., Sun, L., Wang, H., Zhang, Y., Ma, J.: A framework for cardiac arrhythmia detection from IoT-based ECGs. World Wide Web **23**(5), 2835–2850 (2020). https://doi.org/10.1007/s11280-019-00776-9
6. Sarki, R., Ahmed, K., Wang, H., et al.: Convolutional neural network for multi-class classification of diabetic eye disease. EAI Endorsed Trans. Scalable Inf. Syst. e15 (2022)
7. Zhang, Y., Sheng, M., Zhou, R., et al.: HKGB: an inclusive, extensible, intelligent, semi-auto-constructed knowledge graph framework for healthcare with clinicians' expertise incorporated. Inf. Process. Manage. **57**(6), 102324 (2020)
8. Heese, R., Znamirowski, M.: Resource centered RDF data management. In: SSWS, pp. 138–153 (2012)
9. Du, J., Michalska, S., Subramani, S., Wang, H., Zhang, Y.: Neural attention with character embeddings for hay fever detection from twitter. Health Inf. Sci. Syst. **7**(1), 1–7 (2019). https://doi.org/10.1007/s13755-019-0084-2
10. Chen, T., Hu, Y.: Entity relation extraction from electronic medical records based on improved annotation rules and BiLSTM-CRF. Ann. Transl. Med. **9**(18), 1415 (2021)
11. ISO/TC 211: Geographic Information-Metadata-Part 1: Fundamentals. Geneva, Switzerland (2014)
12. Moreau, L., Missier, P., Belhajjame, K., et al.: PROV-dm: the PROV data model (2022-06-08). https://www.w3.org/TR/2013/REC-prov-dm-20130430/

13. Liu, Y., Huang, X., Li, S., et al.: A construction method of power grid monitoring knowledge graph. J. Phys. Conf. Ser. **2166**(1), 012010 (2022)
14. Li, F., Chen, H., Xu, G., et al.: AliMeKG: domain knowledge graph construction and application in e-commerce. In: CIKM, pp. 2581–2588 (2020)
15. Al-Khatib, K., Hou, Y., Wachsmuth, H., et al.: End-to-end argumentation knowledge graph construction. In: AAAI, pp. 7367–7374 (2020)
16. Chen, I., Agrawal, M., Horng, S., et al.: Robustly extracting medical knowledge from EHRs: a case study of learning a health knowledge graph. In: Pacific Symposium on Biocomputing, pp. 19–30 (2019)
17. Kim, T., Yun, Y., Kim, N.: Deep learning-based knowledge graph generation for COVID-19. Sustainability **13**(4), 2276 (2021)
18. Zheng, Z., Liu, Y., Zhang, Y., et al.: TCMKG: a deep learning based traditional Chinese medicine knowledge graph platform. In: ICKG, pp. 560–564 (2020)
19. Sequeda, J., Arenas, M., Miranker, D.: On directly mapping relational databases to RDF and OWL. In: WWW, pp. 649–658 (2012)
20. Spanos, D., Stavrou, P., Mitrou, N.: Bringing relational databases into the semantic web: a survey. Semantic Web **3**(2), 169–209 (2012)
21. Qi, T., Qiu, S., Shen, X., et al.: KeMRE: knowledge-enhanced medical relation extraction for Chinese medicine instructions. J. Biomed. Inform. **120**, 103834 (2021)
22. Trigui, S., Boujelben, I., Jamoussi, S.: SMRE: semi-supervised medical relation extraction. In: ICNLSSP, p. 121 (2017)
23. Kamdar, M., Stanley, C., Carroll, M., et al.: Text snippets to corroborate medical relations: an unsupervised approach using a knowledge graph and embeddings. In: AMIA Summits on Translational Science Proceedings 2020, pp. 288–297 (2020)
24. Wang, Y., Yu, B., Zhang, Y., et al.: TPLinker: single-stage joint extraction of entities and relations through token pair linking. In: COLING, pp. 1572–1582 (2020)
25. Ren, P., Hou, W., Sheng, M., Li, X., Li, C., Zhang, Y.: MKGB: a medical knowledge graph construction framework based on data lake and active learning. In: Siuly, S., Wang, H., Chen, L., Guo, Y., Xing, C. (eds.) HIS 2021. LNCS, vol. 13079, pp. 245–253. Springer, Cham (2021). https://doi.org/10.1007/978-3-030-90885-0_22
26. Lee, J., Park, J., Wang, K., et al.: The use of telehealth during the coronavirus (COVID-19) pandemic in oral and maxillofacial surgery - a qualitative analysis. EAI Endorsed Trans. Scalable Inf. Syst. **18**(e34), (2021)
27. Siuly, S., Alçin, Ö.F., Kabir, E., et al.: A new framework for automatic detection of patients with mild cognitive impairment using resting-state EEG signals. IEEE Trans. Neural Syst. Rehabil. Eng. **28**(9), 1966–1976 (2020)

Automated Knowledge Graph Construction for Healthcare Domain

Markian Jaworsky[1(✉)], Xiaohui Tao[1], Jianming Yong[2], Lei Pan[3], Ji Zhang[1], and Shiva Pokhrel[3]

[1] School of Mathematics, Physics and Computing, University of Southern Queensland, Toowoomba, Australia
{Markian.Jaworsky,Xiaohui.Tao,Ji.Zhang}@usq.edu.au

[2] School of Business, University of Southern Queensland, Toowoomba, Australia
Jianming.Yong@usq.edu.au

[3] School of IT, Deakin University, Waurn Ponds, VIC, Australia
{l.pan,shiva.pokhrel}@deakin.edu.au

Abstract. This research seeks to optimize the process of identifying correlations in common and high severity diseases via the fusion of knowledge graphs and deep learning artificial intelligence. Knowledge graphs can be complicated to construct and resource-intensive, alternatively, knowledge graphs can be seen to legitimize correlation incidence and better explain AI outputs. We propose automation of knowledge graph construction from identifying significant text frequency relations within established knowledge base document structures to identifying inter-feature relations and creating a novel approach for artificial intelligence and machine-learning feature extraction and feature selection. Our knowledge graph construction exploits the structured World Health Organization (WHO) International Classification of Disease (ICD) code chapters, which are specific to a single organ system of the human body. A sorted vector of text-to-chapter frequencies enables Wilcox Rank significance tests to determine the most related features.

Keywords: Chronic illness · Risk factors · Feature selection · Knowledge graphs

1 Introduction

Knowledge Graph-based approaches to artificial intelligence promise to deliver superior performance gains to complex classification problems [12,17]. However, despite evidence-based tactical gains, overall strategies for implementing Knowledge Graph-based solutions need to achieve optimal levels of performance, memory usage, and sustainable maintenance [16]. The common manual selection of knowledge integrated into the knowledge graph construction is a fundamental impedance to knowledge completion and automation.

The study of [8] explains that despite feature selection algorithms being preferred for text-based datasets, they do not consider the relations between features and are subject to data loss.

A. Traina et al. (Eds.): HIS 2022, LNCS 13705, pp. 258–265, 2022.
https://doi.org/10.1007/978-3-031-20627-6_24

In the study of rare diseases, Knowledge graphs promise alternate use to synthetic resampling and upsampling data manipulation methods in predicting rare diseases from datasets with highly imbalanced classes. Li *et al.* [10] explains that while synthetic approaches to data resampling are common approaches to handling imbalanced class data, typical class imbalance ratios range between 1:4 compared to 1:100–1000 for rare diseases. A study on using health survey data to predict self-rated health by Clark *et al.* [5] established that machine-learning models could identify many strong predictor variables for self-rated health. The research was supervised by multiple domain experts who believed that the newly identified features correlated to cancer diagnosis.

The contribution of this paper identifies a robust approach to automation of knowledge graph construction, where most other research has potentially become challenged due to complex, subjective, and time-consuming manual tasks and knowledge collection. The construction of our knowledge graph is automated, as it leverages the structured components of WHO ICD, 26 chapters, arranged by categories and subcategories. Similar diseases affecting a single organ system of the human body can be found in one chapter. Our knowledge graph exploits this arrangement of knowledge, filters survey questions for stop words, creates a sorted vector of text to chapter frequencies, and compares each survey question chapter vector with a Wilcox Rank significance test. Significant features with at least a 95% confidence level populate the knowledge graph and provide a new level of explainability for artificial intelligence and machine-learning algorithms.

The rest of this paper is structured as follows. In Sect. 2, we review related research on using knowledge graphs in healthcare. In Sect. 3, we discuss our framework for developing health survey knowledge graphs using WHO ICD Codes. Section 4 describes in detail the two datasets we have fused to construct a knowledge graph. In Sect. 5, we step through the process of knowledge graph construction and identify the opportunity to configure via truncation or subsets, followed by the use case scenario of applying the knowledge graph in a real-world situation. Finally, Sect. 6 concludes the paper.

2 Related Work

Nicholson & Greene [11] proposed the genuine aspect of reviewing knowledge graphs for biomedical applications. A knowledge graph must consist of meaningful nodes and edges for machine-learning classification to be considered genuine. The review compares different approaches to knowledge graph construction, ranging from manually curated knowledge graphs derived from text to automated processes extracting data from databases.

Knowledge graph embedding is constructing knowledge graph facts into continuous vectors, as explained in the review of Wang, Mao, Wang, & Guo [15]. Facts are also referred to as triplets, written in the notation

$$(h, r, t),$$

where h represents the head entity, r the relation, and t is the tail entity. Each fact also consists of a scoring function that represents the strength of the fact, where relations defined in a knowledge graph outweigh undefined relations. Scoring functions typically represent a distance between the head and tail entities. It is further explained that the knowledge graphs can be categorized as having open-world assumption properties or the closed world. In an open-world assumption, all defined facts are considered true, and anything undefined is considered false. Conversely, a knowledge graph consists of both true and false entity relations in closed world assumption. The review concludes that closed world knowledge graphs are more likely to experience scaling issues and performance constraints.

A knowledge graph-based framework for the recommendation of features is proposed by Polychronopoulos *et al.* [7], in their study of identifying genes that cause resistance to non-small cell lung cancer. Keyword text is used for selecting relevant meta-analysis sources, modeling features are derived from the constructed knowledge graph, a scoring system is calculated, and criteria are set for the gene predictions. The study highlights the importance of knowledge-based classification above correlation, particularly when sample volumes may not be able to determine a pattern in a source dataset.

A major obstacle to the automation of Knowledge graph construction is the completeness of knowledge. The Chen *et al.* [2] review of knowledge graph completeness identify that the vast majority of knowledge graphs are constructed manually and subjectively. The review also points out that 1) knowledge graphs generally consist of nodes, edges, and a scoring function, and 2) the methods to determine the completeness or attempt to complete incomplete knowledge graphs ensure that these three features are consistently populated. Future developments of knowledge graphs include and are not limited to the best approaches for implementation.

Determining if previously unseen knowledge is relevant, by way of being related-to, part-of, or kind-of can be addressed using the model proposed by Tao, Zhong, & Nayak [13]. Establishing an understanding of knowledge structure is referred to as ontology, and can advance healthcare research by determining diseases and treatments can be related to determined to be unrelated, as explained by Tao [14].

Our review of knowledge graph studies indicates that most research depends on the manual selection of articles to be used in constructing a knowledge graph. There exists no standard measure to establish the completeness of knowledge in the selection of articles, publishers, or numbers of articles published in both recent and older years. This situation implies that usage of knowledge graphs requires iterative maintenance to ensure knowledge is up to date and not subject to bias. Therefore we concentrate our knowledge graph construction on an established and recognized data source. Furthermore, identifying a widely accepted complete source of knowledge can be used to map the occurrence of text items in a manually constructed knowledge graph to determine where gaps in knowledge may exist.

3 A Framework for Knowledge Graph Development

We leverage the comprehensive review of the foundation model concept conducted by Bommasani *et al.* [1] to address the knowledge graph completeness challenge. The fundamental component underpinning this review was the training, modeling, adaption, and evaluation via a community consensus of universal datasets. The review highlights the objectives of language comprehension, robotics, vision, reasoning, search, philosophy, understanding, and interaction. Our study leverages the foundation datasets, which are anonymized and have prior ethical approvals, and are tailored for the biomedicine and healthcare, education, and law industries. By basing the knowledge graph on a complete knowledge base, we can automate our knowledge graph construction.

In our knowledge graph implementation, the final procedure of Fig. 1 is to aggregate the edge values of every source node to calculate a respective score. Health survey questions are determined to be significantly related by looping through the number of text items in each question text vector, and when a significant Wilcox ranking is found, the number of matching text items becomes the relevant edge value. We then aggregate the sum of edge values for all the related destination nodes of a given source node.

4 Data Source for Knowledge Graph Learning

An online search tool with categories, concepts, and 1.6 million medical terms is made available by The World Health Organisation[1] the latest revision of the International Classification of Diseases (ICD) codes. With this tool, the possibility of cross-referencing health survey question text to determine relationships between survey questions emerges by matching known symptoms and risk factors assigned to disease subcategories. Health survey question text can be filtered by stop words, and from the frequencies of text appearing in each ICD chapter, the strength of relations between features can be tested for significance. Other motivations for using the WHO ICD codes are the assurance of completeness of knowledge, and low maintenance requirements, due to infrequent revisions.

The annual Behavioral Risk Factor Surveillance System (BRFSS) is anonymized and made publicly available by the United States Centers for Disease Control and Prevention. The survey consists of hundreds of government-approved health survey questions and approximately half a million respondents. The large sample size of the annual survey provides a unique opportunity to establish a ground truth of disease and chronic illness prevalence. Anonymizing respondents' personal information is also a key feature in its usability for performing health studies. In particular, the 2020 BRFSS survey has 279 survey questions and answers. The answers typically have a nominal variable value which can be explained using a codebook[2] to determine an answer meaning.

---

1 https://www.who.int/standards/classifications/classification-of-diseases.

2 https://www.cdc.gov/brfss/annual_data/annual_2020.html.

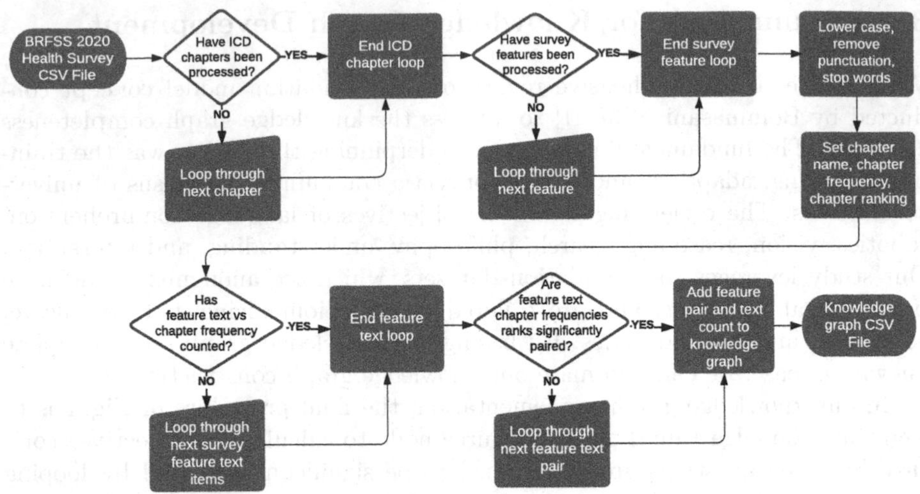

Fig. 1. Knowledge graph construction block diagram

5 Knowledge Graph

Our knowledge graph is exported as a comma-separated value file in its original open-world format and is also aggregated into a format with just the head entity and a respective aggregated score of all relations for that given head entity, and is available for download at the GitHub repository[3]. We use version 4.1.2 of the R Programming language to define BRFSS health survey questions as vectors of individual text items and have also created a text version of the WHO ICD Code chapters for input into the knowledge graph source code. R programming libraries are imported for summarizing the text frequencies inside each of the WHO ICD Code chapter text files, and the R Programming[4] `wilcox.test` function is used to determine if there are significant inter-feature relations between the health survey question text frequencies in each of the WHO ICD Code chapters.

5.1 Construction

According to the Li *et al.* [9] proposal for constructing medical knowledge graphs, manually constructed graphs are unreasonably time-consuming, and the automated alternative is challenging because knowledge is typically derived from unstructured text. The study highlights that the classical knowledge graph contains many triplets, where the combination of head and tail entities, implies a 3_{rd}, their proposal puts forward a quadruplet model, where each knowledge graph entry is also represented by numerical frequency, probability, specificity,

[3] https://github.com/mjaworsky/KnowledgeGraph.

[4] https://www.rdocumentation.org/packages/stats/versions/3.6.2/topics/wilcox.test.

and reliability, which can be used as metrics to filter knowledge graph entries or assist in calculated output functions.

The construction of our knowledge graph is automated, as it leverages the structured components of WHO ICD, 26 chapters, arranged by categories and subcategories. Similar diseases affecting a single organ system of the human body can be found in one chapter. As explained in Fig. 1, our knowledge graph exploits this arrangement of knowledge, filters survey questions for stop words, creates a sorted vector of text to chapter frequencies, and compares each survey question chapter vector with a Wilcox Rank significance test. Significant features with at least a 95% confidence level populate the knowledge graph.

The aggregate scoring function of our knowledge graph provides a method to create an absolute feature ranking of the head entity, provides further insight into the spread of inter-feature relations, and can be exploited with human decision-making to determine a precise selection of features with or without a greater subset of features with outlier properties, or a smaller subset that best represents the larger dataset.

5.2 Case Study

The data preparation in the study of Dinh, Miertschin, Young, & Mohanty [6] predicts the combination of cardiovascular disease and diabetes using the NHANES health survey, removes dataset features where more than 50% of values are missing, and further omits data rows where a selected feature value is missing. Feature selection is based upon previous studies which identified predictor variables of diabetes with the addition of 2 variables, cholesterol and leg length to assist with the classification of cardiovascular disease. In this scenario, the hypothesis in the study could have been simplified by determining if cholesterol and leg length correlate with heart disease.

The construction of a knowledge graph of inter-feature relations to be used for feature selection can provide a more explainable view of the underlying dataset than what is currently derived from an automated deep-learning solution. Automated deep learning feature engineering requires a strategy for optimization and does not provide information about feature extraction or selection. Inter-feature relations, semantics, and dependencies discovered by deep learning models are not traceable and explainable. For these reasons, medical and engineering domain experts have avoided deep learning in favor of standard machine-learning algorithms [3,4].

6 Future Work and Conclusions

Further improvement of our contribution can focus on the prioritization of linear over nonlinear features for feature selection and extraction. As an example, our BRFSS 2020 health survey dataset consists of 279 questions, of which 40 (86%) have nonlinear properties, and only 39 (13%) questions can be considered to have linear variable answers, such as respondent's age, height, and weight.

In this paper, we have presented the construction of a knowledge graph that provides significant inter-feature relations of a health survey by identifying the significant text frequencies within the chapters of the WHO ICD codes. By leveraging an established knowledge base, we can automate the construction of the knowledge graph using a Wilcox rank significance test and discuss ways to analyze the structure of the knowledge graph in order to fine-tune the selection of features that contain the highest and lowest levels of inter-feature relations.

Usage of a knowledge base widely accepted as a complete resource of knowledge can be used to construct a robust knowledge graph. It also has the potential to be used to assess the completeness of other knowledge graphs that have been constructed with a manual selection of individual and potentially unrelated articles. Using the complete knowledge of the WHO ICD Codes, a text frequency search of article titles can scan through each chapter of ICD descriptions and determine if a manually constructed knowledge graph is intentionally focused on a subset of the human body or should contain more generalized human body organ system knowledge.

Our case study demonstrates the utility of the constructed knowledge graph in selecting features for the classification of chronic illness from a high-dimensional health survey. Where artificial intelligence models automate the end-to-end feature engineering and classification process, a knowledge graph of inter-feature relations can provide new insights into the predictive power of features in high-dimensional datasets.

References

1. Bommasani, R., et al.: On the opportunities and risks of foundation models. arXiv preprint arXiv:2108.07258 (2021)
2. Chen, Z., Wang, Y., Zhao, B., Cheng, J., Zhao, X., Duan, Z.: Knowledge graph completion: a review. IEEE Access **8**, 192435–192456 (2020)
3. Chinesta, F., Cueto, E., Abisset-Chavanne, E., Duval, J.L., El Khaldi, F.: Virtual, digital and hybrid twins: a new paradigm in data-based engineering and engineered data. Arch. Comput. Methods Eng. **27**(1), 105–134 (2020). https://doi.org/10.1007/s11831-018-9301-4
4. Ching, T., et al.: Opportunities and obstacles for deep learning in biology and medicine. J. R. Soc. Interface **15**(141), 20170387 (2018). https://doi.org/10.1098/rsif.2017.0387
5. Clark, C.R., et al.: Predicting self-rated health across the life course: health equity insights from machine learning models. J. Gen. Intern. Med. **36**(5), 1181–1188 (2021)
6. Dinh, A., Miertschin, S., Young, A., Mohanty, S.D.: A data-driven approach to predicting diabetes and cardiovascular disease with machine learning. BMC Med. Inform. Decis. Making **19**(1), 1–15 (2019)
7. Gogleva, A., et al.: Knowledge graph-based recommendation framework identifies drivers of resistance in EGFR mutant non-small cell lung cancer. Nat. Commun. **13**(1), 1–14 (2022)
8. Kim, K.: An improved semi-supervised dimensionality reduction using feature weighting: application to sentiment analysis. Expert Syst. Appl. **109**, 49–65 (2018). https://doi.org/10.1016/j.eswa.2018.05.023

9. Li, L., et al.: Real-world data medical knowledge graph: construction and applications. Artif. Intell. Med. **103**, 101817 (2020)
10. Li, X., Wang, Y., Wang, D., Yuan, W., Peng, D., Mei, Q.: Improving rare disease classification using imperfect knowledge graph. BMC Med. Inform. Decis. Making **19**(5), 1–10 (2019). https://doi.org/10.1186/s12911-019-0938-1
11. Nicholson, D.N., Greene, C.S.: Constructing knowledge graphs and their biomedical applications. Comput. Struct. Biotechnol. J. **18**, 1414–1428 (2020)
12. Pham, T., Tao, X., Zhang, J., Yong, J., Li, Y., Xie, H.: Graph-based multi-label disease prediction model learning from medical data and domain knowledge. Knowl.-Based Syst. **235**, 107662 (2022)
13. Tao, X., Li, Y., Zhong, N., Nayak, R.: Ontology mining for personalized web information gathering. In: IEEE/WIC/ACM International Conference on Web Intelligence (WI 2007), pp. 351–358. IEEE (2007)
14. Tao, X., et al.: Mining health knowledge graph for health risk prediction. World Wide Web **23**(4), 2341–2362 (2020)
15. Wang, Q., Mao, Z., Wang, B., Guo, L.: Knowledge graph embedding: a survey of approaches and applications. IEEE Trans. Knowl. Data Eng. **29**(12), 2724–2743 (2017)
16. Zeng, X., Tu, X., Liu, Y., Fu, X., Su, Y.: Toward better drug discovery with knowledge graph. Curr. Opin. Struct. Biol. **72**, 114–126 (2022)
17. Zhang, D., Yang, X., Liu, L., Liu, Q.: A knowledge graph-enhanced attention aggregation network for making recommendations. Appl. Sci. **11**(21), 10432 (2021)

Alcoholic EEG Data Classification Using Weighted Graph-Based Technique

Supriya Supriya(✉), Tony Jan, Nandini Sidnal, and Scott Thompson-Whiteside

Torrens University, Flinders Street, Melbourne, VIC 3000, Australia
{supriya.supriya,tony.jan,nandini.sidnal, scott.whiteside}@torrens.edu.au

Abstract. The analysis and classification of Alcohol Use Disorder (AUD) using non-invasive measurements, such as EEG records from the brain scalp, are of significant importance in neuroscience. Analysis and diagnosis of brain diseases associated with alcoholic subjects using EEG records remain challenging. This study proposes a graph theory-based approach for automated classification of AUD using EEG data. The metrics of the graphs are intrinsically related to the organization of the brain functionality. The main contribution of this study is to evaluate the impact of weighted graph features on AUD classifications based on EEG data. In this study, three different features (average degree, fluctuation difference, and average weighted degree) were extracted from the weighed visibility EEG graph and the performance of the proposed model was evaluated against SVM, k-NN, and Naive Bayes classifiers. The experimental results indicates that the topological features of the weighted EEG graphs supported superior classification performance (97.5%) against the other competing methods.

Keywords: EEG · Alcoholic classification · Weighted visibility graph · Alcohol use disorder (AUD) · EEG-time series analysis

1 Introduction

Alcohol use disorder (AUD) is a morbidity characterized by dysfunction of the central nervous system when alcohol is consumed for a long period [1]. AUD inhibits the ability to regulate the use of alcohol despite adverse consequences in cognitive and mobility impairments, etc. [2]. Chronic heavy consumption of alcohol can deteriorate AUD with aggravated alcohol abuse and dependence. Approximately 3 million deaths occur due to the harmful consumption of alcohol in each year. According to the World Health Organization (WHO), the harmful or heavy consumption of alcohols are the causes of more than 200 different diseases [3].

For effective evaluation of alcoholic conditions, information extraction from neurological data is crucial. Various tools [4–6] were used to evaluate neurological data including magnetic resonance imaging (MRI) and magnetic resonance diffusion tensor imaging (DTI), which helped to identify some vulnerable white matters as well as frontal

A. Traina et al. (Eds.): HIS 2022, LNCS 13705, pp. 266–276, 2022.
https://doi.org/10.1007/978-3-031-20627-6_25

atrophy caused by chronic alcohol use [7, 8]. Positron emission tomography (PET) also helped to identify the response of the brain in an alcoholic state [9]. Electroencephalography (EEG) is an important tool that is often preferred by clinicians and researchers in analyzing neurological data for the detection and treatment of AUD [10]. Clinicians favor EEG as it is non-invasive, convenient, portable, and inexpensive. In addition,, EEG can provide high temporal image resolutions (around ~1 ms).

Once EEG data is collected, a number of different smart classifying models can be used to classify the alcoholics from the collected data. Farsi et al. [11] proposed two deep learning algorithms to identify alcoholics from their EEG signal data. Their first algorithm was based on feature extraction using Principal Component Analysis (PCA) which achieved 86% classification accuracy upon using an Artificial neural network (ANN) as the classifier. Their second algorithm was based on the deep learning on raw EEG signal data, which achieved 93% classification accuracy. Bajaj et al. [12] implemented a novel hybrid approach based on Frequency (T-F) images of EEG data with a non-negative least square classifier (NNLS) to distinguish between alcoholic and control (non-alcoholic) EEG data and achieved 95.83% accuracy. Faust et al. [13] proposed wavelet packet decomposition (WPD) based energy measures for the analysis of alcoholic EEG data and achieved 95.8% accuracy.

Over the past few decades, graph or network theory has played a significant role in analysis of brain structures and functionalities [14–18]. Topological properties of brain EEG graphs are important to identify neurological and various brain disorders [19–21]. Cao et al. [22] proposed a graph-based framework for classifying alcoholic EEG data. Zhu et al. [23] proposed a horizontal-visibility graph-based framework for the classification of EEG data from alcoholics (against the EEG data of control (normal) subjects). The major limitation in these techniques is that they did not consider an important aspect in a graph, that is, weight or edge weight. The weight in a graph plays a crucial role in determining the relationships between different nodes and helps to understand the underlying nature of the graph. The main contribution of this study is to introduce weights in the visibility graph and explore the classification performance of EEG-based AUD.

The key novelty of this study is that the analysis of alcoholic EEG data has never been performed on the visibility graph by introducing a weight in the graph. Before this work, alcoholic EEG data were classified using only horizontal visibility and weighted horizontal visibility graphs. In addition, fluctuation differences features were not used in the analysis of the weighted visibility graph.

In this study, the EEG signals are first mapped to a weighted visibility graph. The weights in the visibility graph play a significant role in EEG signal analysis. Three different features of the graph, namely the average degree, average weighted degree, and fluctuation difference, are extracted. The fluctuation differences features are used for the first time in the visibility graph with weight. Next, the k-NN classifier, Naive Bayes, and SVM classifier with different kernel functions (linear, radio-basis functions (RBF), and polynomial) were used to classify alcoholic and control (normal) subject data. This paper is structured as follows. Section 2 describes various methods with feature extraction. Section 3 discusses the data used in this research study and the experimental results and evaluations. The conclusions are presented in Sect. 4.

2 Methods

This study proposes a weighted visibility graph-based technique for the automated classification of EEG data from alcoholic and control subjects. Figure 1 shows the block diagram of the proposed methodology. As illustrated in Fig. 1, the proposed methodology consists of several steps: mapping of the EEG signals to a weighted visibility graph, extracting three topological features (average weighted degree, average degree, and fluctuation difference), and then employing classification with the help of three different classifiers: SVM with different kernel functions (linear, RBF, polynomial), k-NN and Naive Bayes. Classification performance was evaluated based on three performance metrics: sensitivity, specificity, and accuracy.

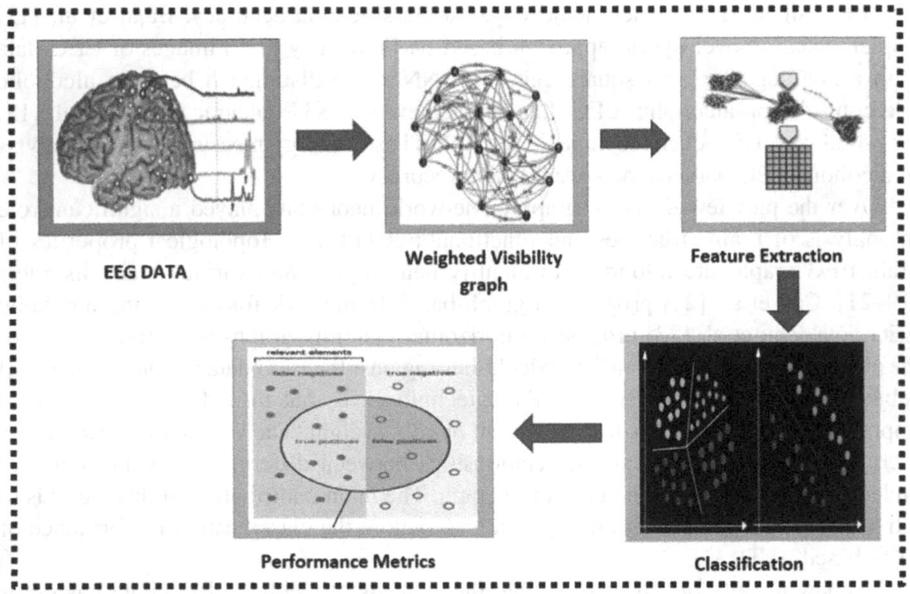

Fig. 1. Block Diagram of the classification of EEG signals from Alcoholic and Control subject, using Weighted Visibility graph.

2.1 Mapping of EEG Data to Complex Network

The first step is to map a time series of $x_{t, \{t = 1, 2, \dots n\}}$ with "n" number of data points to Graph G (N, E), where, each node n_i of a graph corresponds to a data point x_t of the time series. The connection between two nodes is measured by edge ($e_t \in E$), which is based on the following visibility graph equation [26]:

$$x_c < x_a + (x_b - x_a)\frac{c - a}{b - a}, a < c < b \tag{1}$$

where, $x_{a,}x_{band}x_c$ are the time series data points at their corresponding time a, b and c, respectively. If the two nodes satisfy Eq. (1), then an edge is established between them otherwise there is no relationship between them. A more detailed example of this is available in our previous work [18].

The next step is to measure the weight of the edge between the two nodes, which is measured by the following equation, and is directional by nature from a to b.

$$w_{ab} = \left| \frac{x_b - x_a}{b - a} \right|, a < b, \tag{2}$$

where w_{ab} denotes the edge weight between nodes a and b and corresponds to the times series data points x_a and x_b. Finally, a weighted graph is built and named as the weighted visibility graph.

2.2 Feature Extraction of Weighted Visibility Graph

Feature extraction is essential for achieving high classification performance of biomedical signals [24, 25]. The main objective of feature extraction is to identify the most promising set of features that are informative and compact to support computational efficiency of the classifiers. In this study, three distinct topological features were extracted from a weighted visibility graph of alcoholic and control EEG data [27–30]:

2.2.1 Average Weighted Degree

An adjacent matrix of the weighted visibility graph with n nodes is characterized by B_{nXn}, where B_{ij} represents an edge between two nodes i and j. The weighted degree of a node is measured as the sum of the weights of all edges incident on that node [31].

$$wd_a = \sum_{b \varepsilon A(a)} w_{ab} \tag{3}$$

where A(a) denotes the neighborhoods of node a and w_{ab} and is the weight of the links between nodes a and b. The average mean of all total weights that are incident on all the nodes of the network [20].

2.2.2 Average Degree

The average degree of G(N, E) is measured by the ratio of the total number of edges in the graph to the total number of total nodes in a graph. As the edges are directional, the average degree is evaluated as [10]:

$$AD = \left| \frac{E}{N} \right| \tag{4}$$

2.2.3 Fluctuation Difference

The fluctuation difference of a channel plays a crucial role in improving the performance of our classifiers. It is evaluated using the following equation [14]:

$$FD = (w_{max} - w_{min}) \tag{5}$$

where, w_{max} represent the maximum edge weight of a channel corresponding to the maximum fluctuation, and w_{min} denotes the minimum edge weight of the same channel. This helps to increase the classification accuracy of all classifiers used in the experiments.

2.3 Classification

The main aim of classification is to differentiate the unknown observations present in the testing set into their proper categories based on the training of the classifier. In this research, K-Nearest Neighbor (k-NN), Support Vector Machine (SVM), and Naive Bayes classifiers are used for the classification of the extracted topological features of the weighted graph. The reason behind using the k-NN is that it is robust to noisy data while training and very easily handles complex models. SVM encompasses distinct kernel functions, such as linear, RBF, and polynomial, which provide better classification results. Naïve Bayes is fast and does not involve extensive training. Further details on these classifiers are available in [32–34]. The classification performance was measured using accuracy, sensitivity, and specificity parameters [20].

3 Data and Experimental Results

The performance of the proposed model is evaluated on the EEG database, which is available online and encompasses two distinct EEG datasets: an alcoholic person's EEG and a control person's EEG [35]. EEG signals were obtained using 64 electrodes with a sampling frequency of 256 Hz for one second. The dataset used in this study comprised 120 files of each alcoholic as well as control subjects, with 2048 data samples in each file [36]. A detailed description of the EEG database is available in [35] and [36].

Tang et al. [37] mentioned in their research that while mapping time series to graphs, it is not mandatory to use large observations of samples, as the self-similar nature and the quantification of complexity do not require a large number of nodes as observations. In our previous research [28], we observed that the segmentation of the EEG channel does not affect the results. Therefore, in this study, we segmented each channel into two parts. Each channel comprised 2048 data samples, and after segmentation, each segment comprised 1024 data points.

Figure 2 illustrates a comparison of the average weighted features for the alcoholic and control EEG using the notched boxplot. Notches in the boxplot are used to illustrate the variability of the median among the samples. As we can see that the notches of the alcoholic box and control box do not overlap. There were no outliers in the AWD of the control subject data, but there were three outliers in the AWD of alcoholic subject data.

Likewise, Fig. 3 demonstrates the comparison of the average degree (AD) feature for the alcoholic and control EEG using the notched boxplot. There are two outliers in the AD of the control subject data, but one outlier in the AD of the alcoholic subject data. However, the notches of the alcoholic and control boxes did not overlap. Similarly, Fig. 4 illustrates the comparison of the fluctuation difference feature for the alcoholic and control EEG using a notched boxplot. There are no outliers in the fluctuation differences (FD) of the control subject data and alcoholic subject data.

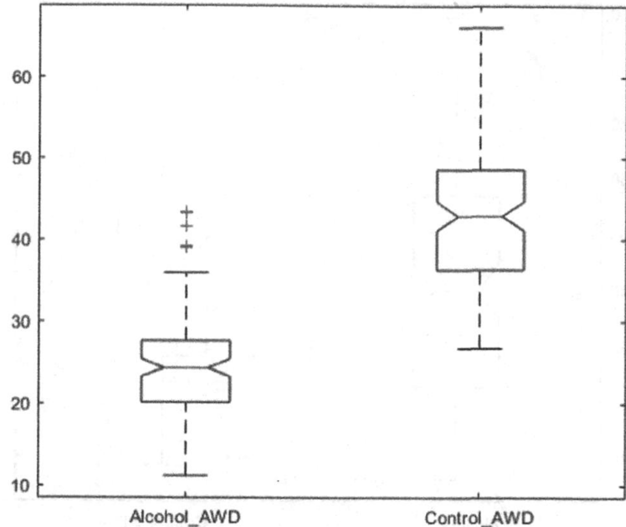

Fig. 2. Notched box plot of Average weighted degree of Alcoholic and Control subject.

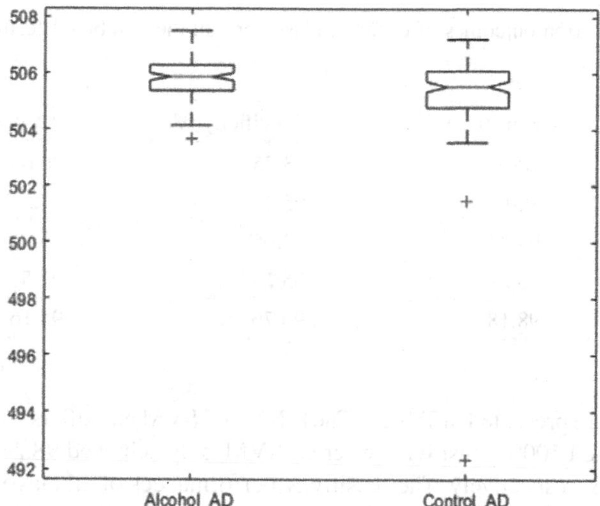

Fig. 3. Notched box plot of average degree of alcoholic and control subject.

As per the described methodology, each channel is mapped to a weighted visibility graph, and three features are extracted: AWD, AD, and FD. Before performing the classification, we took the average of the features of the two segments that correspond to one channel. Then, classification was performed. Different values of the k-NN classifiers were evaluated, but K = 3 performed the classification with highest accuracy. Table 1 illustrates the classification results for the different classifiers obtained by combining the three features.

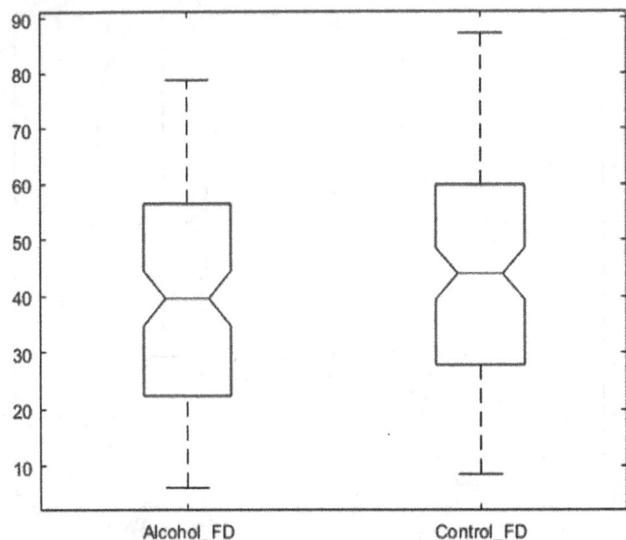

Fig. 4. Notched box plot of fluctuation difference of alcoholic and control subject.

Table 1. Classification outcomes of different classifiers on the combined feature set (AWD + AD + FD)

Classifiers	Sensitivity (%)	Specificity (%)	Accuracy (%)
SVM-Linear	100	93.75	96.66
SVM-RBF	100	95.23	97.5
SVM-Poly	98.24	93.65	95.83
k-NN = 3	100	95.23	97.5
NB	98.18	90.76	94.16

The results are presented in Table 1. The k-NN and SVM classifiers with kernel linear and RBF achieved 100% sensitivity, whereas SVM-poly achieved 98.24% and 98.18% accuracy for NB, respectively. The sensitivity performances of all classifiers were very close to each other. Similarly, the specificity performance of different classifiers was very similar; for SVM-linear, it 93.75% and 95.23% for SVM-RBF, 93.65% for SVM-poly, 95.23% for k-NN, and 90.76% for NB. The SVM-RBF and k-NN classifiers provided higher specificity than the other classifiers. The classification accuracy performance of the different classifiers was: 96.66% for SVM-linear, 97.5% for SVM-RBF, 95.83% for SVM-poly, 97.5% for k-NN, and 94.16% for NB. The SVM-RBF and k-NN classifier provided a higher classification accuracy than the other classifiers.

To validate the classification performance of our proposed method on the experimental dataset, we performed K-fold cross-validation with K = 10. Table 2 shows the classification accuracy results with 10-fold cross-validation and without 10-fold cross-validation. Table 2 clearly shows that the classification accuracy of the 10-fold cross-validation of the different classifiers is very close to our experimental results (without 10-fold cross-validation).

Table 3 presents a comparison analysis of the classification performance of our proposed method with that of some existing state-of-the-art methods. It is clearly demonstrated that our proposed method provides a higher classification accuracy than other methods.

Table 2. Classification accuracy of different classifiers on 10-fold cross validation

Classifiers	Accuracy (%) without 10-fold cross-validation	Accuracy (%) with 10-fold cross-validation
SVM-Linear	96.66	97.5
SVM-RBF	97.5	96
SVM-Poly	95.83	96.3
k-NN = 3	97.5	97
NB	94.16	96

Table 3. Comparative analysis of different methodologies for alcoholic EEG data classification

Authors	Extracted features	Classifiers	Accuracy (%)
Kannathal et al. [38]	CD, LLE, entropy, H	Unique ranges	90%
Faust et al. [13]	WPD—Relative energy	k-NN	95.8%
Ehlers et al. [39]	Correlation dimension	Discriminant analysis	88%
Varun et al. [12]	CoHOG and Eig(Hess)-CoHOG	NNLS	95.83%
Our proposed method	AWD, AD, and FD	SVM-RBF, k-NN = 3	97.5%

Table 3 presents a comparison analysis of the classification performance of our proposed method with that of some existing state-of-the-art methods. It is clearly demonstrated that our proposed method provides a higher classification accuracy as compared to the other methods. In summary, the experimental results of the research disclosed that AWD, AD, and FD features are efficient in classifying alcoholic and control subject using their EEG data. In the future, the proposed methodology can be enhanced by combining the weighted visibility graph technique with a deep learning neural network.

4 Conclusion

In this study, a graph-based approach was applied to the classification of two distinct classes of EEG signals. First, a weight visibility graph is built from EEG data and then three topological features of the graph named average degree, fluctuation difference, and average weighted degree are extracted, and the performance is evaluated with the help of different classifiers. It was observed that SVM-RBF and K-NN = 3 provided better accuracy results than the other classifiers (SVM-linear, SVM-poly, and Naïve Bayes). The results also demonstrated that graph theory plays a crucial role in the analysis of EEG data classification. The experimental results also demonstrate that the proposed method is robust and efficient for the analysis of biomedical EEG signals.

References

1. Diagnostic and Statistical Manual of Mental Disorders: DSM-5, 5th edn. Reference Reviews **28**, 36–37 (2014)
2. Understanding Alcohol Use Disorder | National Institute on Alcohol Abuse and Alcoholism (NIAAA). https://www.niaaa.nih.gov/publications/brochures-and-fact-sheets/understanding-alcohol-use-disorder
3. Alcohol. https://www.who.int/news-room/fact-sheets/detail/alcohol#:~:text=The%20harmful%20use%20of%20alcohol,represents%205.3%25%20of%20all%20deaths
4. Sadiq, M., Akbari, H., Siuly, S., Li, Y., Wen, P.: Alcoholic EEG signals recognition based on phase space dynamic and geometrical features. Chaos Solitons Fractals **158**, 112036 (2022)
5. Hussain, W., Sadiq, M., Siuly, S., Rehman, A.: Epileptic seizure detection using 1 D-convolutional long short-term memory neural networks. Appl. Acoust. **177**, 107941 (2021)
6. Şengür, D., Siuly, S.: Efficient approach for EEG-based emotion recognition. Electron. Lett. **56**, 1361–1364 (2020)
7. Namura, I.: Alcoholic brain damage and dementia viewed by MRI, with special consideration on frontal atrophy and white matter damage in dyslipidemic patients. Psychogeriatrics **6**, 119–127 (2006)
8. Pfefferbaum, A., Sullivan, E.: Disruption of brain white matter microstructure by excessive intracellular and extracellular fluid in alcoholism: evidence from diffusion tensor imaging. Neuropsychopharmacology **30**, 423–432 (2004)
9. Solingapuram Sai, K., Hurley, R., Dodda, M., Taber, K.: Positron emission tomography: updates on imaging of addiction. J. Neuropsychiatry Clin. Neurosci. **31**, A6-288 (2019)
10. Supriya, S., Siuly, S., Wang, H., Zhang, Y.: An efficient framework for the analysis of big brain signals data. In: Wang, J., Cong, G., Chen, J., Qi, J. (eds.) Databases Theory and Applications, vol. 10837, pp. 199–207. Springer, Cham (2018). https://doi.org/10.1007/978-3-319-92013-9_16
11. Farsi, L., Siuly, S., Kabir, E., Wang, H.: Classification of alcoholic EEG signals using a deep learning method. IEEE Sens. J. **21**, 3552–3560 (2021)
12. Bajaj, V., Guo, Y., Sengur, A., Siuly, S., Alcin, O.F.: A hybrid method based on time–frequency images for classification of alcohol and control EEG signals. Neural Comput. Appl. **28**(12), 3717–3723 (2016). https://doi.org/10.1007/s00521-016-2276-x
13. Faust, O., Yu, W., Kadri, N.: Computer-based identification of normal and alcoholic EEG signals using wavelet packets and energy measures. J. Mech. Med. Biol. **13**, 1350033 (2013)
14. Supriya, S., Siuly, S., Wang, H., Zhang, Y.: New feature extraction for automated detection of epileptic seizure using complex network framework. Appl. Acoust. **180**, 108098 (2021)

15. Smit, D., Stam, C., Posthuma, D., Boomsma, D., de Geus, E.: Heritability of "small-world" networks in the brain: a graph theoretical analysis of resting-state EEG functional connectivity. Hum. Brain Mapp. **29**, 1368–1378 (2008)
16. Supriya, S., Siuly, S., Wang, H., Zhang, Y.: Epilepsy detection from EEG using complex network techniques: a review. IEEE Rev. Biomed. Eng. 1 (2021)
17. Sporns, O.: Graph theory methods for the analysis of neural connectivity patterns. In: Kötter, R. (ed.) Neuroscience Databases, pp. 171–185. Springer, Boston (2003)
18. Supriya, S., Siuly, S., Wang, H., Cao, J., Zhang, Y.: Weighted visibility graph with complex network features in the detection of epilepsy. IEEE Access. **4**, 6554–6566 (2016)
19. Supriya, S., Siuly, S., Zhang, Y.: Automatic epilepsy detection from EEG introducing a new edge weight method in the complex network. Electron. Lett. **52**, 1430–1432 (2016)
20. Supriya, S., Siuly, S., Wang, H., Zhang, Y.: EEG sleep stages analysis and classification based on weighed complex network features. IEEE Trans. Emerging Top. Comput. Intell. **5**, 236–246 (2021)
21. Supriya, S., Siuly, S., Wang, H., Zhang, Y.: Automated epilepsy detection techniques from electroencephalogram signals: a review study. Health Inf. Sci. Syst. **8**(1), 1–15 (2020). https://doi.org/10.1007/s13755-020-00129-1
22. Cao, R., Wu, Z., Li, H., Xiang, J., Chen, J.: Disturbed connectivity of EEG functional networks in alcoholism: a graph-theoretic analysis. Bio-Med. Mater. Eng. **24**, 2927–2936 (2014)
23. Zhu, G., Li, Y., Wen, P., Wang, S.: Analysis of alcoholic EEG signals based on horizontal visibility graph entropy. Brain Inform. **1**(1–4), 19–25 (2014). https://doi.org/10.1007/s40708-014-0003-x
24. Hassan, A., Siuly, S., Zhang, Y.: Epileptic seizure detection in EEG signals using tunable-Q factor wavelet transform and bootstrap aggregating. Comput. Methods Programs Biomed. **137**, 247–259 (2016)
25. Siuly, S., Kabir, E., Wang, H., Zhang, Y.: Exploring sampling in the detection of multicategory EEG signals. Comput. Math. Methods Med. **2015**, 1–12 (2015)
26. Lacasa, L., Luque, B., Ballesteros, F., Luque, J., Nuño, J.: From time series to complex networks: the visibility graph. Proc. Natl. Acad. Sci. **105**, 4972–4975 (2008)
27. Wu, J., Sun, L., Peng, D., Siuly, S.: A micro neural network for healthcare sensor data stream classification in sustainable and smart cities. Comput. Intell. Neurosci. **2022**, 1–9 (2022)
28. Supriya, S., Wang, H., Zhuo, G., Zhang, Y.: Analyzing EEG signal data for detection of epileptic seizure: introducing weight on visibility graph with complex network feature. In: Cheema, M., Zhang, W., Chang, L. (eds.) Databases Theory and Applications, vol. 9877, pp. 56–66. Springer, Cham (2016). https://doi.org/10.1007/978-3-319-46922-5_5
29. Alvi, A., Siuly, S., Wang, H.: A long short-term memory based framework for early detection of mild cognitive impairment from EEG signals. IEEE Trans. Emerging Top. Comput. Intell. 1–14 (2022)
30. Sadiq, M.T., Siuly, S., Ur Rehman, A., Wang, H.: Auto-correlation based feature extraction approach for EEG alcoholism identification. In: Siuly, S., Wang, H., Chen, L., Guo, Y., Xing, C. (eds.) HIS 2021. LNCS, vol. 13079, pp. 47–58. Springer, Cham (2021). https://doi.org/10.1007/978-3-030-90885-0_5
31. Antoniou, I., Tsompa, E.: Statistical analysis of weighted networks. Discret. Dyn. Nat. Soc. **2008**, 1–16 (2008)
32. Jiang, W.: Time series classification: nearest neighbor versus deep learning models. SN Appl. Sci. **2**(4), 1–17 (2020). https://doi.org/10.1007/s42452-020-2506-9
33. Wen-ge, F.: Application of SVM classifier in IR target recognition. Phys. Procedia **24**, 2138–2142 (2012)
34. Machado, J., Balbinot, A.: Executed movement using EEG signals through a naive Bayes classifier. Micromachines **5**, 1082–1105 (2014)

35. EEG Database. http://kdd.ics.uci.edu/databases/eeg/eeg.data.html
36. Zhang, X., Begleiter, H., Porjesz, B., Wang, W., Litke, A.: Event related potentials during object recognition tasks. Brain Res. Bull. **38**, 531–538 (1995)
37. Tang, X., et al.: New approach to epileptic diagnosis using visibility graph of high-frequency signal. Clin. EEG Neurosci. **44**, 150–156 (2013)
38. Kannathal, N., Acharya, U., Lim, C., Sadasivan, P.: Characterization of EEG—a comparative study. Comput. Methods Programs Biomed. **80**, 17–23 (2005)
39. Ehlers, C., Havstad, J., Prichard, D., Theiler, J.: Low doses of ethanol reduce evidence for nonlinear structure in brain activity. J. Neurosci. **18**, 7474–7486 (1998)

Health and Medical Data Classification

Optical Coherence Tomography Classification Based on Transfer Learning and RA-Attention

Xiaoyi Lian[1], Lina Chen[1(✉)], Xiayan Ji[1], Fangyao Shen[2], Hongjie Guo[3], and Hong Gao[3]

[1] College of Physics and Electronic Information Engineering, Zhejiang Normal University, Zhejiang 321004, China
chenlina@zjnu.com

[2] College of Mathematics and Computer Science, Zhejiang Normal University, Zhejiang 321004, China
fyshen@zjnu.edu.cn

[3] Faculty of Computing, Harbin Institute of Technology, Harbin 150001, China
hjguo@stu.hit.edu.cn, honggao@hit.edu.cn

Abstract. Macular disease is one of the major causes of blindness. Optical coherence tomography (OCT) is a commonly used ophthalmic diagnostic technique to assist ophthalmologists in their analysis and treatment. However, manual analysis is a time-consuming, heavy and subjective process. In this paper, we propose an improved EfficientNet model for retinal OCT image classification, named TL-RA-EfficientNet. It introduces a Re-Attention module to enable the model to identify the lesions with small areas and fuzzy shapes. During training, a data augmentation strategy is introduced to solve the class-imbalance problem, and a transfer learning strategy is adopted to speed up the convergence of the model. The experimental results on the UCSD dataset show that the average recognition accuracy, sensitivity and specificity of our model are 99.9%, 99.9% and 99.97%, respectively, which are more effective than previous classification methods.

Keywords: Optical coherence tomography · EfficientNet · Transfer learning · Attention mechanism

1 Introduction

Optical coherence tomography (OCT) is one of the most commonly used techniques in clinical ophthalmology. It captures the cross-sectional images of biological tissues at microscopic resolution, and it is a non-invasive and non-contact examination with high resolution and fast imaging. It can provide a useful basis for the diagnosis of retinal diseases, especially macular disease. Clinically, ophthalmologists diagnose diseases according to information such as the shape, thickness and brightness of retinal membrane structure in OCT images [1]. However, manual diagnosis is often a time-consuming, heavy and subjective process [2, 3]. Therefore, developing a computer-aided diagnosis technology is of great significance for the diagnosis and treatment of ophthalmic diseases.

A. Traina et al. (Eds.): HIS 2022, LNCS 13705, pp. 279–290, 2022.
https://doi.org/10.1007/978-3-031-20627-6_26

Recently, deep learning technology has made great achievements in image classification and recognition, which also greatly promotes the development of medical image analysis [4, 5]. In the field of retinal OCT image classification, some deep learning algorithms have been proposed [6, 7]. For example, Awais et al. used the VGG16 model to extract features from different layers of the network and then used different classifiers to classify these features [8]. The accuracy, sensitivity and specificity reached 87.5%, 93.5% and 81%, respectively. Bhowmik et al. used VGG16 and Inception V3 models as baseline networks. Then predict the disease by analyzing the image through the models trained using transfer learning which achieves an accuracy of 94% [9]. Additionally, some studies introduced attention mechanisms to make models focus on retinal lesion areas. For instance, Fang et al. used a lesion detection network designed by itself to generate a soft attention map from the entire OCT image and incorporate it into the classification network [10]. It allowed the network to utilize the information of the lesion-related regions to further accelerate the network training process and enhanced OCT classification with an accuracy of 90.1%. Mishra et al. adopted Multilayer Perturbation Spatial Attention (MPSA) and Multidimensional Attention (MDA) modules to design a new perturbation attention network—PCAM [11]. The network focused on different levels of feature space to extract inter-class discriminative features and achieved an accuracy of 95.3%.

Although these researches have made significant progress in the task of retinal OCT classification, there still exist some problems: 1) The public retinal OCT datasets are usually class-imbalance, which leads to models misjudging the minority class sample as the majority class sample. 2) The number of samples in the retinal OCT dataset is small. Using such a small number of samples to train deep learning models from scratch will lead to slow convergence or even over-fitting. 3) Although most methods paid attention to the key lesion areas for classification, they still easy to ignore lesions with small areas and fuzzy shapes.

To address these issues, in this paper, we proposed an improved EfficientNet [12] model for retinal OCT image classification, referred to as Transfer Learning and Re-Attention based EfficientNet model (TL-RA-EfficientNet). Its contribution can be concluded as the following three aspects. 1) To solve the class-imbalance problem, we design a data augmentation method to generate new samples by flipping original samples horizontally and vertically, so that the number of samples in each class became the same. 2) We introduce a transfer learning module based on a fully open training strategy, which can utilize image prior knowledge from other large image datasets to accelerate the convergence of the model. 3) We propose a Re-Attention (RA) module to select important channels from the feature map again to further identify the lesions with small areas and fuzzy shapes.

The rest of the paper is structured as follows: Sect. 2 describes the detail of the proposed method. Experimental results are conducted in Sect. 3. Section 4 concludes the whole paper and points out future work.

2 TL-RA-EfficientNet Model

In this section, we introduce the proposed model TL-RA-EfficientNet, and the overall framework is depicted in Fig. 1. First, we preprocess the dataset with denoising and data augmentation. Second, we introduce a transfer learning module to provide initial weights for the basic EfficientNet model to accelerate the convergence of it. Third, we add the RA module in the EfficientNet model to make the model pay more attention to the key lesion regions with small areas and fuzzy shapes. More details are as follows.

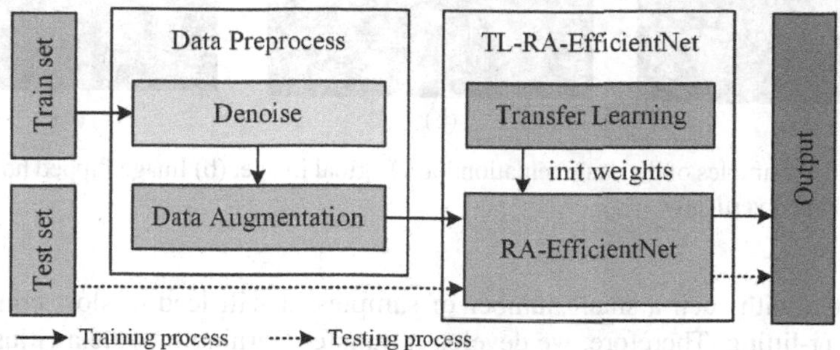

Fig. 1. The overall framework of the proposed TL-RA-EfficientNet model

2.1 Data Preprocess

Denoise. Considering that the assessment of OCT eye disease is connected to the changes in retinal membrane layer form, thickness and contents, the denoising algorithm should maintain the edge and local features of the retina. Therefore, in this paper, the Anisotropic Diffusion method [13] is used to reduce noise from original OCT images, which can be formulated as follows.

$$I_{t+1} = I_t + \lambda(cN_{x,y}\nabla_N(I_t) + cS_{x,y}\nabla_S(I_t) + cE_{x,y}\nabla_E(I_t) + cW_{x,y}\nabla_W(I_t)) \quad (1)$$

where I is the image, t is the number of iterations, λ is the control smoothing coefficient, ∇_I is the partial derivative of the pixel, $cN_{x,y}$, $cS_{x,y}$, $cE_{x,y}$, $cW_{x,y}$ are the thermal conductivity, N, S, E, W are the four directions of the southeast and northwest.

Data Augmentation. To solve the class-imbalance problem of the dataset, we propose a data augmentation strategy. We generate new samples by flipping original images horizontally and vertically. In Fig. 2, we take a DURSEN image as an example. Figure 2(a) is the original DURSEN image, while Fig. 2(b) and Fig. 2(c) are new images obtained after a horizontal and vertical flips, respectively. From them, we can observe that the location of the retinal lesion has changed after flipping, and the flipped image is a new image to the computer. Besides, we use a bilinear interpolation [14] method to convert all images into the size of 224 × 224 × 3 and normalized them.

2.2 Transfer Learning Module

Training a deep learning model usually requires a large number of samples. However, the sample number in OCT datasets is limited. If we train the deep learning model

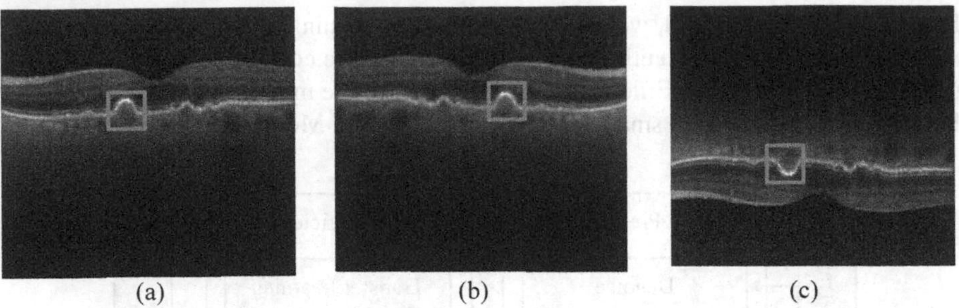

Fig. 2. Image examples of data augmentation. (a) Original image. (b) Image flipped horizontally. (c) Image flipped vertically.

from scratch with such a small number of samples, it will lead to slow convergence or even over-fitting. Therefore, we develop a transfer learning module as illustrated in Fig. 3. The main idea of it is to pre-train the model on a similar large dataset, and then transfer the trained parameters to the target dataset (OCT datasets). It enables the model to have image prior knowledge before proceeding to the target task. In this paper, by taking into consideration of the classification difficulty of the dataset and the complexity of the model, we used the lightweight EfficientNet [12], specifically EfficientNet-B0, as the base model. We pre-train the EfficientNet model on the ImageNet dataset [15], and then initialize the proposed RA-EfficientNet model with these pre-trained parameters. However, we cannot directly apply these parameters to OCT datasets, because there are significant differences between the ImageNet dataset and OCT datasets. Thus, we introduce a fully open training strategy that fine-tunes all parameters of the RA-EfficientNet model on the train set of OCT datasets to fit the classification task.

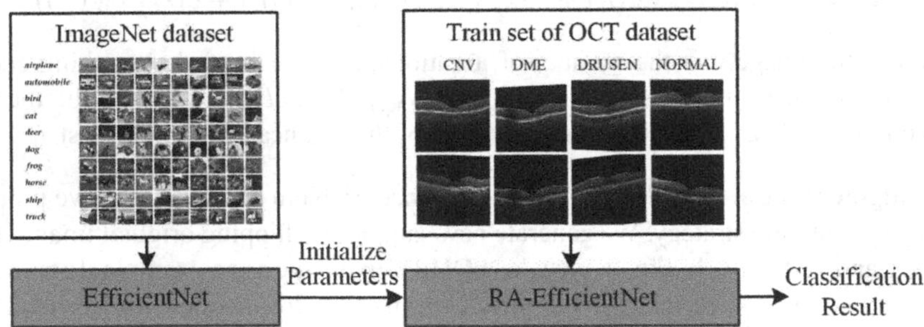

Fig. 3. The framework of the transfer learning module

2.3 RA-EfficientNet

Although there is already an attention mechanism, called Squeeze-and-Excitation module (SE) [16], in the original EfficientNet network, it fails to recognize small and blurred lesions because it will lose channel information with the dimension reduction. To address this issue, we add a RA module after SE to further select important channels from the feature map. It will make the lesion area clearer, even for the small and blurred lesions. The framework of the RA-EfficientNet is shown in Fig. 4.

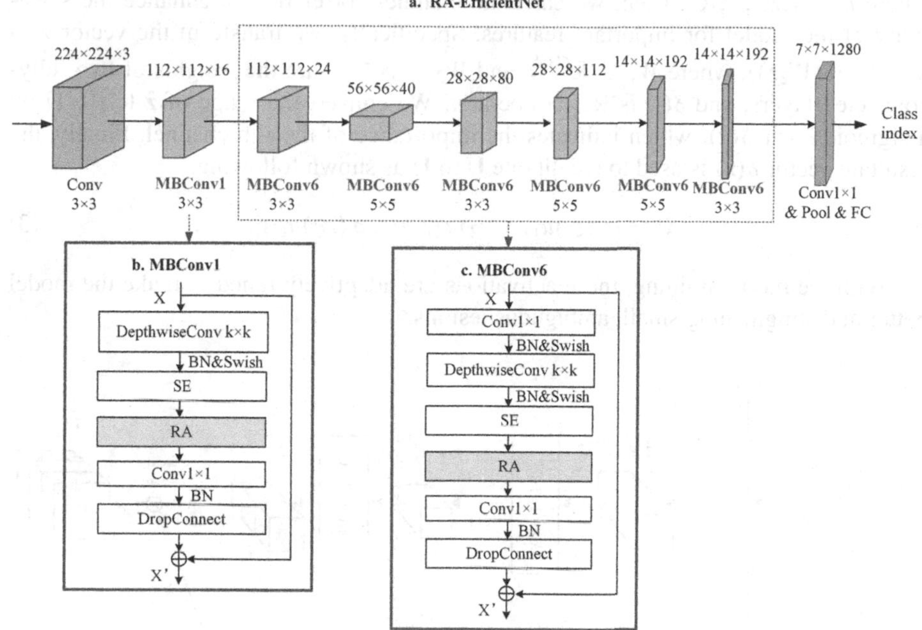

Fig. 4. The framework of the RA-EfficientNet.

In Fig. 4, the input of RA-EfficientNet is with the shape of 224 × 224 × 3. First, the image goes through a mobile inverted bottleneck convolution (MBConv1) block as shown in Fig. 4(b). The MBConv1 block mainly consists of a Depthwise Separable convolution including batch normalization (BN) and Swish, a SE module, a RA module, a 1 × 1 ordinary convolution including BN, and a Dropout layer. The SE module and the RA module will work together to select important channels from the feature map and identify lesions with small areas and ambiguous shapes. Then, it goes through 6 more MBConv6 blocks as shown in Fig. 4(c). The difference between MBConv6 and MBConv1 is that there is an additional convolution with a convolution kernel of 1 × 1. Finally, the output of the last MBConv6 convolution block is sequentially passed through a convolutional layer with 1 × 1 kernel, a global average pooling layer, and a fully connected layer. After that, we obtain the final eye disease category of each sample.

Next, we show the detail of the proposed RA module. As shown in Fig. 5, the input feature map of RA module is denoted as $\mathbf{U} = [u_1, u_2, \cdots, u_C] \in \mathbb{R}^{H \times W \times C}$, where H, W, C are the height, width and channel number of it. First, we use a global average pooling to embed the global spatial information into a vector $\mathbf{z} \in \mathbb{R}^{1 \times 1 \times C}$, which is used to capture the strongest features for each channel. It can be calculated as follows.

$$z_k = \frac{1}{H \times W} \sum_i^H \sum_j^W u_k(i,j) \tag{2}$$

where $k = 1,2, \ldots, C$. Then, we calculate channel correlation to enhance the sensitivity of the model for important features. Specifically, we transform the vector $\mathbf{z}$ to $\hat{\mathbf{z}} = W_1(\delta(W_2 z))$, where $W_1 \in \mathbb{R}^{C \times \frac{C}{2}}$ and $W_2 \in \mathbb{R}^{\frac{C}{2} \times C}$ are the weights of two fully-connected layers, and $\delta(\cdot)$ is ReLU operator. We convert the range of $\hat{\mathbf{z}}$ to [0, 1] by a sigmoid layer $\delta(\hat{\mathbf{z}})$, which indicates the importance of the i-th channel. Finally, the resultant vector $\delta(\hat{\mathbf{z}})$ is used to recalibrate $\mathbf{U}$ to $\hat{\mathbf{U}}$ as shown following.

$$\hat{\mathbf{U}} = [\sigma(\hat{z}_1)u_1, \sigma(\hat{z}_2)u_2, \cdots, \sigma(\hat{z}_C)u_C] \tag{3}$$

With the model training, these activations are adaptively tuned to make the model better at distinguishing small, ambiguous lesions.

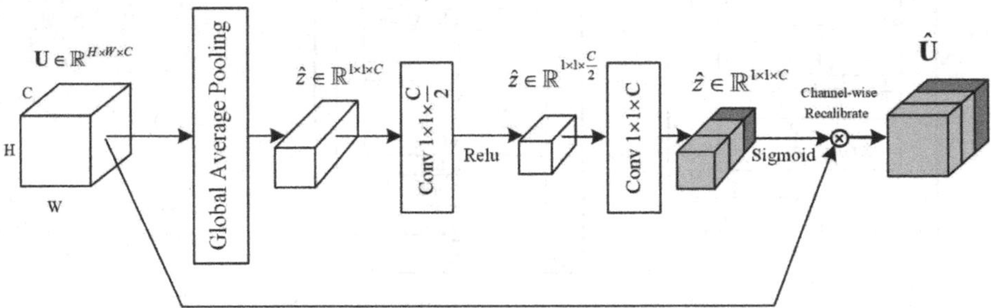

Fig. 5. The framework of the Re-Attention Module

3 Results and Analysis

3.1 Experimental Settings

Dataset. We evaluate the performance of methods on a public dataset provided by the Shiley Eye Institute of the University of California San Diego (UCSD) [17], which contains 84484 OCT B-scans from 4686 patients. It includes three eye disease categories (CNV, DME, DRUSEN) and one NORMAL category. We use the Anisotropic Diffusion method to denoise the image. We apply the data augmentation method as described in Sect. 2.1 to expand the sample number of DME and DRUSEN to 22696. Then we randomly select 22696 samples in the CNV and NORMAL categories. Table 1 shows the sample number before and after data augmentation. We further divide the train set into a training subset and validation subset in a 7:3 ratio. After that, the number of images in the training set, validation set and test set are 15887, 6808 and 250, respectively.

Table 1. Comparison of datasets before and after expansion

Class of eye diseases	UCSD dataset		Expand-UCSD dataset	
	Train set	Test set	Train set	Test set
CNV	37205	250	22696	250
DME	11348	250	22696	250
DRUSEN	8616	250	22696	250
NORMAL	26315	250	22696	250

Experimental Environment and Parameter Settings. The proposed TL-RA-EfficientNet method is implemented using the PyTorch framework with NVIDIA Cuda v10.0 and cuDNN v7.6.5 accelerated library. All experiments are performed under Linux operating system on a machine with GPU NVIDIA GeForce 1080 Ti and 16 GB of RAM.

For training the TL-RA-EfficientNet model, we optimize the network using an SGDM optimizer with a momentum of 0.9, a batch of 64 images per step and an initial learning rate of 0.01. At each iteration, the loss of the model was recorded, and the performance of the model was assessed using the validation subset. During the training process, parameters are adjusted according to the variation trend of the validation subset accuracy and loss function until the model converges. The maximum number of iterations is set as 500 epochs.

3.2 Performance Evaluation

In this section, we investigate the performance of the proposed method and compare it with other four OCT image classification methods, including LACNN [10], PCAM [11], DenseNet201+ANN [18] and GM-OCTnet [19]. To be fair, we compare them on the unmodified UCSD test set. Table 2 shows the experimental results of them. From it, we can observe that our proposed method is superior to other methods in terms of accuracy, sensitivity, specificity and precision. Compared with LACNN, PCAM, GM-OCTnet (g = 4) models, our model exceeds them in terms of accuracy by 9.8%, 4.6% and 3.7%, respectively. Besides, we can draw similar conclusions in terms of sensitivity, specificity and precision. Although all of these models use an attention mechanism, our model performs better than them. It is because our model implements the re-attention mechanism, which not only enables the model to find obvious lesion areas, but also identifies lesions with small areas and blurred shapes. Compared with PCAM and DenceNet201+ANN models with transfer learning module, our model achieves better classification performance. The reason for it may be that our model uses a fully open training strategy to fine-tune all parameters, which is more beneficial to transferring prior knowledge from different but related datasets to the target dataset.

Table 2. Performance of different methods on the UCSD dataset

Model	Accuracy	Sensitivity	Specificity	Precision
LACNN [10]	0.901	0.868	-	0.862
PCAM [11]	0.953	0.9331	-	0.9303
DenseNet201+ANN [18]	0.986	-	0.995	0.986
GM-OCTnet (g = 4) [19]	0.961	-	-	-
TL-SCSE-EfficientNet	0.993	0.993	0.9977	0.9932
TL-MS-CAM-EfficientNet	0.998	0.998	0.998	0.998
TL-RA-EfficientNet (Ours)	**0.999**	**0.999**	**0.999**	**0.9997**

To show the effect of our proposed RA module, we compare it with other existing attention modules, such as SCSE [20] and MS-CAM [21]. We replace the RA module of the TL-RA-EfficientNet with SCSE and MS-CAM and then obtain TL-SCSE-EfficientNet and TL-MS-CAM-EfficientNet models, respectively. Their OCT classification results as shown in Table 2. We find that RA achieves the best performance among these models in terms of accuracy, sensitivity, specificity and precision. The reason may be that the lesion area is only a small part of the overall OCT image. SCSE combine channel and space attention mechanism to focus on the key lesion area. However, as the network deepening, it will make the lesion area smaller and lose more detail about the lesion area. And the complex calculation of the global and local relationship of the channel by MS-CAM will make some information redundancy to affect the model judgment. Therefore, the performance of their models is inferior to ours.

3.3 Effect of Data Augmentation

To verify the effect of the data augmentation method, we compare the performance of EfficientNet on the original and preprocessed UCSD dataset. The results are shown in Fig. 6. We find that the model outperforms better on the preprocessed dataset than that on the original dataset, which increases by 0.7%, 0.7% and 0.6% in terms of accuracy, sensitivity and specificity, respectively. It means that flipping images horizontally and vertically is useful for extending the number of samples, and making different categories balanced can improve the performance of the model.

3.4 Effect of Transfer Learning and Re-attention Modules

To understand the effect of the transfer learning module and RA module in the TL-RA-EfficientNet, we remove one of them at a time and evaluate the performance of the ablated model. The TL-RA-EfficientNet is the full model, the TL-EfficientNet ablates the RA module, and the EfficientNet takes out of both transfer learning and RA modules. The above three experiments are all trained on the preprocessed UCSD dataset. The results of these three models are shown in Table 3. It shows that the TL-RA-EfficientNet model achieves the best performance in terms of accuracy, sensitivity and specificity with all

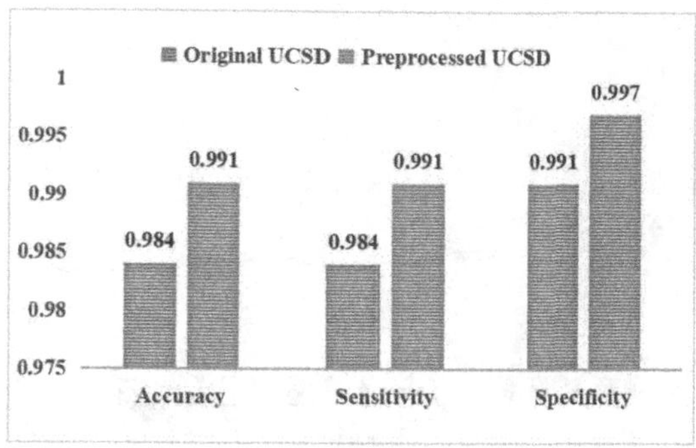

Fig. 6. The results of EfficientNet on the original and preprocessed UCSD dataset.

99.9%, and it takes the least time to train and test. Compared with the TL-EfficientNet, the TL-RA-EfficientNet model improves classification accuracy, sensitivity and specificity by 0.4%, 0.4% and 0.17%, respectively. It indicates that the RA module strengthens the learning ability of the model for important retinal feature maps. Compared performance between the EfficientNet and the TL-EfficientNet, we can observe that the latter model performs better. The training time of the TL-EfficientNet is 16 h shorter than that of the EfficientNet, which means that the transfer learning module enables the model to have some learning ability before the OCT classification, and speeds up the model training.

Table 3. Experimental results of the three models.

Model	Accuracy (%)	Sensitivity (%)	Specificity (%)	Training time (Hour)	Testing time (Second)
EfficientNet	99.1	99.1	99.7	45	11
TL-EfficientNet	99.5	99.5	99.82	29	10
TL-RA-EfficientNet	**99.9**	**99.9**	**99.9**	**25**	**10**

In addition, Fig. 7 shows the cross-entropy loss function curves of the three models. We observe that the green and blue curves decrease faster than the red curve. The reason may be that the transfer learning module makes the model no longer train from scratch, but fine-tune based on the existing parameters, which benefits the model to accelerate the convergence.

To intuitively demonstrate the recognition performance of three models for each eye disease class, Fig. 8 shows their confusion matrices, where the values on the diagonal represent the true positive examples in each class. Taking DME recognition as an example, the EefficientNet model correctly identifies 244 samples as DME, but it wrongly classifies 6 samples as CNV. The TL-EfficientNet model accurately identifies 248 samples and wrongly identifies 2 samples. The TL-RA-EfficientNet can accurately identify all samples. Similar conclusions can be obtained from DURSEN eye disease classes. It indicates that the TL-RA-EfficientNet model effectively improves the recognition rate

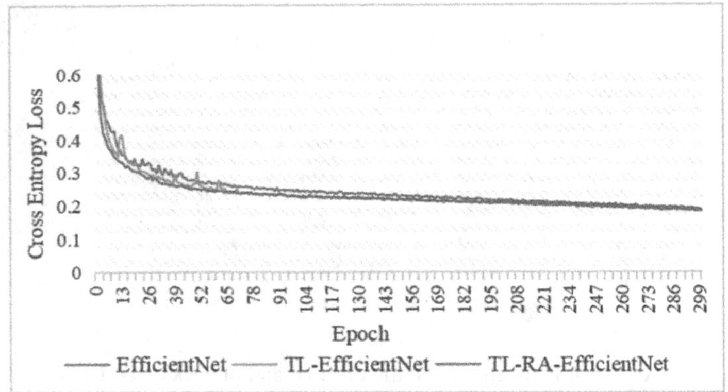

Fig. 7. Cross Entropy Loss curves of the three models.

of DME and DURSEN eye disease. This is mainly due to the contribution of the RA module, which makes small and blurred lesions areas clearer and easier to identify.

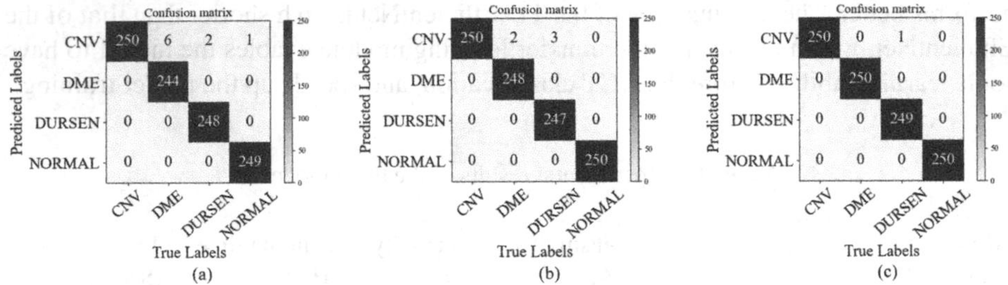

Fig. 8. Confusion matrix of the three models. (a) EfficientNet. (b) TL-EfficientNet. (c) TL-RA-EfficientNet.

4 Conclusions

In this paper, we proposed a TL-RA-EfficientNet model to address the problems of class imbalance and insufficient attention to key lesion areas in retinal OCT image classification tasks. The experimental results show that the data augmentation effectively balances the number of samples from different classes and improves the data quality. The transfer learning module in our model makes full use of the prior knowledge of a large image library, which effectively speeds up the convergence of the model. The RA module enables the model to focus on small and blurred lesions areas and strengthens the learning of important retinal feature maps, thereby further improving the classification accuracy of the model. Therefore, our proposed OCT image classification model with joint transfer learning and attention mechanism is an efficient, reasonable and high-performance algorithm. In future work, we will propose cross-subject OCT image models to meet the clinical requirements of eye disease recognition.

References

1. Kokame, G.T., Omizo, J.N., Kokame, K.A., Yamane, M.L.: Differentiating exudative macular degeneration and polypoidal choroidal vasculopathy using OCT B-scan. Ophthalmol. Retina **5**(10), 954–961 (2021)
2. Goh, J.K.H., Cheung, C.Y., Sim, S.S., Tan, P.C., Tan, G.S.W., Wong, T.Y.: Retinal imaging techniques for diabetic retinopathy screening. J. Diabetes Sci. Technol. **10**(2), 282–294 (2016)
3. Adhi, M., Duker, J.S.: Optical coherence tomography – current and future applications. Curr. Opin. Ophthalmol. **24**(3), 213–221 (2013)
4. Wang, Y., et al.: A DNN for arrhythmia prediction based on ECG. In: Huang, Z., Siuly, S., Wang, H., Zhou, R., Zhang, Y. (eds.) HIS 2020. LNCS, vol. 12435, pp. 146–153. Springer, Cham (2020). https://doi.org/10.1007/978-3-030-61951-0_14
5. Qi, Y., Lin, S., Huang, Z.: Classification of skin pigmented lesions based on deep residual network. In: Wang, H., Siuly, S., Zhou, R., Martin-Sanchez, F., Zhang, Y., Huang, Z. (eds.) HIS 2019. LNCS, vol. 11837, pp. 58–67. Springer, Cham (2019). https://doi.org/10.1007/978-3-030-32962-4_6
6. Puneet, Kumar, R., Gupta, M.: Optical coherence tomography image based eye disease detection using deep convolutional neural network. Health Inf. Sci. Syst. **10**, 13 (2022)
7. Zhang, X., et al.: Mixed pyramid attention network for nuclear cataract classification based on anterior segment OCT images. Health Inf. Sci. Syst. **10**(1), 1–12 (2022). https://doi.org/10.1007/s13755-022-00170-2
8. Awais, M., Müller, H., Tang, T.B., Meriaudeau, F.: Classification of SD-OCT images using a Deep learning approach. In: 2017 IEEE International Conference on Signal and Image Processing Applications (ICSIPA), Kuching, Malaysia, pp. 489–492. IEEE (2017)
9. Bhowmik, A., Kumar, S., Bhat, N.: Eye disease prediction from optical coherence tomography images with transfer learning. In: Macintyre, J., Iliadis, L., Maglogiannis, I., Jayne, C. (eds.) EANN 2019. CCIS, vol. 1000, pp. 104–114. Springer, Cham (2019). https://doi.org/10.1007/978-3-030-20257-6_9
10. Fang, L., Wang, C., Li, S., Rabbani, H., Chen, X., Liu, Z.: Attention to lesion: lesion-aware convolutional neural network for retinal optical coherence tomography image classification. IEEE Trans. Med. Imaging **38**(8), 1959–1970 (2019)
11. Mishra, S.S., Mandal, B., Puhan, N.: Perturbed composite attention model for macular optical coherence tomography image classification. IEEE Trans. AI **3**, 625–635 (2021)
12. Tan, M., Le, Q.V.: EfficientNet: rethinking model scaling for convolutional neural networks. In: 36th International Conference on Machine Learning, Los Angeles, pp. 6105–6114 (2019)
13. Perona, P., Malik, J.: Scale-space and edge detection using anisotropic diffusion. IEEE Trans. Pattern Anal. Mach. Intell. **12**(7), 629–639 (1990)
14. Tezduyar, T.E., Mittal, S., Ray, S.E., Shih, R.: Incompressible flow computations with stabilized bilinear and linear equal-order-interpolation velocity-pressure elements. Comput. Methods Appl. Mech. Eng. **95**(2), 221–242 (1992)
15. Deng, J., Dong, W., Socher, R., Li, L.-J., Li, K., Fei-Fei, L.: ImageNet: a large-scale hierarchical image database. In: 2009 IEEE Conference on Computer Vision and Pattern Recognition, pp. 248–255 (2009)
16. Hu, J., Shen, L., Sun, G.: Squeeze-and-excitation networks. In: 2018 IEEE/CVF Conference on Computer Vision and Pattern Recognition, pp. 7132–7141 (2018)
17. Kermany, D.S., et al.: Identifying medical diagnoses and treatable diseases by image-based deep learning. Cell **172**(5), 1122–1131 (2018)
18. Islam, K.T., Wijewickrema, S., O'Leary, S.: Identifying diabetic retinopathy from OCT images using deep transfer learning with artificial neural networks. In: 2019 IEEE 32nd International Symposium on Computer-Based Medical Systems (CBMS), pp. 281–286 (2019)

19. Chen, S., Chen, M., Ma, W.: Research on automatic classification of optical coherence tomography retina image based on multi-channel. Chin. J. Lasers **48**(23), 109–118 (2021)
20. Roy, A.G., Navab, N., Wachinger, C.: Recalibrating fully convolutional networks with spatial and channel "Squeeze and Excitation." IEEE Trans. Med. Imaging **38**(2), 540–549 (2019)
21. Dai, Y., Gieseke, F., Oehmcke, S., Wu, Y., Barnard, K.: Attentional feature fusion. In: Proceedings of the IEEE/CVF Winter Conference on Applications of Computer Vision (WACV), pp. 3560–3569 (2021)

Intelligent Interpretation and Classification of Multivariate Medical Time Series Based on Convolutional Neural Networks

Tianbo Xu[1], Le Sun[2](✉), Sudha Subramani[3], and Yilin Wang[4]

[1] Engineering Research Center of Digital Forensics, Ministry of Education, Nanjing University of Information Science and Technology, Nanjing, China

[2] Department of Jiangsu Collaborative Innovation Center of Atmospheric Environment and Equipment Technology (CICAEET), Nanjing University of Information Science and Technology, Nanjing 210044, China

LeSun1@nuist.edu.cn

[3] Victoria University, Footscray, Australia

[4] Soochow University, Suzhou, China

Abstract. Physiological signals are bioelectrical signals generated by human organ interactions. These signals can timely reflect the real health status of the human body. With great success in various tasks, there are high expectations for deep learning networks to improve clinical practice. In this paper, we develop a deep neural network to automatically classify arrhythmias recorded by 12-lead electrocardiogram (ECG). And several experiments were conducted on a 12-lead ECG dataset to prove the effectiveness of the method. The mean F1 score of the model is 83.1%, which is 13% higher than the conventional VGG-60. Finally, we interpret the behavior of the model at the patient levels with the SHapley Additive exPlanations (SHAP) method to increase the interpretability of the model.

Keywords: Deep neural network · Classification of arrhythmia · 12-lead electrocardiogram · Model interpretability

1 Introducion

Worldwide, cardiovascular disease (CVD) has become the largest killer of deaths [32]. Statistics show that sudden cardiac death accounts for more than half of all cardiac deaths [18], over 80% of these deaths are associated with cardiac arrhythmias [41]. ECG is a widely used and highly reliable method for diagnosing cardiovascular disease [25,26]. The ECGs automatic monitoring of arrhythmias is of great significance for the early warning and diagnosis of cardiovascular diseases [9]. Currently, ECG is the most widely used method for detecting arrhythmias [3]. A standard ECG has 12 leads, including 6 limb leads

A. Traina et al. (Eds.): HIS 2022, LNCS 13705, pp. 291–302, 2022.
https://doi.org/10.1007/978-3-031-20627-6_27

and 6 chest leads [35] recorded by body surface electrodes. ECG-based automated arrhythmia detection provides important assistance to doctors and provides real-time access to physical health status for patients [20]. Therefore, an automated arrhythmia detection system with high accuracy is of wide commercial value [38].

The current research aspects for heartbeats, the first is based on classic feature extraction methods from machine learning, while the second is based on advanced deep learning approaches [12]. Traditional machine learning methods for heartbeat research rely heavily on manual feature extraction [7,28]. ECG heart rate arrhythmia classification using deep learning algorithms has the following advantages: (1) less preprocessing is required for the signal [37]; (2) features can be extracted automatically [33]. Using the layer-by-layer non-linear representation of deep networks can obtain deep-level features in ECG data [21]. The combination of deep learning and automatic ECG heart rate arrhythmia classification is of great research significance for the clinical prevention of heart disease [10]. Therefore, it can improve the accuracy of ECG heart rate arrhythmia automatic classification algorithms [22,29].

The above work demonstrates many applications of deep learning network architectures widely used in the automatic classification of electrocardiograms. However, there are relatively few studies on deep learning models for physiological signals. The following points should be taken into consideration: (1) ECG signals are periodic [32], and both local and overall characteristics are helpful for the detection of arrhythmias; (2) ECG signal processing is processing time series data [31]; (3) In the design of the model, we should consider the influence of feature extraction on the final model prediction [3].

In this paper, we propose a classification and intelligent interpretation model for ECG data, named H-RESNET. In the meantime, H-RESNET aims to solve the following problems: (1) improve the accuracy of the convolutional deep learning network model in processing ECG data; (2) optimization of the extraction of data features; (3) enhance the interpretability of the model to make people understand the impact of each input of the model on the final output more clearly.

The remainder of the paper is organized as follows: Sect. 2 discusses related work, Sect. 3 describes the H-RESNET system, Sect. 4 discusses the experiments, and Sect. 5 concludes and suggests future research directions.

2 Related Work

Automatic detection of ECG arrhythmias has been extensively studied over the past few years. With the rapid development of machine learning, specific to the characteristics of ECG data, researchers have done a lot of research on ECG according to its characteristics. Sarvan and Özkurt [27] proposed 1-D CNN to conduct QRS detection of arrhythmia in the MIT-BIH (Massachusetts Institute of Technology, Beth Israel Hospital) database. SS and Auxillia [2] proposed a CNN by feature extraction and ECG classification in each CNN unit, and ECG classification can be carried out in a relatively short time. Natesan et al. [16] proposed a deep convolutional network model with data augmentation to increase the accuracy of predicting myocardial infarction. Ma and Liang [15] designed a CNN for 12-lead variable-length ECG signal classification and applied three defense methods to improve the robustness of the CNN for this classification task. Kharshid et al. [6] used a method to classify short-duration single-lead ECG recordings of different sizes. Rai et al. [23] used CNN-LSTM to classify a large amount of medical data, and good results were obtained. Liu et al. [13] proposed a classifier that combines the residual convolutional network (CNN) with the hierarchical attention mechanism. In order to solve the problem of data imbalance between classes, used a new weighted focus loss in model training. Yang et al. [40] proposed an end-to-end deep residual neural network with one dimensional convolution is presented to identify the 12-lead ECGs. Identification of 12-lead electrocardiograms with different durations and sampling frequencies. Tiryaki et al. [36] CNN to classify ECG signals as normal or ST-segment depression episodes with an accuracy of over 92%.

Researchers have also made some progress in deep learning models when ECG data is used for deep model training. Özaltın and Yeniay [17] proposed Net-SVM to converted the ECG signal to two-dimensional image, and the ECG signal is automatically extracted and classifiable. Xiaolin et al. [39] used low-power CNN for edge computing and proposed a new multi-level pruning technique that reduces the complexity of CNN models with negligible performance loss compared to existing pruning techniques. Jiang et al. [11] developed a new end-to-end multi-label heart disease detection framework in which deep CNN models and bidirectional gated recurrence units (GRUs) are combined for learning high-level feature representation of ECG, and a GCN is employed to embed our label graph into inter-dependent cardiac disease classifier. Pardasani and Awasthi [19] designed a parallel CNN with the same architecture in each CNN, including the convolutional layer, batch normalization, activation layer, and dense layer with regularization and exit added. Sun et al. [30] used two stacked bi-directional long and short-term memory networks (Bi-LSTM) and a generative adversarial network (GAN) to create a model to classify supraventricular ectopic beats for better classification performance.

For research on ECG multi-label classification and increased model interpretability. Ran et al. [24] used a 34-layer 1D-deep squeeze-and-excitation network to capture the correlation between the characteristics of heart abnormalities and the heartbeat in the multi-label arrhythmia classification task. Sun et al. [34] proposed a new integrated multi-label classification method. The model consists of a combination of multiple multi-label classification methods, resulting in a higher performing classifier. Ganeshkumar et al. [5] proposed a interpretable CNN model and the ECG classifies the labels and trains them on just one label so that the network can learn the characteristics of multiple labels. Borra et al. [1] proposed a multi-label classification framework for cardiac arrhythmias that integrates feature selection and multi-label classification. Models are selected and analysed with a greater focus on specific features associated with each disease in order to obtain discriminatory information, and the features are highly interpretable. Ferretti et al. [4] used 1-D CNN to explain the behavior of neural networks to increase the interpretability of the model.

3 Methods

3.1 System Overview

The automatic detection of ECG arrhythmias boils down to the classification of a time series of data. This requires an experimental model to correlate ECG data $X = [x_1, \ldots, x_k]$ from a time series to extract the feature. The objective of our proposed model is to minimize the cross-entropy between the reference label and the output, as shown in Formula 1:

$$loss_{cross}(x, c) = -\frac{1}{N}\sum_{x=0}^{X-1}\frac{1}{c}\sum_{c=0}^{C-1} y_{x,c}log(p_{x,c}) + (1 - y_{x,c})log(1 - p_{x,c}) \quad (1)$$

where, $p_{x,c}$ represents the probability of output label C with respect to x, and $y_{x,c}$ represents the value of output label c with respect to x as 1 or 0, and N represents the number of ECG data. The depth learning model is sensitive to input data because the parameter value cannot be controlled in the feature extraction of the data stream. This can result in the final output of different categories being arbitrary and uncontrollable, and makes the values of different categories non-comparable. Features with high values of the input data may be highlighted by the classification headings, and their associated parameters may have very high values.

For multiclassification, each class can be identifiably by considering it as a whole, without the need to discriminate with the help of any information from other courses. This is achieved through a class loss in (Huet al. 2020) [8], which has a new regularisation called H-reg (holistic regularisation).

Formula 2 shows the H-reg algorithm.

$$H - reg = x \sim \mathbb{P}_x^{\mathbb{E}}||\nabla_x f(x)||_2^n \quad (2)$$

where, $\nabla_x f(x)$ represents the importance of each eigenvalue. $\mathbb{E}$ represents the mathematical expectation of two normal forms. The features that also have high input data values may be identified by the classifier as having a greater impact on the final output, and their associated parameter values may therefore have higher parameter values. However, those features with high values may not be important for the final output in terms of identifying the correct input instances, which may reduce the final model output. Therefore, we use the H-reg method to address the above issues, which can improve the accuracy of our model. Formula 2 represents the penalty of the L-2 norm for high eigenvalues and a small penalty for low eigenvalues.

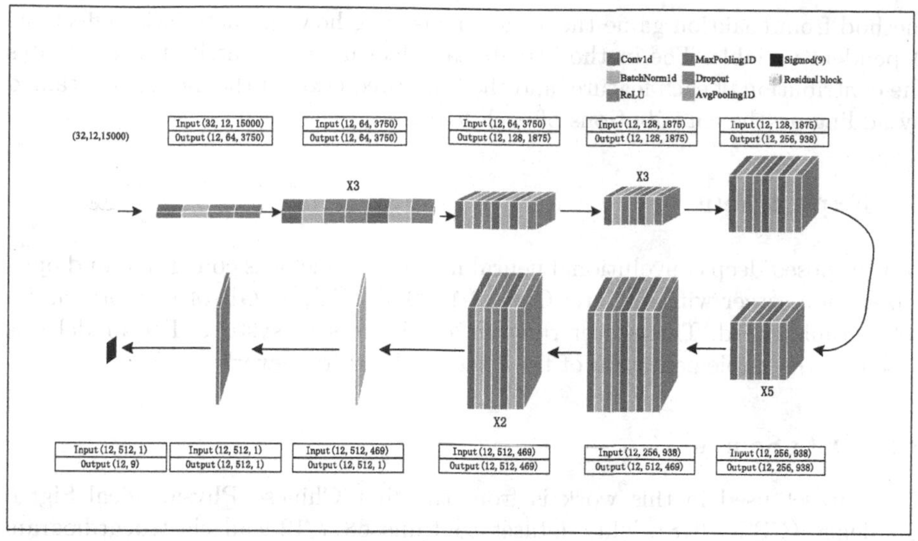

Fig. 1. H-RESNET model framework.

3.2 Proposed H-RESNET Model

The model proposed in this paper is shown in Fig. 1. The model consists of a convolutional neural network. The design of the proposed convolutional neural network is better than the Resnet34 model. The ECG signal is first extracted by Conv1d, BatchNorm1d, ReLU, and Pooling features. The depth features are then extracted using the four superimposed residuals block. In each residual block that follows the model, Conv1d layers, BatchNorm1d layers, Dropout layers and ReLU activation layers are used. The Conv1d layer is used for automatic feature extraction, the BatchNorm1d layer improves training speed and increases classification, the ReLU layer performs non-linear activation to solve the problem of gradient saturation and gradient disappearance, and the Dropout layer reduces overfitting. The trained data is then put through an average pooling layer and a maximum pooling layer, which are used to pull out features. The results of the pooling layer are sent to the output layer, and the Sigmoid activation function is used for classification prediction. After the processing flow in the figure above, the ECG data stream is automatically classified into nine classes after processing by the deep learning model.

3.3 The Interpretability of the Proposed Classification Model

The interpretability of deep convolutional neural network models has been a vexing problem in practical applications. To achieve better performance of deep convolutional models in the diagnosis of cardiac arrhythmias, we have used the SHAP (Lundberg et al. 2017) [14] approach to increase the interpretable predictions of the models. SHAP is a calculation based on Shapley value, an important method from coalition game theory for measuring how characteristics affect the dependent variable. The method treats each feature as a contributor, calculates the contribution of each feature, and the final prediction of the model is obtained by adding up the contributions of each feature.

4 Experiment

Our proposed deep convolutional neural network model was configured and optimized on a server with an Intel Core i9-11900k CPU, 64 GB of memory, and a 3090 graphic card. This server runs on a Windows 10 system. The model was based on the implementation of the Pytorch 1.2.0 framework.

4.1 Data Source

The dataset used in this work is from the first Chinese Physiological Signal Challenge (CPSC2018). This dataset contains 6877 12-lead electrocardiogram recordings. The 12-lead ECGs used in CPSC 2018 include one normal type and eight abnormal types, which are detailed as: (1) Atrial fibrillation (AF) (2) First-degree atrioventricular block (I-AVB) (3) Left bundle brunch block (LBBB) (4) Right bundle brunch block (RBBB) (5) Premature atrial contraction (PAC) (6) Premature ventricular contraction (PVC) (7) ST-segment depression (STD) (8) ST-segment elevated (STE). The records were sampled 500 Hz.

4.2 Pre-processing

ECG signals are susceptible to noise such as baseline drift, inotropic noise, and industrial frequency interference due to their high noise background. Our model uses the wavelet transform for denoising. The flow chart of the wavelet transform is shown in Fig. 2.

As shown in the figure, the raw signal is first preprocessed and then decomposed into 10 scales. Each scale includes low-frequency signals and high-frequency signals. The low-frequency signal is characterized by a low frequency and is relatively stable. Only the wavelet coefficients of the high-frequency signal of each scale need to be processed by the threshold method to eliminate the noise signal with high frequency and low amplitude. Through the inverse wavelet transform, a signal that has been cleaned up and reconstructed is made that is close to the real signal.

4.3 Training Setting

We used the Resnet34 model, which has a very deep model while solving the problem of gradient disappearance or gradient explosion. We chose the Adam optimizer to optimize the whole model. The initial parameters are set to the default parameters and the learning rate is set to 0.0001. The learning rate was

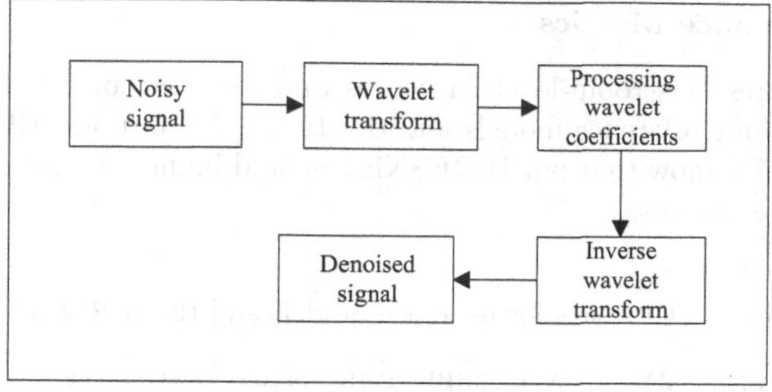

Fig. 2. Wavelet denoising process.

multiplied by a factor of 0.1 for every 10 epochs out of a total of 120 epochs. The loss function uses Formula 1 and Formula 2 as shown in Formula 3.

$$Loss_{(x,c)} = loss_{cross}(x, c) + \lambda \cdot H - reg \tag{3}$$

Dropout is used as a very widely used regularisation method because it is effective in reducing overfitting due to the high number of layers in the model, which helps the model to improve its training accuracy. In this experiment, we used $\lambda = 0.1$ in Formula 3.

4.4 Performance Metrics

We have used typical classifiable metrics for each category in this study, including accuracy, recall and F1 scores. The formula for calculating the accuracy is shown in Formula 4.

$$PRE = \frac{TP}{TP + FP} \tag{4}$$

The calculation formula of recall rate is shown in Formula 5.

$$REC = \frac{TP}{TP + FN} \tag{5}$$

In Formula 4 and Formula 5, TP (True Positive) represents the actual sample of A, and the prediction is also the number of samples of A. FP (False Positive) indicates the number of samples predicted as A samples from other samples. FN (False Negative) indicates that sample A is predicted as the number of samples of other samples. Both accuracy and recall rate are considered comprehensively since F1 scores are the harmonic mean of accuracy and recall rate. Therefore, F1 scores are more convincing than other evaluation criteria. The calculation formula for F1 scores is shown in Formula 6.

$$F1 = \frac{2 * PRE * REC}{PRE + REC} \tag{6}$$

4.5 Performance Metrics

Table 1 compares classroom-level F1 scores and mean accuracy, recall, and F1 scores for the four reference models and the H-RESNET in identifying arrhythmias. The results show that our H-RESNET scored higher than the others in F1 in almost all categories.

Table 1. F1 scores for reference models and the H-RESNET.

Model	SNR	AF	I-AVB	LBBB	RBBB	PAC	PVC	STD	STE	Avg F1
Bi-LSTM	0.739	0.768	0.742	0.706	0.822	0.591	0.807	0.658	0.294	0.742
VGG-60	743	0.889	0.776	0.841	0.910	0.468	0.780	0.721	0.484	0.735
TI-CNN	0.753	0.900	0.809	0.874	0.922	0.638	0.832	0.762	0.462	0.772
Without-hreg	0.791	**0.925**	0.847	**0.920**	0.927	0.752	0.818	0.838	0.524	0.816
Our	**0.824**	0.900	**0.876**	0.772	**0.951**	**0.803**	**0.865**	**0.824**	**0.667**	**0.831**

4.6 Representation of Model Interpretability

The interpretability of deep convolutional neural network models has been a vexing problem in practical applications. With the proposed deep convolutional model in performing diagnostic classification of arrhythmias, we have increased the interpretability of the model through the SHAP method. On the basis of the machine learning model with higher discrimination accuracy, the distribution of feature importance of the SHAP interpretation method has good local and global interpretability, and SHAP interpretation basically contains the information provided by logistic regression. This research method has both discrimination accuracy and index interpretation ability.

Because the SHAP method was directly summed, we calculated the contribution of each of the 12 ECG leads to the final diagnostic category of the model and applied this to a deep learning model to increase the interpretability of the model, as shown in Fig. 3. The criteria for diagnosing AF by ECG are that the three criteria of P-wave disappearance, baseline disappearance, and absolute inequality of the simultaneous RR interval are met simultaneously, most clearly in leads V4 and V5. Separately, the signature features of the RBBB and LBBB are the RSR complex wave in V1 and the deep s-wave in V1. Our model for lead importance in RBBB and LBBB is the same as the standard ECG interpretation for the final identification. From our model plots, it can be seen that for PAC, PVC, lead V1 and II have the highest contribution to the final impact. STD and STE are generally present in acute coronary syndromes, where the cardiac portion of the syndrome often exhibits poor oxygenation. From an average point of view, leads V1 and V2 were the most important leads out of 12 leads. We also observed a low contribution of some leads (III, aVL), such a clinical presentation may be due to the influence of characteristic interactions between ECG leads.

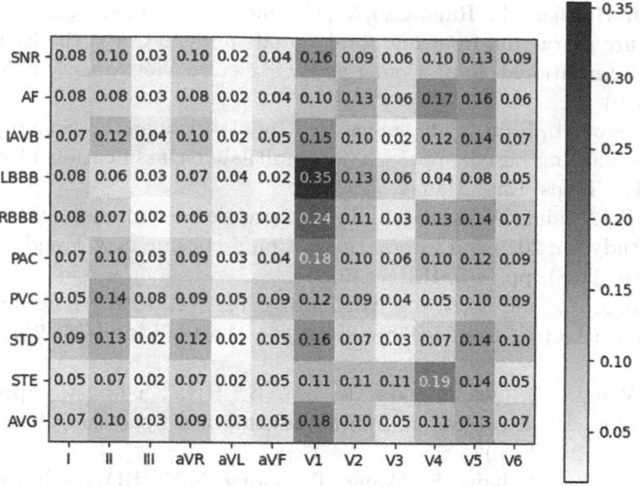

Fig. 3. Contribution of the 12-lead to the model output prediction after training by H-RESNET.

5 Conclusion

We propose a novel framework called H-RESNET for 12-lead electrocardiography data classification. The proposed H-RESNET framework uses H-reg method to optimize the extracted features and train the extracted data based on the advantages of the Resnet34 deep learning model. We used this new framework, H-RESNET, to classify nine arrhythmias with a mean F1 score of 0.831, 13% higher than the reference CNN model. The SHAP approach was used to improve the interpretability of the model. H-RESNET performs well in solving the multi-classification problem of 12-lead ECG signals. It provides an example for other signal processing problems in time series. In the future, we hope to conduct more tests on other datasets, especially experiments to improve the performance of our H-RESNET.

References

1. Agrawal, A., Chauhan, A., Shetty, M.K., Gupta, M.D., Gupta, A., et al.: ECG-iCOVIDNet: interpretable AI model to identify changes in the ECG signals of post-covid subjects. Comput. Biol. Med. **146**, 105540 (2022)
2. Dhakshaya, S., Auxillia, D.J.: Classification of ECG using convolutional neural network (CNN). In: 2019 International Conference on Recent Advances in Energy-Efficient Computing and Communication (ICRAECC), pp. 1–6. IEEE (2019)
3. Du, J., Michalska, S., Subramani, S., Wang, H., Zhang, Y.: Neural attention with character embeddings for hay fever detection from Twitter. Health Inf. Sci. Syst. **7**(1), 1–7 (2019)

4. Ferretti, J., Barbiero, P., Randazzo, V., Cirrincione, G., Pasero, E.: Towards uncovering feature extraction from temporal signals in deep CNN: the ECG case study. In: 2020 International Joint Conference on Neural Networks (IJCNN), pp. 1–7. IEEE (2020)
5. Ganeshkumar, M., Ravi, V., Sowmya, V., Gopalakrishnan, E., Soman, K.: Explainable deep learning-based approach for multilabel classification of electrocardiogram. IEEE Trans. Eng. Manag. (2021)
6. Hamdan, S., Awaian, A., Almajali, S.: Compression techniques used in IoT: a comparitive study. In: 2019 2nd International Conference on new Trends in Computing Sciences (ICTCS), pp. 1–5. IEEE (2019)
7. He, J., Rong, J., Sun, L., Wang, H., Zhang, Y., Ma, J.: A framework for cardiac arrhythmia detection from IoT-based ECGs. World Wide Web **23**(5), 2835–2850 (2020)
8. Hu, W., Wang, M., Qin, Q., Ma, J., Liu, B.: HRN: a holistic approach to one class learning. In: Advances in Neural Information Processing Systems, vol. 33, pp. 19111–19124 (2020)
9. Huang, S., Liu, A., Zhang, S., Wang, T., Xiong, N.N.: BD-VTE: a novel baseline data based verifiable trust evaluation scheme for smart network systems. IEEE Trans. Netw. Sci. Eng. **8**(3), 2087–2105 (2020)
10. Jiang, H., Zhou, R., Zhang, L., Wang, H., Zhang, Y.: Sentence level topic models for associated topics extraction. World Wide Web **22**(6), 2545–2560 (2019)
11. Jiang, Z., Almeida, T.P., Schlindwein, F.S., Ng, G.A., Zhou, H., Li, X.: Diagnostic of multiple cardiac disorders from 12-lead ECGs using graph convolutional network based multi-label classification. In: 2020 Computing in Cardiology, pp. 1–4. IEEE (2020)
12. Lee, J., Park, J.S., Wang, K.N., Feng, B., Tennant, M., Kruger, E.: The use of telehealth during the coronavirus (Covid-19) pandemic in oral and maxillofacial surgery-a qualitative analysis. EAI Endorsed Trans. Scalable Inf. Syst. e10–e10 (2022)
13. Liu, Y., et al.: Multi-label classification of 12-lead ECGs by using residual CNN and class-wise attention. In: 2020 Computing in Cardiology, pp. 1–4. IEEE (2020)
14. Lundberg, S.M., Lee, S.I.: A unified approach to interpreting model predictions. In: Advances in Neural Information Processing Systems, vol. 30 (2017)
15. Ma, L., Liang, L.: Enhance CNN robustness against noises for classification of 12-lead ECG with variable length. In: 2020 19th IEEE International Conference on Machine Learning and Applications (ICMLA), pp. 839–846. IEEE (2020)
16. Natesan, P., Gothai, E., et al.: Classification of multi-lead ECG signals to predict myocardial infarction using CNN. In: 2020 Fourth International Conference on Computing Methodologies and Communication (ICCMC), pp. 1029–1033. IEEE (2020)
17. Özaltın, Ö., Yeniay, Ö.: ECG classification performing feature extraction automatically using a hybrid CNN-SVM algorithm. In: 2021 3rd International Congress on Human-Computer Interaction, Optimization and Robotic Applications (HORA), pp. 1–5. IEEE (2021)
18. Pandey, D., Wang, H., Yin, X., Wang, K., Zhang, Y., Shen, J.: Automatic breast lesion segmentation in phase preserved DCE-MRIs. Health Inf. Sci. Syst. **10**(1), 1–19 (2022)
19. Pardasani, R., Awasthi, N.: Classification of 12 lead ECG signal using 1D-convolutional neural network with class dependent threshold. In: 2020 Computing in Cardiology, pp. 1–4. IEEE (2020)

20. Peng, D., Sun, L., Zhou, R., Wang, Y.: Study QoS-aware fog computing for disease diagnosis and prognosis. Mob. Netw. Appl. 1–8 (2022)
21. Qu, Z., Chen, S., Wang, X.: A secure controlled quantum image steganography algorithm. Quantum Inf. Process. **19**(10), 1–25 (2020)
22. Qu, Z., Sun, H., Zheng, M.: An efficient quantum image steganography protocol based on improved EMD algorithm. Quantum Inf. Process. **20**(2), 1–29 (2021)
23. Rai, H.M., Chatterjee, K., Mukherjee, C.: Hybrid CNN-LSTM model for automatic prediction of cardiac arrhythmias from ECG big data. In: 2020 IEEE 7th Uttar Pradesh Section International Conference on Electrical, Electronics and Computer Engineering (UPCON), pp. 1–6. IEEE (2020)
24. Ran, A., Ruan, D., Zheng, Y., Liu, H.: Multi-label classification of abnormalities in 12-lead ECG using deep learning. In: 2020 Computing in Cardiology, pp. 1–4. IEEE (2020)
25. Sarki, R., Ahmed, K., Wang, H., Zhang, Y.: Automated detection of mild and multi-class diabetic eye diseases using deep learning. Health Inf. Sci. Syst. **8**(1), 1–9 (2020)
26. Sarki, R., Ahmed, K., Wang, H., Zhang, Y., Wang, K.: Convolutional neural network for multi-class classification of diabetic eye disease. EAI Endorsed Trans. Scalable Inf. Syst. e15–e15 (2022)
27. Sarvan, Ç., Özkurt, N.: ECG beat arrhythmia classification by using 1-D CNN in case of class imbalance. In: 2019 Medical Technologies Congress (TIPTEKNO), pp. 1–4. IEEE (2019)
28. Singh, R., Zhang, Y., Wang, H., Miao, Y., Ahmed, K.: Investigation of social behaviour patterns using location-based data-a Melbourne case study. EAI Endorsed Trans. Scalable Inf. Syst. **8**(31), e2 (2020)
29. Siuly, S., et al.: A new framework for automatic detection of patients with mild cognitive impairment using resting-state EEG signals. IEEE Trans. Neural Syst. Rehabil. Eng. **28**(9), 1966–1976 (2020)
30. Sun, L., Wang, Y., Qu, Z., Xiong, N.N.: BeatClass: a sustainable ECG classification system in IoT-based eHealth. IEEE Internet Things J. **9**(10), 7178–7195 (2021)
31. Sun, L., Yu, Q., Peng, D., Subramani, S., Wang, X.: FogMed: a fog-based framework for disease prognosis based medical sensor data streams. CMC-Comput. Mater. Continua **66**(1), 603–619 (2021)
32. Sun, L., Zhong, Z., Qu, Z., Xiong, N.: PerAE: an effective personalized autoencoder for ECG-based biometric in augmented reality system. IEEE J. Biomed. Health Inform. **26**(6), 2435–2446 (2022)
33. Sun, L., Zhou, R., Peng, D., Bouguettaya, A., Zhang, Y.: Automatically building service-based systems with function relaxation. IEEE Trans. Cybern. (2022)
34. Sun, Z., Wang, C., Zhao, Y., Yan, C.: Multi-label ECG signal classification based on ensemble classifier. IEEE Access **8**, 117986–117996 (2020)
35. Supriya, S., Siuly, S., Wang, H., Zhang, Y.: Automated epilepsy detection techniques from electroencephalogram signals: a review study. Health Inf. Sci. Syst. **8**(1), 1–15 (2020)
36. Tiryaki, E., Sonawane, A., Tamil, L.: Real-time CNN based ST depression episode detection using single-lead ECG. In: 2021 22nd International Symposium on Quality Electronic Design (ISQED), pp. 566–570. IEEE (2021)
37. Vimalachandran, P., Liu, H., Lin, Y., Ji, K., Wang, H., Zhang, Y.: Improving accessibility of the Australian my health records while preserving privacy and security of the system. Health Inf. Sci. Syst. **8**(1), 1–9 (2020)
38. Wang, Y., Sun, L., Subramani, S.: CAB: classifying arrhythmias based on imbalanced sensor data. KSII Trans. Internet Inf. Syst. (TIIS) **15**(7), 2304–2320 (2021)

39. Xiaolin, L., Panicker, R.C., Cardiff, B., John, D.: Multistage pruning of CNN based ECG classifiers for edge devices. In: 2021 43rd Annual International Conference of the IEEE Engineering in Medicine & Biology Society (EMBC), pp. 1965–1968. IEEE (2021)
40. Yang, S., Xiang, H., Kong, Q., Wang, C.: Multi-label classification of electrocardiogram with modified residual networks. In: 2020 Computing in Cardiology, pp. 1–4. IEEE (2020)
41. Yu, Q., Sun, L.: LPClass: lightweight personalized sensor data classification in computational social systems. IEEE Trans. Comput. Soc. Syst. (2022)

ECG Signals Classification Model Based on Frequency Domain Features Coupled with Least Square Support Vector Machine (LS-SVM)

Rand Ameen Azeez[1], Sarmad K. D. Alkhafaji[2], Mohammed Diyk[2,3,4](✉), and Shahab Abdulla[3]

[1] Iraqi Ministry of Education, Thi-Qar, Iraq
[2] Department of Computer Sciences, College of Education for Pure Sciences, University of Thi-Qar, Nasiriyah, Iraq
{Dr.sarmad,Mohammed.diykh}@utq.edu.iq, mohammed.diykh@usq.edu.au
[3] UniSQ College, University of Southern Queensland, Springfield, Australia
Shahab.abdulla@usq.edu.au
[4] Information and Communication Technology Research Group, Scientific Research Centre, Al-Ayen University, Nasiriyah, Iraq

Abstract. The electrocardiogram (ECG) is used to inspect the electrical activity of the heart through which experts can detect heart disorders. Mainly medical experts manually examine ECG patterns; however, manual inspection of ECG signals takes significant amount of time and effort as well as is prone to errors. As a result, researchers have started to design automatic models for ECG patterns classification. In this paper, we propose a novel ECG signals classification model that utilises frequency characteristics of ECG signals coupled with a least-squares support vector machine (LS-SVM). An Optimization Triple Half Band Filter Bank (OTHFB) is used to decompose ECG signals into 6 bands delta δ, theta θ, alpha α, beta1 $\beta 1$, beta2 $\beta 2$, and gamma γ. Then nine statistical features named *{max, min, mean, mode, std, variance, skewness, rang, median}* are extracted from each band and sent to the LS-SVM. The obtained results showed that the extracted features from the bands alpha α, beta1 $\beta 1$, beta2 $\beta 2$, gamma γ gave a high classification accuracy compared bands delta δ, theta θ. The results showed that the proposed model achieved a high accuracy compared with the previous studies. An accuracy of 96% was obtained by the proposed model.

Keywords: ECG · OTFB · Statistical features · LSSVM

1 Introduction

Electrocardiograms (ECG) signals have been widely utilised to detect arrhythmias and other heart-related disorders [1–5]. The medical studies showed that ECG signals reflect abnormalities in electrical activity of heart. Classifying ECG patterns accurately can deliver a great importance for patients with heard disorders [5, 6]. Over the last few

A. Traina et al. (Eds.): HIS 2022, LNCS 13705, pp. 303–312, 2022.
https://doi.org/10.1007/978-3-031-20627-6_28

decades, there are surge demands for designing automatic classification ECG models to interpret and understand behavioural patterns of ECG signals.

Recently, ECG signals have been employed in different application such as disease detection, human identification [7–9]. Several commercial, and government systems use ECG signals for health monitoring and human identification [9–11].

Recently many researchers have designed machine learning based models to analyse ECG signals. Several machine learning algorithms such as linear discriminant analysis (LDA), support vector machine (SVM), and K-means have been employed [19–23]. Recently, deep learning approaches have designed and become a trend to detect abnormalities in biomedical signals. For example, Al Alkeem, et al. [11] identified individuals using a combination of ECG, fingerprint, and face attributes. The extracted features were sent to neural networks model. Hamza et al. [5] used ECG signals as an identification system. Three ECG features were employed to identify individuals including entropy, cepstral coefficient, and ZCR. In that study, a SVM classifier was utilised to identify individuals.

Arteaga-Falconi et al. [12] designed a conventional neural network (CNN) model coupled with a one-class SVM. They used a wavelet transform to analyse ECG signals. In that study, each ECG segment was transferred into an image form. The resulted images were forwarded into CNN model. Wang et al. [13] applied a band pass Butterworth filter with cut-off frequencies spanning from 1 to 40 Hz. A multi-scale differential feature was employed in that study and combined with one-dimensional multi-resolution local binary patterns to pulled out ECG attributes. Four datasets were used to evaluate the suggested model in that research. Although the approaches listed above function well, the ECG properties have not been thoroughly investigated. This work provides a novel ECG classification approach based on frequency features and the Least Square Support Vector Machine (LS-SVM). ECG signals are partitioned into intervals. Each interval is passed through optimal triple filter bank. As a result, each ECG interval is decomposed into six bands. Then, nine statistical features are extracted from each band to construct the final feature vector. Finally, the extracted features are sent into the LS-SVM.

2 Methodlgy and ECG Data

2.1 ECG Dataset

ECG dataset from the physio net organization was utilised in this paper to evaluate the performance of the proposed model [14]. The dataset is publicly available on the following URL https://physionet.org/content/mitdb/1.0.0/. The ECG recording were gathered from 47 subjects. We used all ECG records in our study. The ECG signals were sampled at 1000 Hz.

2.2 Proposed Model

This research proposed a new framework to classify ECG signals. We employed a Butterworth low-pass filter with a 128 Hz cut-off frequency to filter ECG signals. Frequency domain features are extracted ECG signals. in this paper, each ECG signals is segmented into intervals. Then, each ECG segment was decomposed into six bands using an Optimization Triple Half Band Filter Bank (OTHFB). Nine statistical attributes named {max, min, mean, mode, std, variance, skewness, rang, median} are extracted from each band. The extracted features from each ECG segment are sent into LS-SVM. Several statistical metrics are used to evaluate the performance of the proposed model. Figure 1 depicts the proposed model of ECG classification.

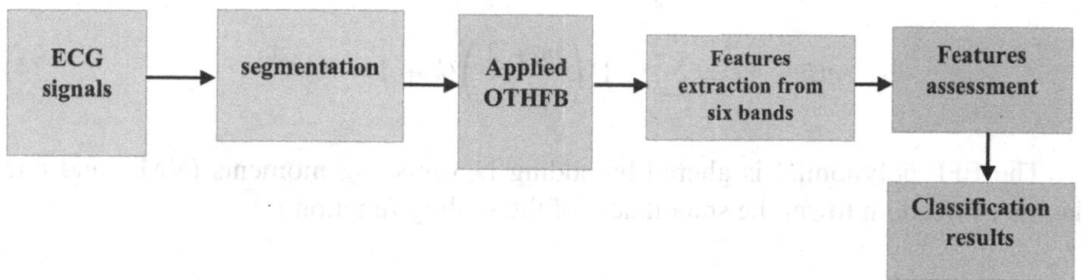

Fig. 1. The proposed framework of ECG classification

2.3 ECG Segmentation

Each ECG signal is segmented into epochs using fiducial points as a reference. The start and end of each heartbeat are identified by the credit points LP and TP. We applied a differentiation detection method in [6] to segment ECG signal. For example, suppose an ECG signal of s m data points $X = \{x_1, x_2, x_3, \ldots., x_n\}$. Using LP and TP, the signal X was divided into n segments with each one contains k data points.

2.4 Optimization Triple Half Band Filter Bank (OTHFB)

A triplet half-band filter bank is utilised to extract frequency features from ECG signals [19]. The THFB is expressed as

$$H_0(z)G_0(z) + H_0(-z)G_0(-Z) = 2 \tag{1}$$

$H_0(z)$ and $G_0(z)$ are the analysis and synthesis low pass filters. The low pass filter and high pass filter for the THFB are calculated as follows:

$$H_0(z) = \frac{1+P}{2} + \frac{1}{2}L_1(Z)(1 - pL_0(z)) \tag{2}$$

where L_1 and L_0 are kernel functions of the THFB which are produced from the half band polynomial $Pi(z)$ of order K, $Pi(z) = 1 + Li(z)$ *for* $I = 0; 1; 2$.

These half-band filters and kernels are non-causal filters that meet the PR requirement. The shape parameters of p0, p1, and p2 are computed as follows: p0 = p1 = ((1 + P))/2 and p2 = ((1 − p))/((1 + p)) where p's range is between 0 and 1.

In this study, the Euler-Fresenius polynomials (EFP) are used with THFB. The EFP coefficients are computed recursively. The EFP is described as follows:

$$E(z) = \sum_{k=0\, e(k+1)z}^{m} -k \tag{3}$$

where M stands for polynomial order and may be calculated as follows:

$$e(k+1) = \sum_{k=0}^{n}(-1)\binom{m+2}{m}(k+1-m)^{m+1} \tag{4}$$

The EFP polynomial is altered by adding N vanishing moments (VMs) and one degree of freedom to get the smoothness of the scaling function i.

$$p(z) = (1+z)^n = E(z)\sum_{k=0}^{l} \alpha k^{z-k} \tag{5}$$

The order of P(z) is K = M + N + L, and L = K = 2, 1. The time-frequency half-band filter that has been optimized is defined as

$$\mathrm{Q(z)} = \mathrm{P(z)}\sum\nolimits_k \beta kRk(z) \tag{6}$$

where _k is the degree of freedom to be evaluated. R k is an interpolator with a polynomial specification. In this situation, we utilized k = L = 2.

The OTHFB half-band filters L0(z); L1(z); L2(z) are adjusted using the balanced-uncertainty (BU) measure to balance in time and frequency localisation. BU measurements are optimized to yield the value of L/2.

$$\upbeta = \Delta\omega^2 + \mathrm{k}^2\Delta\mathrm{t}^2 \tag{7}$$

where Δt^2 and $\Delta\omega^2$ are the time and frequency localization parameters, respectively.

$$\Delta t^2 = \frac{1}{\sum q(n)}\sum_{k=0}^{n} n^2 q^2(n) \tag{8}$$

$$\Delta\omega^2 = \frac{\pi 2}{3} + 4\sum\nolimits_{n=0}^{\mathrm{k}-1}\sum\nolimits_{\mathrm{m=n+1}}^{\mathrm{k}-1}\frac{(-1)^{(\mathrm{m-n})}(a)}{\mathrm{U(m-n)}}\mathrm{q(m)q(n)}^n \tag{9}$$

where q(n) is the impulse response as calculated by Eq. (7). We got the following by inserting (9) and (10) in (8):

$$\beta = \frac{\pi}{2} + \frac{\sum \mathrm{n} \sum \frac{\mathrm{m}(-1)^{\mathrm{m-n}}}{(\mathrm{m-n})^2\mathrm{q(m)q(n)}} + \mathrm{k}^2 \sum \mathrm{n}\ \mathrm{n}^2\mathrm{q}^2(\mathrm{n})}{\sum_{\mathrm{n}}^{\mathrm{m}} \mathrm{q}^2(\mathrm{n})} \tag{10}$$

2.5 Classification

The LS-SVM classifier is used in this paper to classify ECG signals. The extracted features were sent to the LS-SVM and all results were recorded.

2.6 Performance Evaluation Measurements

The following statistical metrics are used to evaluate the proposed model [23–25]

$$Accuracy = \frac{TP + TN}{TP + FN + TN + FP} \tag{11}$$

$$Sensitivity = \frac{TP}{TP + FN} \tag{12}$$

$$Specificity = \frac{TN}{TN + FP} \tag{13}$$

$$False\ Positive\ Rate\ (FPR)\ or\ fall - out$$

$$FPR = \frac{FP}{FP + TN} \tag{14}$$

where true positive (TP) is the number of correct classifications of all subsets, true negative (TN) is the number of correct classifications of all subsets, false positive (FP) is the number of incorrect classifications of all subsets, false negative (FN) is the number of incorrect classifications of all subsets.

3 Experimental Results

The performance of the proposed framework is evaluated using several metrics. The extracted features from ECG signals using Optimization Triple Half Band Filter Bank (OTHFB). Were investigated to find the most powerful features. Nine statistical features were extracted from each band and tested individually. The results showed that the extracted features from bands alpha α, beta1 $\beta 1$, beta2 $\beta 2$, gamma γ recorded a high classification accuracy. Table 1 shows the classification results based on each band. It can be noticed that the classification accuracy was improved when the features from four bands combined together. Bands delta δ, theta θ, alpha α, beta1 $\beta 1$ beta2 $\beta 2$, gamma γ.

Table 1. ECG Classification accuracy of the proposed model

Band	Accuracy	Sensitivity	Specificity
delta δ	65%	61%	62%
theta θ	60%	59%	60%
alpha α	78%	76%	76%
beta1 $\beta 1$	83%	83%	82%
beta2 $\beta 2$	86%	85%	86%
gamma γ	87%	86%	85%
alpha α, beta1 $\beta 1$ beta2 $\beta 2$, gamma γ	97%	96%	97%

3.1 Performance Evaluation Based on 10 Cross Validations

In this experiment, we used a 10-fold validation metric. ECG dataset was divided into 10 groups, and at each experiment, one group was used for the testing and the others for the training. Figure 1 reports the classification rates based on 10-cross validation. An average of accuracy of 94% was obtained (Fig. 2).

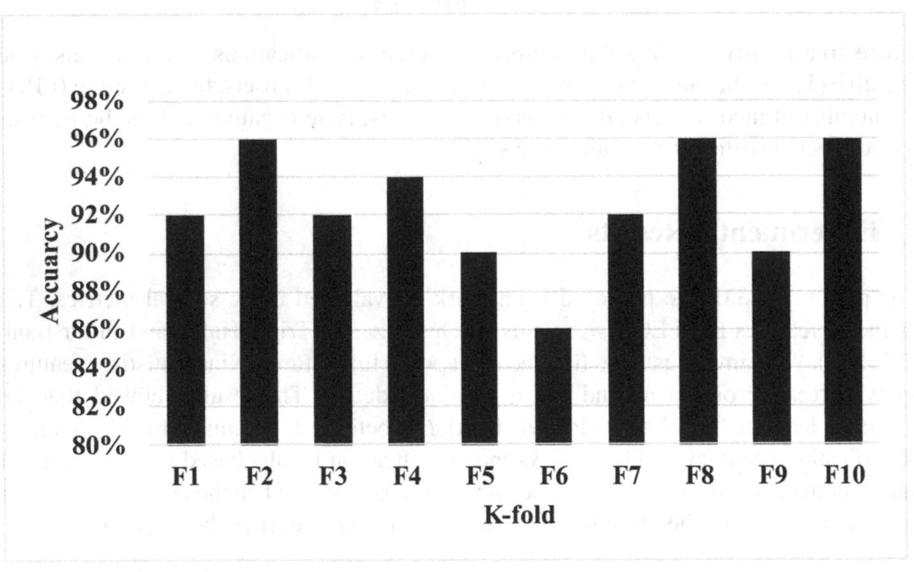

Fig. 2. A 10-fold cross-validation accuracy of the proposed method

3.2 Classification Results Based on Different Kernel Functions

In this study, we tested different kernels of LS-SVM. Table 2 reports the classification results obtained based on different kernel functions. The RBF kernel scored the highest accuracy 96% compared with other kernel function. However, poiy-kernel recorded 88% the lowest accuracy rate.

Table 2. Classification results based on different kernel functions

Type kernel	Accuracy	Sensitivity	Precision	Specificity	F-measure
Lin_kernel	0.92	0.82	0.90	0.92	0.90
Poly-kernel	0.93	0.87	0.91	0.92	0.88
RBF-kernel	0.96	0.96	0.96	0.95	0.95

Note: Lin = Linear kernel; Poly = Polynomial kernel; RBF = Radial Basis Function kernel.

Table 3. Classification results based on different gam and sig2 values

Gam	sig2	Accuracy	Sensitivity	Precision	Specificity	F-measure
100	0.2	0.82	0.81	0.80	0.83	0.82
100	100	0.89	0.88	0.87	0.86	0.88
1000	100	0.92	0.844	0.89	0.88	0.87
70	4	0.87	0.74	0.89	0.88	0.85
20	20	0.91	0.7838	0.90	0.90	0.89
10	0.1	0.96	0.95	0.96	0.95	0.96

The gam and sig2 parameter which were used to optimize the LS-SVM were tested. The LS-SVM was trained with several sets of gam and sig2 parameters to get the best results. The highest results were obtained when Gam = 10 and sig2 = 0.1. Table 3 reports the obtained results based on different LS-SVM parameters.

3.3 Performance Evaluation Based on Different Classification Models

The performance of the proposed ECG classification model was tested with several classification algorithms, including k-means, support vector machine, Naïve Bayes and k-nearest. The extracted features from ECG using the OTHFB were forwarded to k-means, support vector machine, Naïve Bayes and k-nearest as well as to the LS-SVM. A 10-cross validation metric was used, and all obtained results were recorded and used for comparison. Table 4 reports the classification results based on five classification algorithms. The obtained results demonstrated that the LS-SVM surpassed the k-means, support vector machine, Naïve Bayes and k-nearest. However, the SVM scored the second highest accuracy rate of 93% while k-means obtained the lowest rate of 84%.

3.4 Comparisons with Previous Studies

The proposed model was compared with previous approaches in literature. Based on the comparison results, the proposed model obtained a high classification result compared

Table 4. Performance evaluation based on several classification model

	Accuracy	Sensitivity	Specificity
Naïve bayes	65%	61%	62%
k-nearest	88%	87%	87%
SVM	93%	92%	90%
k-means	84%	85%	83%
LS-SVM	97%	96%	97%

with other studies. Table 5 reports the comparisons results. Hanilçi et al. [28] adopted a handcrafted features with CNN. They recorded 88% accuracy which is lower than our model. Agrafioti et al. [26] suggested a k-nearest with Butterworth filter technique to classify ECG signals. They obtained 92.3% while our model recorded 96%. We can notice that the proposed model outperformed previous studies.

Table 5. Comparisons among the proposed model and previous approaches

Author	Approach	Accuracy
Agrafioti et al. [26]	Frequency technique based on KNN	90%
Agrafioti et al. [27]	Butterworth bandpass filter method with KNN, k-means	92.3%
Lourenço et al. [28]	Chaos theory with SVM	81.73%
Hanilçi et al. [29]	CNN based on handcrafted features	88%
Proposed model	Time and frequency-based approaches with LS-SVM	96%

4 Conclusions

In this study, we proposed an ECG signals classification model. The OTHFB was utilised to extract representative features to classify ECG signals. We carefully examined the influence of features extract from each band ECG classification system. Several experiments were designed, and it was found that statistical features from bands alpha α, beta1 $\beta 1$ beta2 $\beta 2$, gamma γ gave a high classification accuracy A least support vector machine was employed to classify ECG signals. Although the proposed model achieved a high classification accuracy, further assessment is required to evaluate the proposed model with a large data set. An addition several classifiers, and features selection models can be integrated with the proposed model to improve the classification results.

References

1. Wu, W., Pirbhulal, S., Sangaiah, A.K., Mukhopadhyay, S.C., Li, G.: Optimization of signal quality over comfortability of textile electrodes for ECG monitoring in fog computing based medical applications. Future Gener. Comput. Syst. **86**, 515–526 (2018)

2. Hammad, M., Wang, K.: Parallel score fusion of ECG and fingerprint for human authentication based on convolution neural network. Comput. Secur. **81**, 107–122 (2019)
3. Bai, T., et al.: A lightweight method of data encryption in BANs using electrocardiogram signal. Futur. Gener. Comput. Syst. **92**, 800–811 (2019)
4. Peris-Lopez, P., González-Manzano, L., Camara, C., de Fuentes, J.M.: Effect of attacker characterization in ECG-based continuous authentication mechanisms for Internet of Things. Future Gener. Comput. Syst. **81**, 67–77 (2018)
5. Hamza, S., Ayed, Y.B.: SVM for human identification using the ECG signal. Procedia Comput. Sci. **176**, 430–439 (2020). https://doi.org/10.1016/j.procs.2020.08.044
6. Hong, S., Zhou, Y., Shang, J., Xiao, C., Sun, J.: Opportunities and challenges of deep learning methods for electrocardiogram data: a systematic review. Comput. Biol. Med. **122**, 103801 (2020)
7. Rabinezhadsadatmahaleh, N., Khatibi, T.: A novel noise-robust stacked ensemble of deep and conventional machine learning classifiers (NRSE-DCML) for human biometric identification from electrocardiogram signals. Inform. Med. Unlocked **21**, 100469 (2020). https://doi.org/10.1016/j.imu.2020.100469
8. Klonowski, W.: Fractal analysis of electroencephalographic time series (EEG signals). In: Di Ieva, A. (ed.) The Fractal Geometry of the Brain, pp. 413–429. Springer, New York (2016). https://doi.org/10.1007/978-1-4939-3995-4_25
9. Namazi, H., Jafari, S.: Age-based variations of fractal structure of EEG signal in patients with epilepsy. Fractals **26**(04), 1850051 (2018)
10. Hjorth, B.: EEG analysis based on time domain properties. Electroencephalogr. Clin. Neurophysiol. **29**(3), 306–310 (1970)
11. Al Alkeem, E., et al.: Robust deep identification using ECG and multimodal biometrics for industrial Internet of Things. Ad Hoc Netw. **121**, 102581 (2021). https://doi.org/10.1016/j.adhoc.2021.102581
12. Arteaga-Falconi, J.S., Al Osman, H., El Saddik, A.: ECG and fingerprint bimodal authentication. Sustain. Cities Soc. **40**, 274–283 (2018). https://doi.org/10.1016/j.scs.2017.12.023
13. Wang, K., Yang, G., Huang, Y., Yin, Y.: Multi-scale differential feature for ECG biometrics with collective matrix factorization. Pattern Recogn. **102**, 107211 (2020). https://doi.org/10.1016/j.patcog.2020.107211
14. Moody, G.B., Mark, R.G.: The impact of the MIT-BIH arrhythmia database. IEEE Eng. Med. Biol. Mag. **20**(3), 45–50 (2001)
15. Stehman, S.V.: Selecting and interpreting measures of thematic classification accuracy. Remote Sens. Environ. **62**(1), 77–89 (1997)
16. Powers, D.M.W.: Evaluation: from precision, recall and F-measure to ROC, informedness, markedness and correlation. arXiv preprint arXiv:2010.16061 (2020)
17. Sammut, C., Webb, G.I.: Encyclopedia of Machine Learning. Springer, New York (2010). https://doi.org/10.1007/978-0-387-30164-8
18. Brooks, H., et al.: WWRP/WGNE joint working group on forecast verification research. In: Collaboration for Australian Weather and Climate Research. World Meteorological Organisation (2015)
19. Majeed, R.R., Alkhafaji, S.K.: ECG classification system based on multi-domain features approach coupled with least square support vector machine (LS-SVM). Comput. Methods Biomech. Biomed. Eng. 1–8 (2022)
20. Khare, S.K., Bajaj, V., Sengur, A., Sinha, G.R.: Classification of mental states from rational dilation wavelet transform and bagged tree classifier using EEG signals. In: Artificial Intelligence-Based Brain-Computer Interface, pp. 217–235. Academic Press (2022)
21. Khare, S.K., Bajaj, V.: A hybrid decision support system for automatic detection of Schizophrenia using EEG signals. Comput. Biol. Med. **141**, 105028 (2022)

22. Sharma, S., Khare, S.K., Bajaj, V., Ansari, I.A.: Improving the separability of drowsiness and alert EEG signals using analytic form of wavelet transform. Appl. Acoust. **181**, 108164 (2021)
23. Alsafy, I., Diykh, M.: Developing a robust model to predict depth of anesthesia from single channel EEG signal. Phys. Eng. Sci. Med. **45**, 793–808 (2022). https://doi.org/10.1007/s13246-022-01145-z
24. Diykh, M., et al.: Texture analysis based graph approach for automatic detection of neonatal seizure from multi-channel EEG signals. Measurement **190**, 110731 (2022)
25. Diykh, M., Miften, F.S., Abdulla, S., Saleh, K., Green, J.H.: Robust approach to depth of anaesthesia assessment based on hybrid transform and statistical features<? show [AQ ID= Q1]?>. IET Sci. Meas. Technol. **14**(1), 128–136 (2020)
26. Agrafioti, F., Gao, J., Hatzinakos, D., Yang, J.: Heart biometrics: theory, methods and applications. Biometrics **3**, 199–216 (2011)
27. Agrafioti, F., Hatzinakos, D.: Signal validation for cardiac biometrics. In: 2010 IEEE International Conference on Acoustics, Speech and Signal Processing, pp. 1734–1737. IEEE, March 2010
28. Lourenço, A., Silva, H., Fred, A.: ECG-based biometrics: a real time classification approach. In: 2012 IEEE International Workshop on Machine Learning for Signal Processing, pp. 1–6. IEEE, September 2012
29. Hanilçi, A., Gürkan, H.: ECG biometric identification method based on parallel 2-D convolutional neural networks. J. Innov. Sci. Eng. **3**(1), 11–22 (2019)

Cluster Analysis of Low-Dimensional Medical Concept Representations from Electronic Health Records

Fernando Jaume-Santero[1,2], Boya Zhang[1], Dimitrios Proios[1,2], Anthony Yazdani[1], Racha Gouareb[1], Mina Bjelogrlic[1,3], and Douglas Teodoro[1,2](✉)

[1] Department of Radiology and Medical Informatics, University of Geneva, Geneva, Switzerland
{fernando.jaume,boya.zhang,dimitrios.proios,anthony.yazdani, racha.gouareb,douglas.teodoro}@unige.ch

[2] Business Information Systems, University of Applied Sciences and Arts of Western Switzerland (HES-SO), Geneva, Switzerland

[3] Medical Information Sciences Division, Diagnostic Department, University Hospitals of Geneva, Geneva, Switzerland
mina.bjelogrlic@hcuge.ch

Abstract. The study of existing links among different types of medical concepts can support research on optimal pathways for the treatment of human diseases. Here, we present a clustering analysis of medical concept learned representations generated from MIMIC-IV, an open dataset of de-identified digital health records. Patient's trajectory information were extracted in chronological order to generate +500k sequence-like data structures, which were fed to a word2vec model to automatically learn concept representations. As a result, we obtained concept embeddings that describe diagnostics, procedures, and medications in a continuous low-dimensional space. A quantitative evaluation of the embeddings shows the significant power of the extracted embeddings on predicting exact labels of diagnoses, procedures, and medications for a given patient trajectory, achieving top-10 and top-30 accuracy over 47% and 66%, respectively, for all the dimensions evaluated. Moreover, clustering analyses of medical concepts after dimensionality reduction with t-SNE and UMAP techniques show that similar diagnoses (and procedures) are grouped together matching the categories of ICD-10 codes. However, the distribution by categories is not as evident if PCA or SVD are employed, indicating that the relationships among concepts are highly non-linear. This highlights the importance of non-linear models, such as those provided by deep learning, to capture the complex relationships of medical concepts.

Keywords: Electronic health records · Patient trajectory · Embeddings · Clustering · Representation learning

A. Traina et al. (Eds.): HIS 2022, LNCS 13705, pp. 313–324, 2022.
https://doi.org/10.1007/978-3-031-20627-6_29

1 Introduction

Electronic health record (EHR) data can be used in secondary applications to monitor, diagnose and predict the future state of a patient, providing personalized health care, while exploring new treatments for human diseases [9]. Nonetheless, an important challenge to overcome when using EHR data is their heterogeneous composition and high dimensionality, since they usually include a plethora of concept types, such as patient demographics, hospital administrative information, diagnoses, procedures, lab tests and medications, in the most varied formats (categories, free-text, numerals, etc.) [4,19,20]. These features can be semantically normalised in knowledge-based systems and treated as categorical values [18,20]. However, the manual curation process is expensive, often limiting its application to the whole extend of the EHR datasets. Features extraction via automatic derivation using natural language processing models, also called concept embeddings, have been suggested as an alternative [1,2,16,17].

Concept embeddings in natural language are aimed to be semantic, meaning that similar concepts should be characterized by geometrical proximity in the vector space. Previous studies [2] suggest that rule-based algorithms designed by medical experts are limited in terms of scalability, as well as in predictive capacity compared to data-driven concept embeddings obtained with neural networks. This has led to a significant increase in research that utilizes deep learning to extract information from EHR [17] using static-vector models [2], as well as, deep contextualized models [15]. In turn, the study of semantic relations among medical concept embeddings has gained popularity in the last few years, providing for example insights into the biomedical domain while preserving the anonymity of personal information [3].

In this paper, we aim to assess the complexity nature of concept relations in low-dimensional vector spaces created by embedding models. After preprocessing EHR data to create admission-wise data structures, clinical events for a given patient were provided to a representation learning model based on the word2vec algorithm [13] to create low-dimensional representations of the medical concepts. The study presented herein is divided into three main parts: *i)* selection and pre-processing of EHR datasets (Subsect. 2.1), *ii)* generation and validation of medical concept embeddings (Subsects. 2.2 and 3.1), and *iii)* clustering analysis of low-dimensional medical concept representations (Subsect. 3.2).

2 Methodology

Clinical information of +382k patients was extracted from the Medical Information Mart for Intensive Care - version 4 (MIMIC-IV) [7], an open dataset of de-identified digital health records from the Beth Israel Deaconess Medical Center with +523k hospital admissions that span between 2008 and 2019. Previous studies in medical informatics have already used MIMIC-IV [6,12,14], validating the use of this database for digital health-related topics. In our study, EHR data of every patient's admission were chronologically extracted and converted into sequence-like data structures ready to be processed by the word2vec model. Medical concept embeddings were further dimensionally reduced for analysis and visualization purposes. Figure 1 shows a flowchart of the methodology followed in this study.

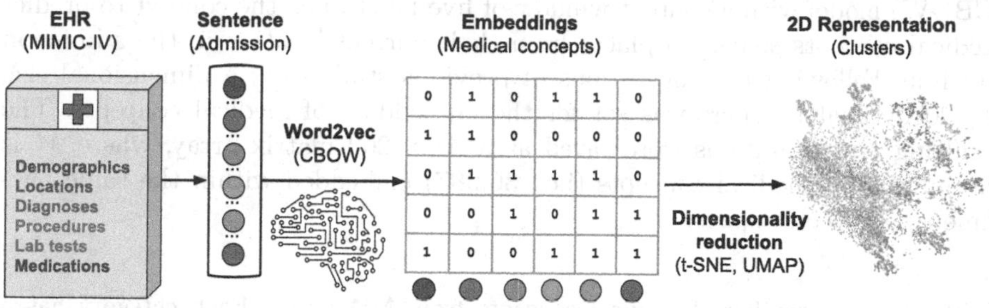

Fig. 1. Workflow scheme illustrating the process followed in the study. Colored dots represent medical concepts of different categories, that are embedded into a 200-dimensional vector space, and visualized after dimensionality reduction. (Color figure online)

2.1 Data Pre-processing

More than 35,000 medical concepts within 6 different categories (i.e., demographics, locations, diagnoses, procedures, lab tests, and medications) were extracted from the MIMIC-IV database (see Table 1 for detailed information). These concepts were then mapped to standard biomedical terminologies (e.g., ICD-10 codes for diagnoses and procedures, and Generic Sequence Number for medications) or to local terminologies, such as for hospital locations (e.g., *PACU* instead of *Post-anesthesia care unit*). Patient's age was also normalized into four labels according to the admission's starting date and their first registered age. For each patient's admission, the corresponding medical concepts were chronologically placed into text arrays forming word2vec compatible sequence-like data structures (or sentences). Note that, to reduce the number of concepts per admission-sequence, for laboratory results only lab tests with abnormal results (i.e., above or below normal ranges) were included in the final corpus, setting the average number of medical concepts per admission to 60 ($\sigma = 66$). Moreover, as diagnoses are billed on hospital discharge, they do not have a temporal order of appearance, and therefore they were put together in each sequence by level of importance after demographic data. The complete dataset was split into three subsets for training, validation, and testing purposes, with 521.2k, 1.3k, and 1.3k admissions, respectively.

2.2 Word2vec Embeddings

To obtain medical concept embeddings, a word2vec model was trained with the MIMIC-IV dataset. Word2vec is a natural language processing technique that utilizes shallow fully-connected neural networks to learn representations of different labels from large text datasets [13]. The information of each concept is embedded into a unique numeric array of a pre-determined dimension, which allows the assessment of semantic relationships with a quantitative mathematical framework. In our case, word2vec was trained as a Continuous Bag of Words (CBOW) model with a context window of five labels, i.e., the context to predict medical concepts spans ± 5 places from their current location in the admission timeline. Following the suggestions of previous studies [2], a dimensional size of 200 decimal numbers was set for the embedding of medical concepts. The resulting representations were saved as a $M \times 200$ matrix array, where M is the number of medical concepts (i.e., 36,987) embedded within the same low-dimensional vector space.

Table 1. Classification of medical concepts from MIMIC-IV. Each category has a determined number of different medical concepts whose embbedings are generated by a word2vec model. * local terminology.

Category	Concepts	Terminology
Demographics*	14	Gender, age, ethnicity, status
Location*	36	Hospital location
Diagnosis	19,735	ICD-10 CM
Procedure	11,503	ICD-10 PCS
Lab test*	929	MIMIC-IV ItemID
Medication	4,770	Generic Sequence Number

3 Results and Discussion

3.1 Medical Concept Prediction

For this study, we employed the properties of numerical vectors to evaluate the predictive power of medical concept embeddings over different clinical categories. A subset of hospital admissions for 1000 out-of-sample patients, i.e., not present in the training dataset, was used to evaluate diagnosis, procedure, and medication predictions. It is noteworthy to mention that patients could be admitted to the hospital more than once, and therefore the number of admissions is usually higher than the number of patients (i.e., around 1.3k in our case). Within this framework, all concepts associated with a given category (e.g., ICD-10 CM codes for diagnoses) were subtracted from the admission-sequence and used as true labels to be predicted. The remaining concepts within each sequence were aggregated together using the weighted average to generate embeddings that represent patients in the vector space. Individual weights were inversely proportional to the frequency of label appearance across the entire corpus, assigning lower values to highly repeated concepts. The similarity of these admission representations with the embeddings of the true labels was subsequently evaluated by means of the cosine distance, creating a ranking of most similar concepts. The predictive power was estimated using the top-k accuracy, where a successful outcome was registered when at least one of the hidden true labels was ranked within the k-most similar concepts.

Table 2 shows the top-10 and top-30 accuracy for prediction of diagnoses, procedures, and medications using word2vec models trained with different representations of patient's admission-sequences created from the MIMIC-IV dataset. While the *sorted* dataset displays locations, procedures, medications, and lab tests in chronological order of intervention, the *shuffled* one contains the same medical concepts per admission, randomly shuffled without a specific order. One more dataset - *mixed* - was also created by concatenating the sorted and shuffled datasets, generating a semi-sorted text corpus with twice the number of concepts. Superior predictive performances for diagnoses and medications were achieved with the model trained using the shuffled dataset, whereas the prediction of procedures (i.e., ICD-10 PCS codes) was highest when the model was trained with the mixed one. On the other hand, a significantly lower accuracy is obtained for the prediction of diagnoses when the sorted dataset is employed. The drop in performance is consistent with the fact that when all diagnoses are masked from the test dataset, most of the context necessary to describe the concepts is also removed. Note that in the sorted dataset, diagnoses are grouped together after the demographic information, which forces the model to learn their relationships from previous diagnoses. This does not happen with the shuffled dataset, where diagnoses can be located at any position of the sequence, having labels from different categories as neighbours. Overall, the medical concept embeddings have a high predictive power with a top-10 accuracy over 47%, and a top-30 accuracy over 66%, for all three categories. This is quite remarkable taking into account that predictions were enforced to match true labels, e.g., ICD-10 CM codes were predicted with the same number of characters as they were billed by the hospital administration, i.e., nearly 20k different concepts. It is also noteworthy to mention that similar results were obtained for different validation and test datasets.

On the other hand, a less strict experiment has also been analyzed for diagnoses and procedures, where the accuracy on successful concept prediction has been constrained to the initial characters of the ICD-10 codes. Figure 2 shows a significant increase of more than 15% on top 5, 10, and 30 accuracy in both cases when three (or less) ICD-10 characters had to be predicted, indicating that word2vec embeddings are able to capture the general relationships among different medical concepts. In terms of applicability, this high accuracy on category prediction indicates that small but reliable NLP models such as word2vec could be useful to aid in determining general type of injuries or diseases in patients.

Table 2. Top 10/30 accuracy on predicting exact labels of diagnoses, procedures, and medications over 1000 out-of-sample patients. Word2vec (CBOW) was trained with three different datasets: EHR preserving patient timeliness (sorted), shuffled, and a combination of both (mixed).

Category	Accuracy@10			Accuracy@30		
	Sorted	Shuffled	Mixed	Sorted	Shuffled	Mixed
Diagnosis	4.28	**47.07**	15.61	8.16	**66.48**	30.11
Procedure	50.23	52.85	**58.86**	63.02	70.26	**77.20**
Medication	22.55	**65.45**	44.09	32.64	**80.55**	62.27

3.2 Cluster Analysis of Medical Concepts

To obtain a qualitative understanding of medical concept relationships, the embeddings of diagnoses, procedures, and medications were further dimensionally reduced using non-linear visualization algorithms, such as t-SNE and UMAP [10,11]. These techniques provide a 2-dimensional representation of the vector space, aggregating similar concepts closer to each other, while separating significantly dissimilar sub-groups. Note that diagnosis and medication embeddings were obtained from the model trained with the shuffled dataset, whereas procedure vectors were generated with the model trained using the mixed dataset, as it showed higher predictive power for that category. To evaluate the capacity of these embeddings on capturing the semantic meaning of different medical concepts, these 2-D representations were depicted with distinctive colors associated with their corresponding code topics as shown in Fig. 3. Diagnoses with the same first ICD-10 CM letter belong to the same medical topic, e.g., codes staring with the letter "O" are diagnoses related to *pregnancy*, *childbirth*, and *puerperium*, while in procedures, the second ICD-10 PCS digit determines the part of the body where a surgical procedure takes place. In this case, 2-dimensional representations and their corresponding colors show a clear correspondence among groups of concepts in the low-dimensional vector space and the topics associated with their true label.

Figure 3a & 3b show that similar diagnoses are grouped together matching the sub-categories of ICD-10 codes. While specific diagnoses (e.g., *pregnancy* and *childbirth*) are aggregated within a limited region (orange dots), more general diagnoses such as those involving *injury* and *poisoning* (i.e., codes staring with S or T) are situated all across the vector space. A similar distribution is observed for surgical interventions, indicating that procedure embeddings capture to some extent the information regarding the part of the body where surgical operations should take place (e.g., red dots in Fig. 3c & 3d correspond to surgeries of the respiratory system).

On the other hand, prescribed medications in MIMIC-IV are labelled using generic sequence numbers that do not give information about their components. Therefore, to associate types of medication with embedding locations within the 2-dimensional vector space, drug names were mapped to their correspond-

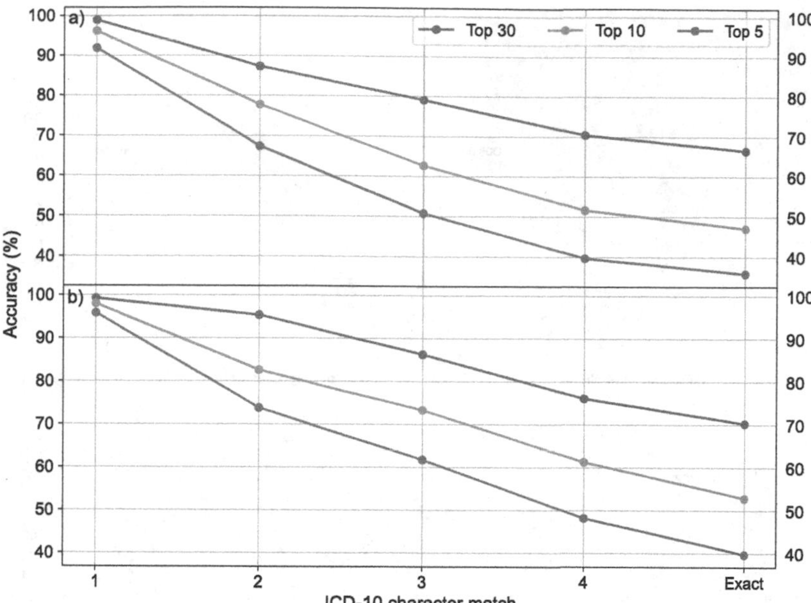

Fig. 2. Top 5, 10, and 30 accuracy on predicting ICD-10 codes for (a) diagnoses and (b) procedures. Medical concept representations have been obtained from a word2vec model trained with the shuffled dataset. Accuracy on concept prediction has been calculated for successful matches of 1, 2, 3, and 4 ICD-10 characters, as well as, an exact match with the target.

ing Anatomical Therapeutic Chemical (ATC) codes, where the first letter indicates the anatomical main group (e.g., ATC drug codes starting with "C" were designed for the cardiovascular system). It is noteworthy to mention that only 56.2% of the medications in the dataset were successfully mapped to ATC codes, reducing the overall number of displayed concepts in Fig. 3e & 3f from 4,770 to 2,681. Nevertheless, similar concept aggregations are still present for some medications (e.g., C-starting ATC codes form a blue point aggregation), suggesting a consistent match between medication embeddings and their associated anatomical main group even when this information was not present during the training process, as word2vec models were trained with generic sequence numbers.

This topic distribution is not as evident when linear methods, such as Principal Component Analysis (PCA) or Singular Value Decomposition (SVD), are employed to reduce the vector space or to generate linear concept embeddings. A cluster analysis over medical concepts was performed to quantitatively assess the performance mismatch between linear and non-linear approaches. The k-means algorithm [5] was applied separately over diagnosis, procedure, and medication embeddings to group the concepts into 50 different clusters. These clusters were subsequently assigned to a medical topic using the majority vote rule, i.e., if most diagnoses within a given cluster started with letter "O", that cluster was

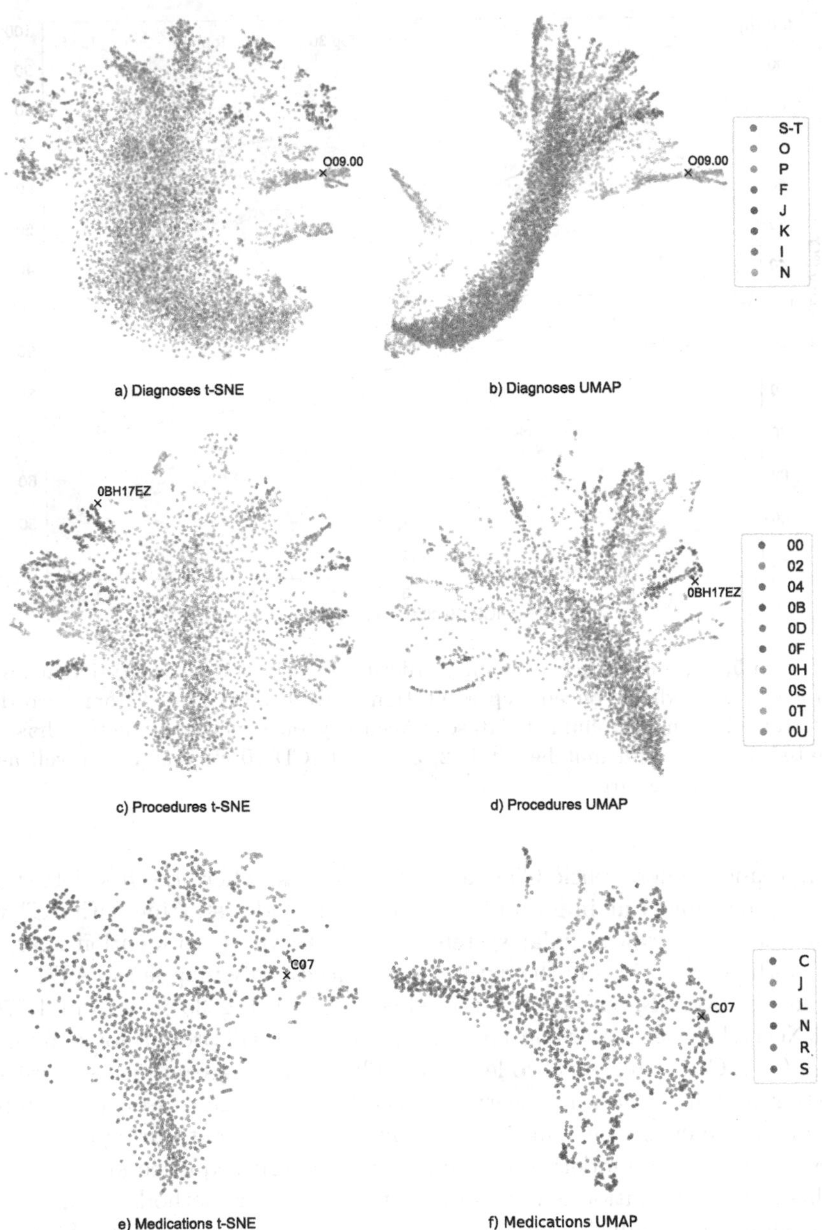

Fig. 3. 2-dimensional representation of diagnoses (a, b), procedures (c, d), and medications (e, f) using t-SNE (left) and UMAP (right). Medical concepts are depicted as dots using colors associated with the first (and second for procedures) characters of ICD-10 CM (diagnosis), ICD-10 PCS (procedures), and ATC (medication) codes. Crosses show example codes for clarification purposes. ICD-10 CM *O09.00* is associated with supervision of pregnancy with history of infertility in an unspecified trimester. ICD-10 PCS *0BH17EZ* is related to insertion of endotracheal airway into trachea, via natural or artificial opening. ATC *C07* refers to beta-blocking agents.

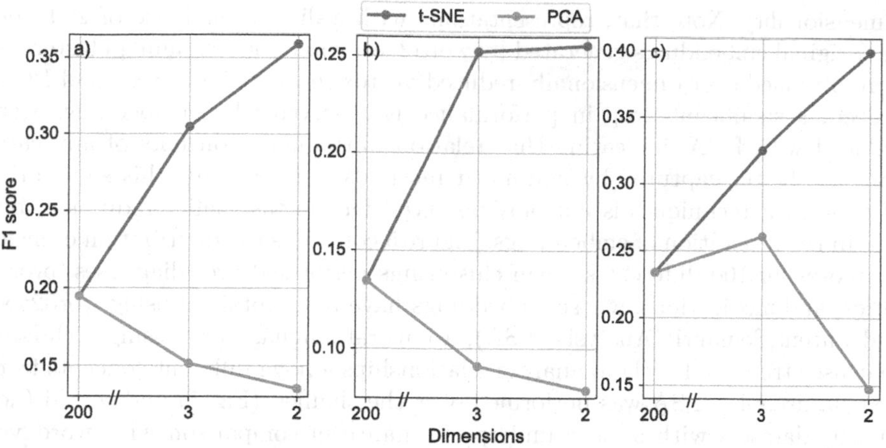

Fig. 4. Mean F1-scores of k-means clusters with respect to true labels of (a) diagnoses, (b) procedures, and (c) medications as a function of the vector dimensionality. Blue (orange) lines represent medical concepts after dimensionality reduction (with sizes 2 and 3) using t-SNE (PCA). (Color figure online)

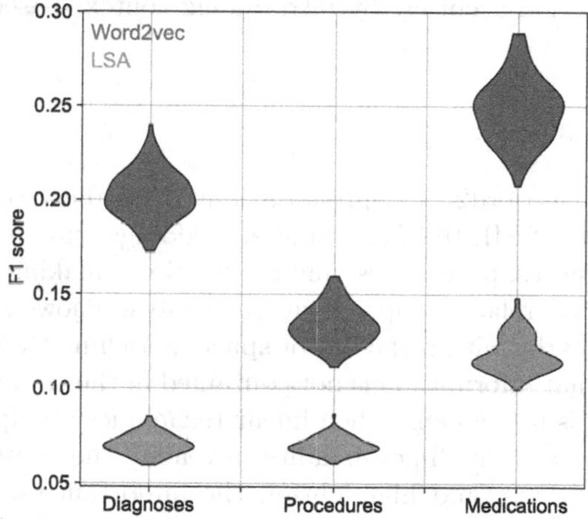

Fig. 5. Distribution of F1-scores for 100 k-means clusterings compared with respect to the true labels of diagnoses, procedures, and medications. Blue (orange) violins represent the kernel density estimation of F1-scores averaged over all category sub-groups for embeddings generated with word2vec (LSA). (Color figure online)

associated with the "O" ICD-10 CM sub-category. This allowed for the comparison of true label locations with clusters that minimize the squared Euclidean distance among embeddings.

Figure 4 shows the F1-scores (averaged over all sub-categories) of the clusterings obtained for diagnoses, procedures, and medications, as a function of their dimensionality. Note that, representations with a dimensional size of 200 were the original embeddings generated by word2vec, while the remaining clusterings were obtained over dimensionally-reduced vector spaces using t-SNE and PCA. Indeed, a significant drop in performance is observed when embeddings were reduced with PCA, indicating that relationships among concepts of any category are better captured by non-linear methods. Interestingly, this superiority of non-linear techniques is not only observed for dimensionality reduction, but also in the generation of embeddings. Figure 5 compares the distribution of mean F1-scores for 100 different k-mean clusterings performed over diagnoses, procedures, and medications, whose embeddings have been obtained using word2vec, and Latent Semantic Analysis (LSA), a natural language processing technique that uses truncated SVD to analyze relationships among different concepts from text datasets [8]. LSA was performed over the shuffled (Fig. 5) and sorted (not shown) datasets with a clear underperformance in comparison with word2vec embeddings trained with the shuffled (diagnoses and medications) and mixed (procedures) corpora. This reveals the non-linear nature of the relationships among medical concepts even within the same category, stressing the need for novel machine learning architectures beyond log-linear models. In this sense, deep contextual language models could solve current word2vec limitations in terms of linearity and prediction accuracy by introducing context-based representations of medical concepts.

4 Conclusions

We generated robust word2vec representations of medical concepts extracted from digital records of MIMIC-IV. These embeddings exhibited a high predictive power for diagnoses, procedures, and medications, making them suitable for the study of semantic relationships. A cluster analysis showed that similar concepts are located nearby within the vector space, matching their respective topic codes, even when that information is not contained in the training dataset. However, this behavior is not evident when linear techniques are applied to generate embeddings or reduce their dimensionality, revealing the complex relationships among medical concepts, and highlighting the importance of using non-linear models, such as neural networks, in order to capture their semantic meaning and relationships. Future studies could therefore be focused on the comparison of static-vector and context-dependent medical representations from different NLP models.

References

1. Choi, E., Bahadori, M.T., Schuetz, A., Stewart, W.F., Sun, J.: Doctor AI: Predicting Clinical Events via Recurrent Neural Networks (2016). https://proceedings.mlr.press/v56/Choi16.html
2. De Freitas, J.K., et al.: Phe2vec: automated disease phenotyping based on unsupervised embeddings from electronic health records. Patterns **2**(9), 100337 (2021). https://doi.org/10.1016/j.patter.2021.100337

3. Flamholz, Z.N., Crane-Droesch, A., Ungar, L.H., Weissman, G.E.: Word embeddings trained on published case reports are lightweight, effective for clinical tasks, and free of protected health information. J. Biomed. Inform. **125**, 103971 (2022). https://doi.org/10.1016/j.jbi.2021.103971. https://www.sciencedirect.com/science/article/pii/S1532046421003002
4. Glynn, E.F., Hoffman, M.A.: Heterogeneity introduced by EHR system implementation in a de-identified data resource from 100 non-affiliated organizations. JAMIA Open **2**(4), 554–561 (2019). https://doi.org/10.1093/jamiaopen/ooz035. https://pubmed.ncbi.nlm.nih.gov/32025653
5. Hartigan, J.A., Wong, M.A.: Algorithm AS 136: a K-means clustering algorithm. J. R. Stat. Soc. C: Appl. Stat. **28**(1), 100–108 (1979). https://doi.org/10.2307/2346830. Full publication date 1979
6. Hua, R., Liu, X., Yuan, E.: Red blood cell distribution width at admission predicts outcome in critically ill patients with kidney failure: a retrospective cohort study based on the MIMIC-IV database. Ren. Fail. **44**(1), 1182–1191 (2022). https://doi.org/10.1080/0886022X.2022.2098766. pMID: 35834358
7. Johnson, A.E., Bulgarelli, L., Pollard, T.J., Horng, S., Celi, L., Mark, R.G.: MIMIC-IV (version 1.0) (2021). https://doi.org/10.13026/s6n6-xd98
8. Landauer, T.K., Foltz, P.W., Laham, D.: An introduction to latent semantic analysis. Discourse Process. **25**(2–3), 259–284 (1998). https://doi.org/10.1080/01638539809545028
9. Li, Z., Roberts, K., Jiang, X., Long, Q.: Distributed learning from multiple EHR databases: contextual embedding models for medical events. J. Biomed. Inform. **92**, 103138 (2019). https://doi.org/10.1016/j.jbi.2019.103138. https://www.sciencedirect.com/science/article/pii/S1532046419300565
10. van der Maaten, L., Hinton, G.: Visualizing data using t-SNE. J. Mach. Learn. Res. **9**(86), 2579–2605 (2008). http://jmlr.org/papers/v9/vandermaaten08a.html
11. McInnes, L., Healy, J., Saul, N., Großberger, L.: UMAP: uniform manifold approximation and projection. J. Open Source Softw. **3**(29), 861 (2018). https://doi.org/10.21105/joss.00861
12. Meng, C., Trinh, L., Xu, N., Enouen, J., Liu, Y.: Interpretability and fairness evaluation of deep learning models on MIMIC-IV dataset. Sci. Rep. **12**(1), 7166 (2022). https://doi.org/10.1038/s41598-022-11012-2
13. Mikolov, T., Sutskever, I., Chen, K., Corrado, G.S., Dean, J.: Distributed representations of words and phrases and their compositionality. In: Advances in Neural Information Processing Systems, pp. 3111–3119 (2013)
14. Nowroozilarki, Z., Pakbin, A., Royalty, J., Lee, D.K., Mortazavi, B.J.: Real-time mortality prediction using MIMIC-IV ICU data via boosted nonparametric hazards. In: 2021 IEEE EMBS International Conference on Biomedical and Health Informatics (BHI), pp. 1–4 (2021). https://doi.org/10.1109/BHI50953.2021.9508537
15. Rasmy, L., Xiang, Y., Xie, Z., Tao, C., Zhi, D.: Med-BERT: pretrained contextualized embeddings on large-scale structured electronic health records for disease prediction. NPJ Digit. Med. **4**(1), 86 (2021). https://doi.org/10.1038/s41746-021-00455-y
16. Schneider, E.T.R., et al.: BioBERTpt - a Portuguese neural language model for clinical named entity recognition. In: Proceedings of the 3rd Clinical Natural Language Processing Workshop, pp. 65–72. Association for Computational Linguistics (2020). https://doi.org/10.18653/v1/2020.clinicalnlp-1.7
17. Si, Y., et al.: Deep representation learning of patient data from electronic health records (EHR): a systematic review. J. Biomed. Inform. **115**, 103671 (2021)

18. Teodoro, D., et al.: Interoperability driven integration of biomedical data sources. Stud. Health Technol. Inform. **169**, 185–189 (2011). https://doi.org/10.3233/978-1-60750-806-9-185. https://www.ncbi.nlm.nih.gov/pubmed/21893739
19. Teodoro, D., Pasche, E., Gobeill, J., Emonet, S., Ruch, P., Lovis, C.: Building a transnational biosurveillance network using semantic web technologies: requirements, design, and preliminary evaluation. J. Med. Internet Res. **14**(3), e73–e73 (2012). https://doi.org/10.2196/jmir.2043. https://pubmed.ncbi.nlm.nih.gov/22642960, 22642960[pmid]
20. Teodoro, D., Sundvall, E., João Junior, M., Ruch, P., Miranda Freire, S.: ORBDA: an openEHR benchmark dataset for performance assessment of electronic health record servers. PloS One **13**(1), e0190028–e0190028 (2018). https://doi.org/10.1371/journal.pone.0190028. https://pubmed.ncbi.nlm.nih.gov/29293556, 29293556[pmid]

Author Index

Printed in the United States
by Baker & Taylor Publisher Services